Dentists Who Care:
Inspiring Stories of Professional Com

Dentists Who Care:
Inspiring Stories
of
Professional Commitment

James T. Rule, DDS, MS

Professor Emeritus
Department of Pediatric Dentistry
Dental School
University of Maryland
Baltimore, Maryland

and

Muriel J. Bebeau, PhD

Professor
Department of Preventive Sciences
University of Minnesota School of Dentistry
Minneapolis, Minnesota

Quintessence Publishing Co, Inc

Chicago, Berlin, Tokyo, London, Paris, Milan, Barcelona, Istanbul,
São Paulo, New Delhi, Moscow, Prague, and Warsaw

To Joanne Thompson Rule, my personal moral exemplar

To Ella Margaretha Bohlsen Duin (1904–2003): model parent, exemplary teacher

Library of Congress Cataloging-in-Publication Data

Rule, James T.
  Dentists who care : inspiring stories of professional commitment / James T. Rule, Muriel J. Bebeau.
    p. ; cm.
  ISBN 0-86715-451-9 (softcover)
  1. Dentists—United States—Biography. 2. Dentists—Professional ethics.
  [DNLM: 1. Dentists—Biography. 2. Professional Role—Biography.] I. Bebeau, Muriel J. II. Title.
  RK41.R85 2005
  617.6'0922—dc22
                          2004025258

quintessence
books

©2005 Quintessence Publishing Co, Inc

Quintessence Publishing Co, Inc
4350 Chandler Drive
Hanover Park, Illinois 60133
www.quintpub.com

Editor: Lindsay Harmon
Production: Patrick Penney
Cover design: Dawn Hartman

Printed in Canada

Table of Contents

Preface

Dentistry, like all professions, needs a moral identity that sustains its existing membership and also attracts honorable young men and women who seek a calling that is compatible with their standards. This book attempts to contribute to the ongoing development of such a moral identity. It contains stories and accompanying commentaries about 10 dentists who were identified by their colleagues as moral exemplars for acting upon ideals that are fundamental to their profession. Whereas all dental professionals are expected to act in accordance with their profession's central values, these particular individuals have gone to exceptional lengths to act on behalf of the interests of others.

Most of the exemplars profiled in this book have spent their lives as community practitioners, and a few have been academics. Some are nationally known, while others have local or regional reputations. Some have dramatically visible accomplishments, while others are identified primarily as caring, thoughtful people.

The initial stimulus for this book was the result of experience gathered during the writing of the book *Ethical Questions in Dentistry* (Quintessence, 2004), in which dental practitioners in the field offered actual ethical dilemmas that they had encountered personally. Their enthusiasm and interest as participants in these discussions led to the conviction that extended interviews with dentists about values and moral issues would be valuable as the basis for another book.

Further support for the book emerged during a 1996 meeting of the Professional Ethics in Dentistry Network* (PEDNET) that was held in San Diego to discuss the major ethical issues facing dentistry in the new millennium. One of the presenters was Dr Gerald Winslow,

dean of Religion at Loma Linda University. He expressed his surprise, as a newcomer to the field of dental ethics, that he had not heard stories about dentists who might be thought of as "moral heroes"–people who stood for, and acted upon, ideals that were beyond their own self-interest. In his view, moral role models can play an important part in the development of a moral tradition, something he thought was relatively deficient in dentistry. Medicine, he felt, was ahead of dentistry in that regard and could readily point to numerous individuals who are known for moral leadership within their community. Dentistry also had them, he felt sure, but where were they?

Our judgment is that Dr Winslow is correct: While dentistry has many enriching traditions, its moral tradition would be enhanced if stories about some of its moral heroes were publicly known.

Not only does this book present the stories of 10 such dentists, but the stories are bookended by opening and closing chapters that contextualize and synthesize them. The book begins with an account of how the exemplars were nominated, selected, interviewed, and written about–as well as the various lenses applied to make meaning of the stories. It concludes with a chapter that captures the essence of the messages in their stories.

The book can be read in two different ways. One approach, for the casual reader, is simply to enjoy the narratives about 10 interesting, talented, and caring individuals whose actions help define dentistry's moral identity. The other approach is to actively reflect on the meaning of the stories. As an aid to the latter approach, the reader will find questions included at the end of each chapter. For educators and study group leaders, Appendix A provides a series of useful suggestions for getting the most from this book.

---

*As of 2005, PEDNET has been renamed the American Society for Dental Ethics.

Acknowledgments

This book would not have been possible without the financial support provided by the University of Maryland's Department of Pediatric Dentistry, which covered most of the costs associated with traveling to various locations across the country. Dr Rule is also indebted to the University of Maryland for its generous sabbatical policies, which greatly enhanced the interview process.

Before work on this book began, Dr Gerald Winslow, dean of the Faculty of Religion at Loma Linda University, made an invaluable contribution by pointing out the important function that "moral heroes" could play as role models in the development of a moral tradition.

We deeply appreciate the willingness of the exemplars to participate in this project and feel enriched by our exposure to their stories and their views of professional life. Dr Rule feels especially privileged to have had hours of fascinating and meaningful discussion with them.

Our appreciation also extends to those who took the time to make the nominations, and to those who were nominated but not selected, virtually all of whom were very meritorious nominees. Many of their stories would have been equally worthwhile.

Several people assisted us in the preparation of this book. Ann Higgins-D'Alessandro, professor of psychology at Fordham University, shared her interview questions. The American College of Dentists established a special committee, consisting of Drs B. Charles Kerhove, Jr; Robert E. Mecklenburg; and James L. Palmisano, to assist with selection of the exemplars. John F. Rule helped with transcription of two of the interviews and provided editorial support. Students in Dr Bebeau's graduate seminar on the psychology of morality read the stories and made useful comments on the stages and phases of identity formation as they had come to understand them.

Finally, Drs Andrew E. Allen of Brunswick, Maine, and William E. Stein of Aitken, Minnesota, both members of the American College of Dentists, reviewed the stories and commentaries and provided helpful insights into how this book might be used.

Dentists Who Care: Their Selection and Interviews

This book, as described in the preface, is an attempt to contribute to the ongoing development of dentistry's moral identity. In it, we present stories and commentaries about 10 dentists whose life experiences collectively demonstrate the various roles that dentists are called upon to play during their professional lives.

Each of the exemplars does not represent every role; rather, their individual accomplishments emphasize certain roles rather than others. The point to be made here is that no one expects that all dentists will become exemplary leaders in community projects, champions of a cause, or researchers, teachers, or academic leaders. However, dentists *are* expected to contribute to community welfare, involve themselves in worthwhile endeavors, and see to it that their profession is being run properly—in other words, to assume responsibilities and obligations that go beyond their own self-interest. We are convinced that a broad and inclusive concept of one's professional responsibilities has intrinsic value for everyone—laypeople and professionals alike.

We also believe that stories such as the ones in this book can help both dentists and those entering the dental profession to better understand the essence and scope of the various roles and their attendant responsibilities. Many dentists look back with affection at colleagues who, as role models, have made important contributions to their development as professionals. Some

of these role models are catalysts for clinical excellence, a forward-thinking philosophy of practice, or a concept of professionalism. Others represent paradigms for relationships with their patients. Like role models from all walks of life, the dentists profiled in this book share a common link: concern for the interests of others. And like other role models, our exemplars have a broad assortment of talents and personal priorities, not to mention the occasional flaw. Collectively, they represent a picture of the dental profession that is attractive and uplifting but also realistic.

We think that the timing for such an assemblage of stories is good, if not somewhat overdue. Among the public, the credibility of dentists may well be in decline. The 2003 Gallup Poll[1] on honesty and ethics in American professions placed dentistry fifth, below nurses, physicians, pharmacists, and veterinarians. While fifth is not bad, it is several steps down from the top two or three, where it stood for decades. Additionally, in one of his monthly commentaries in the *Journal of the American Dental Association*,[2] Gordon Christensen suggested five reasons why the public's attitude towards dentistry may be changing: "having a commercial, self-promotional orientation; planning and carrying out excessive treatment; charging high fees without justification; providing service only when it is convenient; [and] refusing to accept responsibility when treatment fails prematurely."

The dentists who appear in these stories have altogether different perspectives from those represented in Christensen's troubling conclusions. They are not primarily focused on themselves. Instead, they are guided by compassion and concern for others. Notions of personal responsibility are high on their list of priorities. Furthermore, some of them feel that their profession has changed them for the better. One speaks of how his practice has enhanced his ability to care about other people, another of how it has made him feel a sense of gratitude to his community. Others have used their practices as a home base for launching and even funding projects in the larger community.

Role models can be an important influence on the formulation of one's values and ideals, and most of our exemplars were greatly influenced by their own role models. Quite obviously, other factors can also be influential, for instance, family, religious institutions, school, community and social organizations, and professional organizations.[3] Indeed, these factors are all represented in the stories of our exemplars.

Furthermore, we suggest that stories such as those in this book may help promote the acquisition of a moral identity and serve as possible agents for change in one's behavior. To that end, we have provided suggestions for ways in which educators and study group leaders can use this book to encourage active reflection on the meaning of the stories (Appendix A). Whether these outcomes will prove to be true for readers of this book remains to be seen. What is clear, however, is that collectively these dentists represent the highest ideals of their profession.

The 10 stories that follow present a diverse picture of the many aspects of the dental profession. Each story is self-contained. While they may be read in any sequence, the order of the chapters was chosen according to the venue of the activity for which the exemplars were nominated.

The first five stories feature private practitioners whose sphere of activity revolved around the office in which they worked. To be sure, their pursuits varied widely. In Brainerd, Minnesota, Jack Echternacht was heavily involved in projects of great benefit to his community, the most noteworthy of which was a decades-long battle to promote water fluoridation. Hugo Owens used his private practice in Chesapeake, Virginia, as a vehicle for a career as a community leader, especially in the area of civil rights. In Manhattan, Kansas, Brent Benkelman focused primarily on his commitment to his patients to order to make their experience as stress-free

as possible. Jack Whittaker developed his practice in Bowling Green, Ohio, as a model for treating low-income children and influenced changes in state policies for Medicaid reimbursement. And Janet Johnson (a pseudonym) participated dramatically in the self-regulation component of her profession by reporting her supervisor, who was mistreating patients in a hospital dental clinic.

The sixth and seventh stories, while also featuring private practitioners, describe dentists with extraordinary organizational skills who expressed their talents beyond the walls of their offices. Jerry Lowney practiced orthodontics in Norwich, Connecticut, but created a major dental and medical program for the poorest of the poor in Haiti. And Donna Rumberger used her leadership position in organized dentistry in New York City to show how dental societies can function effectively as agents for helping others.

The last three stories are those of academic dentists: a teacher, an administrator, and a researcher. Camille Capdeboscq became a legendary figure for his ability to inspire confidence in his students and instill a sense of dignity in each encounter with them, despite being the toughest grader in Louisiana State University's operative dentistry department. During her 16 years as dean of Howard University College of Dentistry, Jeanne Sinkford was widely known for her principled approach to getting things done. And Irwin Mandel, while carving out an international reputation in salivary research at Columbia University, served as a symbol of integrity in research and as a prototype for thoughtful mentoring of rising scientists.

Criteria for Selection

This project began in 1996 with the establishment of criteria by which the moral exemplars were selected. The criteria presented below are modeled after those of Anne Colby and William Damon in their book *Some Do Care*.[4] Not every person who was selected necessarily displayed all the criteria.

1. "A sustained commitment to moral ideals or principles that include a generalized respect for humanity; or a sustained evidence of moral virtue."

The idea of a "sustained commitment" is implicit in one's notion of a moral exemplar. It is someone whose actions are there to be observed and evaluated over a long haul. With one dramatic exception (Johnson), this was true for all or our exemplars. Their nominations were viewed by their colleagues as "lifetime achievement awards." Almost all who were nominated were at least in their 60s.

The phrase "generalized respect for humanity" was included because, as Colby and Damon put it, "Not just any principle counts as a moral one: Principles that cause harm or injustice to some people are excluded," so as to "weed out fanatics who are passionately dedicated to immoral goals." Among our nominees, both those selected and not selected, there were no fanatics.

2. "A disposition to act in accord with one's moral ideals or principles, implying also a consistency between one's actions and intentions and between the means and ends of one's actions."

This criterion has two components. One is that it was not enough to have lofty ideas; one needed also to act upon them. The other component, that of consistency between means and ends, was designed primarily to eliminate people who "do more harm than good because of the destructive means they employ." We believe that all of our choices meet that criterion.

3. "A willingness to risk one's self-interest for the sake of one's moral values."

As Colby and Damon suggest, to fulfill this criterion, martyrdom is not required. The natural circumstances of our exemplars' lives varied substantially. For some, their life choices provided only subtle risks. For others, the risks were palpably overt. None of them, however, appeared to consider their actions in terms of risk versus benefit. They appeared to be undeterred by the complicating factors that could easily have been anticipated.

4. "A tendency to be inspiring to others and thereby to move them to moral action."

Colby and Damon point out that "one does not perform moral acts in isolation." This criterion was easily seen in all of our moral exemplars in dentistry. Some of them operated primarily within their community, and for them the scale of their effect was smaller than those with a national or international orientation. However, for all of them the quality of inspiration to others was present.

5. "A sense of realistic humility about one's own importance relative to the world at large, implying a relative lack of concern for one's own ego."

This criterion means that the exemplars' perspective on their work is tempered by an understanding that their accomplishments were made possible by the efforts of the people around them, the influence of their own role models, the unique circumstances of their working conditions, and, sometimes, blind chance. All of our exemplars made it clear during the interviews that they had such understandings, and almost all of them expressed concern at the outset about whether they qualified as a moral exemplar. Furthermore, we agree with Colby and Damon's observations that they "are dedicated to missions, values, or persons beyond their own self-aggrandizement. They are not taken, therefore, by the majesty of their own power or the sweep of their own influence."

Nominations and Selection

The above criteria and a request for nominations by letter, not to exceed two pages, were published in a September 1996 issue of the *ADA News*. The nominating letter was to fully develop the reasons why the nominee met the criteria. To be eligible, nominees were required to be living and either active or retired members of the profession. If retired, they were required to have previously been an active member of the profession. Past or current active involvement in the profession was required in order to avoid having nominations of individuals who were dentists but primarily active in another profession.

Additional nominees were obtained in other ways as well. Requests for nomination were distributed to members of the American College of Dentists (ACD) who attended the 1996 annual meeting. (It should be noted that membership in the ACD was not a requirement for nomination.) Because our request for nominations via the *ADA News* and the ACD resulted in no nominations of women, we also made telephone requests for nominations to all officers of the American Association of Women Dentists from the previous 5 years. Finally, additional nominations—including some that were selected—were an unexpected byproduct of calls that we made within the dentistry network to gather corroborative evidence in support of other nominees.

Every attempt was made to select the exemplars from a diverse group of nominees from the standpoint of gender, race, and professional activities, as well as balance between practitioners and academics.

We had decided that we would attempt to identify 10 individuals as moral exemplars in dentistry who not only fit the criteria but also exhibited exceptional commitment to one or more of the ordinary responsibilities of the dentist. As the nominations came in, it was evident that they fell into certain categories of professional activity. First, there was the division between academia and practice. We decided that the balance should be tipped clearly toward those in community practice. Therefore, we decided to limit the academic exemplars to three: one who would represent moral exemplars in teaching, another in academic administration, and a third in research. Among the other seven, all of whom either are or were practitioners, the breakdown was as follows: Four of them represented moral leadership in the community, albeit with very different representations of the nature of the community. The remaining three exemplars fell into different categories. One we classified as a "good practitioner" for the way he treated his patients. Another showed moral leadership in her involvement with organized dentistry. And the last one demonstrated monitoring responsibility toward her profession in her activities as a whistle-blower.

All selections except three were made by the coauthors using the Colby-Damon criteria. The exceptions, which were cases where there was some uncertainty about which were the best choices, were made with the help of a three-member panel of the American College of Dentists.*

A total of 46 nominations were received. Only a few failed to meet the criteria. When this occurred, it was usually because the nominee, while showing admirable courage in standing up for his or her beliefs, championed a cause that was deemed to be of questionable merit.

Interviews

The interviews followed a pattern of ethnographic conversations and explored the exemplars' personal beliefs and values, as well as factual information about their lives and the basis for their nomination. They included a series of open-ended questions concerning specific events or stages in the life of the exemplar. The questions were supplemented by probe questions, as needed, in order to acquire the necessary depth and to ensure the dependability of information through the use of narratives, stories, examples, and additional evidence. A framework for the interview, adapted from a protocol developed by Ann Higgins-D'Alessandro, is included in Appendix B.

The interviews were conducted in the communities of the selected exemplars over a period of 3 to 5 days. Each day's interview lasted from 1 to 3 hours, at the convenience of the interviewee. The total length of the interviews varied from 5 to 10 hours. The meetings took place in a variety of settings, including the exemplar's home and/or office, a hotel room, and at one point or another, all of them in a restaurant. In some instances, a spouse was present for part or all of the interview, in others not—all according to the interviewee's preferences. Occasionally, additional information was obtained through interviews of spouses, colleagues, employees, and patients. All interviews were recorded.

The interviews provided a narrative that explored the reasons why each exemplar was nominated and how he or she viewed the factors that influenced his or her moral development. The focus was on the meaning the exemplars assigned to events in their lives as well as how they saw their moral identity developing.

From time to time during the interviews, the coauthors talked about the content of the discussions with the exemplars and reflected on additional questions to ask and impressions to verify.

Writing Process

Transcripts were made from the tapes for all of the interviews except for the last two. The transcripts were used as the basis for writing the stories. In the absence of transcripts, extensive verbatim notes taken from the tapes by Dr Rule or John F. Rule were used instead. The first draft of each story was written by Dr Rule and edited by Dr Bebeau.

The final version of each story was sent to the exemplar for comment and correction. At times several exchanges of drafts were made. No versions of the story were published without the nominees' consent.†

---

*The panel consisted of Drs B. Charles Kerhove, Jr, Robert E. Mecklenburg, and James L. Palmisano.

†All the stories and commentaries except for that of Dr Johnson were published as a series in the journal *Quintessence International* between 2000 and 2004.

Once the story had been approved by the exemplar, it was reviewed independently by the authors, who summarized the exemplar's virtues, expectations, and dimensions of a moral identity. Discussions were held to achieve consensus regarding interpretations. Based on these interpretations, a commentary was written by Dr Bebeau and edited by Dr Rule. The commentaries were not sent to the exemplars for review.

During the writing of the commentaries and chapter 12, we derived meaning from the stories through the use of three different lenses:

Lens 1: The Special Characteristics of Professions

This lens is derived from the sociologic study of the special characteristics of the "learned professions." It provides grounding for the ethic of all professions and for the expectations that we as patients or clients and as members of society have of the professional and the profession.[5,6] The distinctive features of the "learned professions" generate a kind of internal morality or grounding for expectations and obligations (Appendix C). We look to see how each exemplar has internalized and acted upon these expectations and obligations. But knowing what is expected is not synonymous with living the moral life. We also ask what motivated the exemplar to act upon the obligations. We are curious about the particular virtues that define the character of the exemplar and, by extension, the character of the "good dentist."

Lens 2: The Virtues of Medical Practice

The second lens through which we read the stories is an account of the virtues in medical practice. Having defined the "good practitioner" in terms of the ends of the professional practice–healing, helping, and caring–Pellegrino and Thomasma[7] describe in detail particular virtues that are "internal to the practice of the health professional" (Appendix D). Their list includes fidelity to trust, benevolence, compassion and caring, intellectual honesty, competence, prudence, and effacement of self-interest.

Lens 3: The Evolving Moral Self

In examining important events of an exemplar's life, we applied a third lens whereby we looked for the shifts in identity formation that are characteristic of a "developmental trajectory" that ends with the mature moral identity described by Blasi[8] and Kegan[9] as the goal of development. Whereas the interview process was not designed specifically to assess stages of identity formation for each exemplar, the general descriptions provided a point of reference for reflection on the stories and are the basis of some of the general conclusions we have drawn. Appendix E provides a brief synopsis of the stages and transition phases of identity formation as experienced from late adolescence to full maturity.

Notes on the Exemplars

Nominees Who Declined

When the stories were sent to the exemplars for their approval, two declined to participate. In the first instance, the withdrawal was based on the nominee's concern over how the story was portrayed. Despite prolonged attempts on both sides to compromise on the presentation of the story, the negotiations eventually failed and permission to publish was withdrawn. A new nominee was found as a replacement.

The second person who withdrew permission after reading the story was the whistle-blower. She had reported a colleague for significant ethical violations, and her actions had been vindicated by a severe penalty levied by the state board of dentistry. However, her personal experiences during and after the activities of the state board were extremely painful. Seeing the story in written form raised fears that the trauma of those years would be relived. Because we believed that the telling of the story would be worthwhile, however, 2 years after her permission was withdrawn, we rewrote the story in an anonymous format. Besides changing her name, we also changed the circumstances of her life and the events that precipitated her action. In doing so, we attempted to make the seriousness of the events parallel to and comparable with those in the original story. When the second story was sent to her for review, it was approved. At that time, some additional reflections on the initial event were added.

A third nominee had also declined to participate, this time prior to the interview. The nominee, an African-American man, declined because of prior time commitments he had made for a writing project of his own.

Characteristics of the Exemplars

As one might expect, being recognized as a moral exemplar by one's peers is something of a "lifetime achievement award." Except for the whistle-blower, whose age is withheld in the interest of preserving anonymity, at the time of the interview, one was in transition between the fifth and sixth decades, five were in their 60s, two in their 70s, and one in his 80s. The retirement profile of this group is somewhat different from that of most dentists. They are working well beyond the usual ages for retirement–and by their own comments, most of them are enjoying it immensely. This is true despite the fact that some of them entered dentistry largely by chance or by circumstances that excluded other possibilities.

Another characteristic, along with age, that was not represented equally in all parameters was geography. We would have preferred to select exemplars from all corners of the country, but our nominees happened to be skewed eastward. Of the nine upon whom we can report, three were from the Midwest, two from the south, one from the Washington, DC, area, and three from the Northeast. None was from the western states, although both the exemplar who withdrew permission and the one who declined to be interviewed would have qualified as westerners.

The political inclination of the exemplars was also a factor that happened by chance. Questions about politics were never raised by the interviewer. Nevertheless, some of the exemplars included it in their discussions. Drs Lowney, Mandel, and Owens clearly stated their affiliations with the Democratic party, as did Dr Benkelman with the Republican party. Although Dr Whittaker's political accomplishments took place during a Republican administration in Ohio, we have no clue as to his personal political leanings. We could only speculate on the rest.

All but one of the exemplars thought of himself or herself as religious. Those who did spoke of religious teaching with varying degrees of enthusiasm. Four, in particular, discussed the great influence of religion in their formative years, and for one it was a material factor in his commitment to the group he served.

Two other points should be made. One is that we recognized at the outset that the world was not composed of perfect people. Neither should the readers of this book expect to find perfection among those selected as moral exemplars in dentistry. Jerry Lowney, for example, at times has been taken to task for singlemindedness as he pushes for his agenda at the Haitian Health Foundation. Camille Capdebosque gave lower grades than anyone else in the operative dentistry department. Jeanne Sinkford might be thought of as uncompromising in her upholding of academic standards. Jack Whittaker has been condemned for his criticism of dentists who refuse to treat Medicaid patients. Yet the balance, we feel, tips overwhelmingly toward the good they do on behalf of others.

Finally, it is equally clear that in selecting the exemplars presented here, we did not exhaust the supply of such people within the dental profession. Based on the articles we see in dental journals, newsletters, and newspapers, the activities of many dentists across the country could have qualified them as moral exemplars as well.

References

1. Public rates nursing as most honest and ethical profession. Available at www.gallup.com/poll/content/?ci=9823. Accessed 7 February 2005.
2. Christensen GJ. The credibility of dentists. J Am Dent Assoc 2001;132:1163–1165.
3. Pellegrino E. Virtues in medical ethics. Presented at the University of Maryland at Baltimore Biomedical Ethics Center, Baltimore, 1996.
4. Colby A, Damon W. Some Do Care: Contemporary Lives of Moral Commitment. New York: Free Press, 1992:29–32.
5. Hall RH. The professions. In: Occupations and the Social Structure, ed 2. Englewood Cliffs, NJ: Prentice-Hall, 1975: 63–135.
6. Bebeau MJ, Kahn J. Ethical issues in community dental health. In: Gluck GM, Morganstein WM (eds). Jong's Community Dental Health, ed 5. St Louis: Mosby, 2003:425–445.
7. Pellegrino ED, Thomasma DC. The Virtues in Medical Practice. New York: Oxford University Press, 1983.
8. Blasi A. Moral identity: Its role in moral functioning. In: Krutines W, Gerwitz J (eds). Morality, Moral Behavior, and Moral Development. New York: Wiley, 1984:128–139.
9. Kegan R. The Evolving Self: Problem and Process in Human Development. Cambridge, MA: Harvard University Press, 1982.

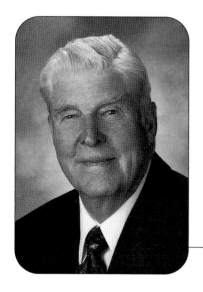

2

John E. Echternacht

Practitioner and Community Leader

For Minnesota dentists with long memories, Dr Jack Echternacht is a legendary figure. He graduated from the University of Minnesota School of Dentistry in 1943. Except for a 3-year enlistment in the Navy during World War II, he has made his home and his professional life in Brainerd, on the edge of Minnesota's lake country. A few years after he started his general practice, reports began to appear about the striking reduction of dental caries in children's teeth when fluoride was placed in the drinking water. Excited by these prospects for better oral health, Dr Echternacht led a Chamber of Commerce initiative in 1954 to introduce fluoride into Brainerd's water supply. What seemed at first an easy victory turned into a 30-year struggle. Dr Echternacht's determination, persistence, and leadership during this fight for fluoridation led to his selection as a moral model in dentistry.

John Echternacht (called Jack by everyone who knows him) lives on Gull Lake on the outskirts of Brainerd, Minnesota, a town of 12,000 citizens approximately 150 miles north of Minneapolis. The Mississippi, a small river there, runs through Brainerd. In early November 1996, during the 5-day interview process, the outdoor thermometer never moved from 11°F. On the first day, one third of the lake was frozen. Five bald eagles circled above, watching ducks swimming at the edge of the ice. By the fourth day, ice covered the lake—no water, no ducks, and no eagles.

Inside the wood-beamed house, over his family room fireplace, 31 of approximately 400 birds he has mounted over the years are displayed. Jack's presence and his choices of companion pieces added extra insurance against the cold.

Being with Jack Echternacht is an experience in security. Listening to his slow, deep voice as he discussed the important circumstances of his life, I (JTR) was enveloped in a feeling of trust. If I were one of his patients, I would say, "Go right ahead. Do it."

The Brainerd Fluoridation Story

In 1946 Jack Echternacht was discharged from the Navy and drove with his father through Minnesota looking for a place to practice. They first considered New Ulm, a German community in the western part of the state, judging that with a name like Echternacht, it would be a good match. Their judgment was sound, but their timing was wrong. There was no office space available. Next they drove northwest to Fergus Falls, and found nothing there either. But in Brainerd, right on the edge of the lake country, they discovered an office. As one who loved to fish and had always wanted to live on a lake, Jack couldn't have been happier, and so he began his practice.

By 1954 Dr Echternacht was an established figure in the Brainerd community. His practice was thriving, and he had quickly built a reputation for community involvement. That reputation and his outgoing manner soon earned him an invitation to join the Junior Chamber of Commerce, and he readily agreed. He now had a source of "thought leaders" to help him promote the use of fluoride. By this time research had been published showing that fluoridated drinking water offered huge benefits. Landmark studies involving thousands of schoolchildren had been underway since 1945 in Grand Rapids, Michigan; Kingston-Newburgh, New York; and Grantsburg, Ontario. The studies had been planned to last for 10 years, but the gains were so great–cavity reductions of 60%–that public health agencies were already formulating policy, and some local jurisdictions had already fluoridated their drinking water. Dentifrice manufacturers also had been at work. The first tube of Crest was about to be sold.

In 1954 the National Junior Chamber of Commerce chose for its annual project the fluoridation of all municipal water supplies in the United States. Since Jack was active in the Junior Chamber, it was logical that he would lead the effort in Brainerd. Expecting an easy acceptance, he drafted a proposal to fluoridate the water supply and took it to the city council. Without much discussion it was approved–temporarily, as it turned out.

In short order, Jack received a certificate of merit: "In recognition of unselfish service as chairman of the fluoridation of city water of the Brainerd Junior Chamber of Commerce." The decision-making phase was finished. However, no word came from the city council about the implementation phase. After 3 months of silence, Jack called the council and learned that the project had been shelved because the Water and Light Board, which represented the community power structure, had said no. The council had no interest in overriding the Water and Light Board.

Dr Echternacht was dumbfounded. In response, he initiated a campaign to educate the council on the benefits of water fluoridation. He attended council meetings, wrote letters to the *Brainerd Daily Dispatch*'s Open

Forum, gave talks at parent-teacher association meetings, and distributed literature in his office and wherever he could find willing recipients. Nothing happened. He learned that his efforts had been stalled by the work of a small but effective group of antifluoridationists.

The leader of the antifluoridationist movement in Brainerd was Irene Johnson. Possessed with dedication, an independent spirit, and what the newspapers were to call "a legendary will," she made Jack Echternacht's life memorable for most of the next 30 years. Dr Echternacht and Mrs Johnson became polar figures in the fluoridation fight. The conflict attracted both statewide and national interest. At one point, NBC, an American television news network, broadcast a story on Brainerd's fluoridation controversy, featuring interviews with both Jack and Irene Johnson. The air of antagonism was so sharp that at no time did they ever appear together.

According to newspaper accounts, Irene Johnson asserted that Jack Echternacht had been dispatched to Brainerd as a "pusher assigned by the American Dental Association" to smooth the way for the introduction of fluoride. "There's one in every community," she said. "Good looking, respectable, a community leader. Just like Echternacht." To make matters worse, he was of German descent. "Just like all Germans," she said, "Jack Echternacht is going to get his way. Or else."

For Irene Johnson and the group she led, Jack's efforts to put fluoride in the water were both infuriating and alarming. From their perspective, besides killing rats, fluoride caused cancer, kidney failure, nail biting, hypertension, hair loss, mongolism, skin rashes, sterility, miscarriage, brittle bones, and disfigured teeth. Furthermore, Irene added, it was all part of a communist plot to introduce harmful mass medication.

Antifluoridationists were especially irritated about having no choice other than to drink fluoridated water. They said it was another example of the loss of political liberty. For a time, the Johnsons displayed a poster on their front door that showed a dentist shoving a garden hose into the mouth of a helpless patient, with the admonition: "Don't let them push fluoridation down your throat." Frustrations ran high. Mrs Johnson's husband said, "If they try to put that stuff in our water, we'll get out the guns." He pointed out that many people in Brainerd, including Irene, carried guns. "When she goes out to meetings at night, she always takes along her gun. They don't call her Pistol-Packin' Mama for nothin'."

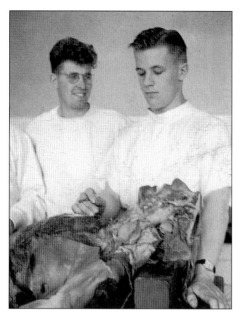

Jack *(left)* and John Lee in the freshman gross anatomy lab.

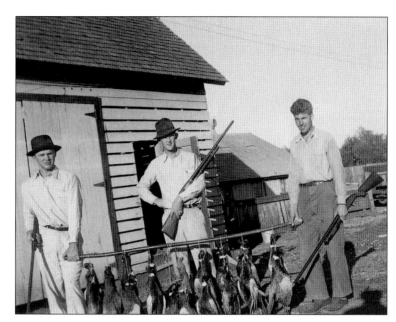

Jack *(right)* shoots pheasants on his father's farm with dental school classmates Chris Bendickson and Jim Eubanks.

When Mrs Johnson first heard about Dr Echternacht's success in winning fluoridation approval by the city council, she was alarmed. In response, she circulated a petition against fluoridation that was supported by more than 4,000 signatures, approximately 40% of the town's population at the time. Typical of this feeling was the message on a sign on the main route into town that read, "World's Best Drink: Brainerd's Pure, Cold, Deep Well Water." For the Brainerd citizens, the slogan was reality, and they did not want their water ruined by Dr Echternacht. Letters opposing fluoridation began to appear in the Open Forum section of the newspaper. It seemed that for every profluoridation letter that was published, three appeared in opposition. Mrs Johnson was in full gear. Her activities were sustained by the organization Minnesotans Opposed to Forced Fluoridation (MOFF), which she founded.

Looking back at the activities of the antifluoridationists, Jack realizes now how naïve he was. He saw the issue strictly from the standpoint of fluoride's benefits. The reduction of caries was dramatic. The addition of such small amounts of fluoride to the water, and at such small cost, produced almost unbelievable results. Furthermore, it was not as if Brainerd's water supply was completely fluoride free to begin with. From natural sources, it already contained 20% of what was needed for optimal benefits. Adding a little more would do so much good. How could anyone not be convinced?

Most people, however, were not convinced and showed it by supporting the already formidable antifluoridationists. Jack felt the bite of their disregard for objectivity, honesty, and civility. Furthermore, there were few people on whom Jack could rely for help. Although the other Brainerd dentists had signed their names to a public statement supporting fluoridation, none was willing to work for the cause. The strident nature of the opposition was such that most dentists were concerned about losing patients if they became involved. In addition, activism was unpleasant. In Jack's words, "Every time you put your head up, there were four or five of these anti-people who would take a swipe at you."

The personal attacks on his name that appeared in the Open Forum were also of great concern to his wife, Flo, whom he had married in his last year of dental school. In one form or another, the struggle dominated his thoughts and competed for time that was important to him in raising his three children. Even in his college days, he had dreamed about the importance of family commitments in his future life. In fact, the availability of time for family was a key reason he chose dentistry over medicine. The life of a country physician in rural Minnesota could be burdened by routine off-hour obligations. His life might not be his own. The irony of his current situation was that now, as a dentist, he faced the same issue.

The ugliness of the conflict became worse. Jack began receiving anonymous calls at all hours of the night. His visits to the city council became charged with hostility. Later, when the fluoride issue was being considered at the Minnesota State Legislature, Jack attended one of the critical meetings. As he walked down an aisle, a man from Brainerd absurdly stuck out his foot and tried to trip him. On another occasion, while Dr Echternacht was sitting at his lab bench working on a crown, a stranger walked in and suggested that he be careful which streets he walked on. One snowy night, when he could not drive home, he slept in his reception room. In the middle of the night he heard a loud noise. He thought the furnace had backfired. The next morning he found a bullet hole in his reception room window.

Jack continued to work for fluoridation. He was constantly on call to set the record straight. When anything was said against fluoridation, Jack would find evidence to refute it. When the opposition claimed that the American Medical Association did not approve of fluoridation, Jack got a letter from its president saying they did approve. When his opponents stated that the Minnesota Medical Association (MMA) was opposed to fluoridation, Jack showed that the MMA had gone on record favoring it on May 27, 1952. It was the same with the American Dental Association and the American Public Health Association. Jack always went to the source. When MOFF declared that J. Edgar Hoover was against fluoridation, Jack telegraphed the FBI director and received an airmail letter from him dated November 28, 1961, that stated:

> Fluoridation is a legislative matter and I have always followed the policy of not injecting the FBI or myself into situations involving local or Federal legislation. Therefore, I want to assure you that I did not make the statement attributed to me which you quoted.

> "Every time you put your head up, there were three or five of these anti-people who would take a swipe at you."
>
> *Dr Echternacht on antifluoridationists*

The opposition suggested that fluoride pills be given voluntarily by those parents who chose to do so. Jack presented the studies that showed the poor compliance rate with such approaches. In preparation for his first trip to the city council, Jack had asked a pharmacist to add the proper amount of fluoride to a big jug of city water. He brought the jug and some waxed paper cups to the meeting. He also brought a jug of the pure, unfluoridated "world's best drink." Everyone was served both drinks, and no one could tell the difference. Jack thought that his lesson in objectivity had convinced them. But no opinions were changed.

At one point Jack even took action against a friend, the editor of the *Brainerd Daily Dispatch*. Jack, along with Dr Bob Uppgaard, a dentist from the nearby town of Pequot, reported the *Dispatch* to the Minnesota Press Council, complaining that more press space was given to the antifluoridationists than to the profluoridationists. The press council agreed. The ruling had no effect whatsoever on the editor. Jack, however, lost a friend.

Fluoridation in Brainerd was put to a vote in 1961, and Jack was there to advocate for fluoride. It lost, 2,846 to 1,427. In 1967 fluoridation of the public water supplies became a state law, but Brainerd refused to comply. At that point, Jack could only follow the legal proceedings through a contact in the Attorney General's office. In 1971, the State Health Department formally requested that Brainerd comply with state law. Brainerd still refused to comply. An attempt was made in the state legislature to exempt Brainerd from the law. The attempt was unsuccessful. Another referendum was held in 1974, and fluoridation lost again. Later that year, a district court ordered that Brainerd's water be fluoridated. The state supreme court heard an appeal, but upheld the judgment. The appeal was then taken to the US Supreme Court, which refused to hear the case. In 1978 a governor's panel conducted an exhaustive study. Still nothing happened.

In 1979 Jack and three other members of a group named "The Committee for Responsible Government in Brainerd" inserted into the *Brainerd Daily Dispatch* a quarter-page "Open Letter to the Legislature, Courts, and People of Minnesota with Respect to Fluoridation." A few days later Irene Johnson and 19 other signatories responded with a quarter-page rebuttal entitled "Enough Is Enough." In it they asked, "Who are these four unctu-

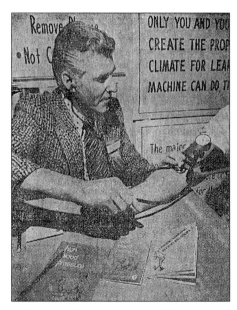

Dr Echternacht encourages dentists to use the "newest" preventive health approach at a meeting of the Minnesota Dental Association in 1974. (From the *Minneapolis Tribune*, April 2, 1974.)

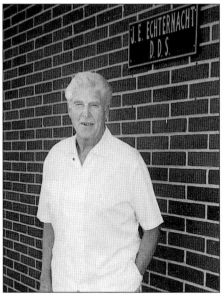

Jack Echternacht on his last day at the office.

ous, arrogant, self-appointed elitists . . . ?" and, "Who anointed these four shamans with the holy oils and ordained them to ridicule and denigrate the good elected officials [of Brainerd]?" Under pressure from the Department of Health, a judge set a deadline of October 19, 1979, for the city council's decision to fluoridate. The council took no action. Finally on October 24, 1979, the council's opposition folded under a contempt citation that carried penalties of $250 per day. The fines were too much to handle. The council voted to fluoridate, and 3 months later fluoride was added to the water. On February 7, 1980, the director of the Brainerd Water and Light Department pushed a pumphouse switch and rotated a valve that allowed fluoride to enter what Brainerd citizens hoped would continue to be the "world's best drink." Ultimately, Mrs Johnson was correct: Jack Echternacht did get his way.

The Jackson County Freelance

In my initial telephone call, I (JTR) had told Dr Echternacht that we wanted to understand both the people in his life and the circumstances that led ultimately to his nomination as a moral exemplar. Knowing something about the extraordinary length of his involvement, I was particularly interested in what gave him the taste for engagement and the stubbornness to persist.

As soon as I arrived for our first meeting, he told me that he had been thinking about his father ever since my call. Estell Ira Echternacht was a memorable man, the type of person about whom stories were told. One of these stories kept Jack going.

When Jack was 7 years old, the family moved from Estherville, Iowa, to Alpha, Minnesota, population 200, some 25 miles from Estherville just across the state line. Mr Echternacht had been a salesman who aspired to be a farmer. He had first worked for the Reed-Murdoch Grocery Company, and then became a salesman with the Buster Brown Shoe Company. The job kept him on the road, and he hated it. Consequently, when given the opportunity to buy 260 acres of prime farmland in Minnesota, he did not hesitate. After only a brief taste of farming, Estell told his wife that if he ever had to go back on the road again, she'd find him "swinging from the rafters."

The Echternachts' home in Estherville was comfortable, but their new place in Alpha was not much more than "a chicken shed with a pot-bellied stove and bed bugs." Though Jack's father had invested in some Oklahoma oil stock, which had turned a modest profit, the proceeds went directly into the farm, and money was still in short supply. Once, when they could not pay their utility bills, their electricity was turned off, adding to the distress of his older sister, who had a patent foramen ovale (a manageable congenital heart defect in today's medicine). Life was not easy, and she became increasingly ill.

It turned out that their inability to pay their electric bills was not entirely of their own doing. The town telephone operator, who was always current on the activities of the citizens, had overheard someone giving Jack's dad the good news about the stock. Before long, the rumor had spread around town that his father had come into some big money. This news was unsettling to a group of three men who were Alpha's self-appointed power structure: the owner of the bank, one of his clerks, and the proprietor of the hardware store. They saw the supposed Echternacht affluence as potentially disrupting the equilibrium of their authority. Adding to their concern was their belief that Estell was Jewish. The name "Echternacht" sounded Jewish to them, and he had a prominent nose, dark eyes, and dark hair. Not only were their views discriminatory, they were also wrong. Mr Echternacht was not Jewish. Nevertheless, to set things "right," they pressured the electric company to charge the Echternachts exorbitant rates. When Jack's father discovered that he was being charged three times more for electricity than anyone else, he was furious.

Mr Echternacht confronted the electric company and the Alpha power brokers with the inequity, but they refused to back down. He went to the county attorney, who refused to take a stand on Estell's behalf. Angry and energized by the injustice, he fought back. He paid every electric bill under protest. More important, believing in the power of public opinion and public pressure, he decided to publish a newspaper, his grade school education notwithstanding. An editor friend in Estherville gave him advice, and Estell got it rolling. He called the newspaper *The Jackson County Freelance*. It was four pages long, and its theme was expressed in the following unattributed quotation: "Truth, crushed to earth, shall rise again; the eternal years of God are hers. But error, wounded, writhes in pain and dies among its worshipers."

The *Freelance* was short on news and long on editorials about honesty and public responsibility. Seven-year-old Jack and his father drove all around the county distributing the papers. In less than a year, the electric

> From his father, Jack learned fortitude, which became his own vehicle for principled action. From his mother, he learned the rudiments of compassion.

Commentary

Dr Echternacht's story is inspiring for at least two reasons. First, as Jack reflected on his actions and the models in his life that shaped him, he illustrated many of the important virtues of the health care professional described by Pellegrino and Thomasma.[1] Second, as he spoke about his views of and satisfactions with dentistry, he revealed a remarkable commitment to professional ideals and obligations. His disposition is to habitually act to benefit others through both professional actions and community service.

Jack recalled a single event that, upon reflection, he believes shaped his disposition to persevere in pursuit of a "just cause." His role model for sustained principled action in the face of adversity was his father. Like his father, Jack displayed what Pellegrino and Thomasma refer to as fortitude, rather than courage. The action was not necessarily heroic, in the sense of risking physical harm, though the elements of physical harm certainly presented themselves as the saga unfolded.

Fortitude, or moral courage, "is the virtue that renders an individual capable of acting on principle in the face of potential harmful consequences without either retreating too soon from that principle or remaining steadfast to the point of absurdity."[1p111]

From his father, Jack learned fortitude, which became his own vehicle for principled action. From his mother, he learned the rudiments of compassion, which is so essential for the health care professional. As Pellegrino and Thomasma asserted, "Compassion is the character trait that shapes the cognitive aspect of healing to fit the unique predicament of this patient."[1p79] As the "good physician" co-suffers with the patient, a bond is created through which symptoms of the condition are filtered. Through the fellowship in experience, the particular circumstances are understood, enabling the professional to bring technical and scientific competence to the patient's predicament. The early development of this compassion became evident as Jack reflected on the loss of his sister.

company lowered his rate and the *Freelance* went out of business. Years later, long after Jack's father died, his mother was at a hotel restaurant in Spirit Lake, Iowa, waiting to be shown to a table. She and a man sitting in the lobby looked familiar to each other, and he introduced himself. He was one of the men, the bank clerk, who had acted against their family. He apologized, saying that his actions had been coerced by the others, but that he had regretted his involvement in that sad affair ever since.

Jack went through high school, college, dental school, a stint in the US Navy, and his first 8 years of practice without ever thinking of *The Jackson County Freelance*. The memory did not surface until himself was under fire. He felt great admiration for his father. For the first time he fully appreciated his father's position and the principled stand his father had taken. This story from his childhood became a reservoir of tenacity and fortitude that he drew upon 25 years later.

A More Subtle Contributor

Jack tells this story of his father's initiative and aggressiveness with relish and pride. He loves to tell it. Nevertheless, he is troubled that his father's self-fulfilling behavior was hard on his mother, Nelda. Nelda was an outgoing person who thrived on friendships with others.

Estell, however, loved his home, and that's where he wanted to be. So they stayed at home. Nelda was religious and enjoyed going to church. Estell, however, remained home on Sundays because the church leaders were the ones who had given him trouble. Consequently, Nelda rarely went to church.

During all of the hardships associated with their new life in Alpha, Jack never saw his mother angry or resentful. In fact, she hated conflict of any kind: She was a peaceloving person who was also an effective peacemaker. She was fairminded. When Jack needed comfort and understanding, he headed for the kitchen. She was a wonderful mother. Estell Echternacht was Jack's hero, but Nelda was the parent he adored.

Jack sees himself as more like his mother than his father. He definitely characterizes himself as peaceloving. As for conflict, he avoids it. "But, if there's a just cause involved," he says, "that's another matter. Then we go to war."

The poignancy of Jack's memories of his mother is enhanced because of the sad and progressive episode of his sister's illness. By the time Jean was 15, she was bedridden. For 2 years, until Jean's death, Jack's mother could only nurse her and watch her get progressively worse. Throughout this terrible experience, his mother remained the same and was always there for him. Even so, Jack, just entering adolescence, remembers seeing her age during those stressful 2 years.

Both of his parents, his mother especially, grieved terribly over Jean's illness and death. Although Jack also

Both of his parents, his mother especially, grieved terribly over Jean's illness and death. Jack felt that his parents had been hurt so much that he had to do everything possible to bring more joy into their lives. In the Echternacht family, that meant the fulfillment of one's potential. "So that was the driving force in my life," Jack said, "trying to be the best I could be. I had an advantage over a lot of fellows in that respect." Jack recognized the lesson of compassion, the gift of intellectual competence, and the value placed on making the most of that gift. Pellegrino and Thomasma remarked that "the virtuous person is impelled by his virtue to strive for perfection—not because it is a duty, but because he seeks perfection . . . in whatever he is engaged in. He cannot act otherwise. It is part of his character. He is disposed habitually to fill out the potential for moral perfection inherent in his actions because he wishes to be as close to perfection as possible . . . realizing all the while that he cannot get there and, in that realization, being prevented from the vices of self-righteousness and hubris."[1p166]

The merging of competence and compassion is evident as he talked about his work. "When he entered his office, he absorbed himself completely with his patients and the procedures themselves. The concerns of the outside world would vanish." He spoke of the joy of both the technical and interactive parts of practice and his own disassociation from the monetary rewards. He described himself as divorced from the business aspects of his practice. His satisfaction comes from an internal motivation rather than from external rewards.

Much of his motivation for community service is based on his conviction that he is obligated to pay back the community for what it has provided him and his family. Whereas he began his professional life with a more minimalist view of professional service—the provision of care for those who can pay for services—his gregarious personality prompted him to engage in community activity. As he did so, his conception of professional service broadened to embrace a duty to engage in public action. He attended to the scientific advances in his profession and then persisted in activities to benefit the oral health of the community,

grieved, it was the effect of Jean's tragedy on his parents that had a defining impact on him. Jack felt that his parents had been hurt so much that he had to do everything possible to bring more joy into their lives. In the Echternacht family, that meant the fulfillment of one's potential. "So that was the driving force in my life," Jack said, "trying to be the best I could be. I had an advantage over a lot of fellows in that respect."

Entering a Profession

> "Dentists and physicians are servants of the people. . . . There's a great deal of satisfaction derived from that."
>
> *Dr Echternacht on the role of dentists*

Growing up in the Echternacht household, Jack came to know not only how much his father loved farming, but also how difficult and unpredictable it was. The Echternachts raised Hereford cattle and fed them for market. In the winter, the work was brutal. When the cattle reached a certain weight, they were shipped to Chicago. Sometimes the stockyards paid prime price; sometimes the price was poor. Jack's father had no control over market prices, nor could he influence the weather or the price of grain. Jack thought there must be something that was more responsive to his efforts.

By the time Jack graduated from high school, he was convinced that farming was not in his future, but he was not yet prepared to be that frank with his father. So Jack did not go directly into college. He took a year off, his publicly stated objective being to make a decision whether to take over his dad's farm or to go to college. It was a self-imposed choice; his father had not asked. Looking back, Jack thinks that the real reason he stayed home that year was because of a feeling of guilty obligation to his father. It was Jack's good luck that the year of 1935 to 1936 happened to be the hottest summer and coldest winter in living memory. People still talk about the winter of '36. Consequently, no one was surprised when Jack said he did not choose to feed 125 Herefords every cold winter morning for the rest of his life.

Two men were influential in giving him alternatives to farming. One was a physician and the other a dentist. Both were family friends, and both were seemingly giants, about 6 feet 4 inches tall and big in other ways as well. Both were great sportsmen and crack shots. When they bought their guns, they had to get the stocks remade to fit them. As a young boy, Jack thought it would be ideal to be like either one of them, including their professional career choices. Years later, when it came time to make a decision, Jack's images of an uncomplicated family life directed him toward den-

even when his colleagues retreated from the cause. Then, as he matured as a professional and citizen, his vision and activity expanded to encompass a responsibility to benefit the community above and beyond what might be expected of a health care professional. He began to see himself not only as a dentist, but also as a citizen responsible for the welfare of his community.

As remarkable as is his persistence in the face of adverse public reaction, even greater is his persistence to promote collegiality among his colleagues even when they neglect what is arguably the collective responsibility of the profession—to promote the oral health of the community. For many professionals, the reluctance of colleagues to give tangible support to a "just cause" would engender feelings of anger, resentment, and alienation. Instead, Dr Echternacht treated his colleagues to an annual hunting trip.

What makes persistence in pursuing professional obligations virtuous? Pellegrino and Thomasma wrote, ". . . a virtuous person is not virtuous because her actions are judged admirable by those around her. . . . Rather, we deem a person virtuous because she does perceive, and act, habitually in a

way that exhibits the habitual disposition to perfection that, as humans, we perceive to be consistent with what it is to be a good person."[1p22] Thus, we consider Dr Echternacht a virtuous person not because his actions are judged admirable by those around him—indeed, Irene Johnson would not judge his actions to be admirable. Instead, we find him virtuous because he perceived, and acted, habitually in a way that exhibited consistency with what he believed to be a good and responsible professional. Some might question the "ethics of action," asking whether the strategy used was the most effective strategy to bring about public acceptance. As Dr Echternacht reflected on his own actions, he remarked about his naïveté in believing that reason and proof were the antidote to the opposition's stance.

Of interest in Dr Echternacht's character is that his disposition to habitually act to benefit others extended beyond his role as dentist and member of a profession. As his own fortune grew, he was moved to actions that benefited his community in many other ways. Many ethicists argue that the beneficence is supererogatory, rather than obligatory. In reflecting on Dr Echternacht's

tistry, which he assumed would be less demanding of his personal time.

For some students, attending dental school is at least as traumatic as 5 AM feedings in sub-zero temperatures. Jack, however, loved dental school and almost everything about it. As most dental students will admit, mastering the technical aspects of dentistry is often difficult. Consistency in the performance of even minimally satisfactory work evades the novice. The demonstration of technical skill becomes vitally linked to one's feeling of self-worth. Until one's hands are under control, dental education can be an emotional roller coaster. For Jack, there were mostly peaks and few valleys.

The most satisfying of Jack's many high points came during a freshman dental anatomy lab. The instructor, while widely admired, was of the loud and critical variety. The class assignment was to carve a mandibular right lateral incisor from a block of simulated tooth material. Students waiting to have their projects graded stood in line, dreading the sarcastic critique. Jack remembers that the student ahead of him was told, "When you go home tonight, I want you to go across the Washington Avenue Bridge, and I want you to take this and throw it as far as you can." Jack was next. The instructor just sat there and didn't say a word. Finally, he said, "This is the best carving I've seen in 20 years." The rest of his dental school career was no different. He graduated first in his class.

Views and Satisfactions About Dentistry

Jack conducted a general practice, and he loved it. He did extractions, other minor surgery, crown and bridge, operative dentistry, and a lot of periodontal treatment. When he entered his office, he absorbed himself completely with his patients and the procedures themselves. The concerns of the outside world would vanish. Jack said, "I just felt at peace. I liked my patients. I had a good relationship with them. And I felt I was doing something for them. I think that's the wonderful thing about dentistry. You can relieve people of pain and discomfort, and you can prevent it." Part of what satisfied Jack was the manual activity itself. He enjoyed lab work, and he waxed and cast all his own gold crowns. "If a patient canceled," Jack said, "or if I had a little time between patients, I always had something to do. Go into the laboratory and carve a crown, or cast one, or polish one. It was just great, and I loved to work with it."

When Jack thinks about the beliefs and moral values that describe him best, his frame of reference is his profession. After 52 years as a dentist, how could he think otherwise? In fact, Jack feels that one's personal and professional value systems are integrated. "You can't have two sets of values and be consistent in what you do." The values he feels most strongly about include the

perception of community service, we see that he conceptualizes as obligatory what others might characterize as "beyond the call of duty." He said, "I believe that if one lives in a community and makes his livelihood from it, he should return that benefit by participating in the activities of the community to better it in any way that he can." At the end of the story, when commenting on the Salvation Army's request for bell ringers, he again used the language of obligation: "Don't you think I ought to do that?" In response to his wife's objection, "No, really. Don't you think I should?"

Dr Echternacht fulfills Pellegrino and Thomasma's characterization of a virtuous person in that he "places the point of separation between moral acceptability and moral unacceptability of a decision to act at a different place than would one who acts solely from principle, rule, or duty. The virtuous person will interpret the span of duty . . . more inclusively and more in the direction of perfection of the good end to which the action is naturally oriented."[1p166] He is impelled to strive for perfection, not because it is a duty but because he cannot act otherwise. It is part of his character.

As we completed the story of Dr Echternacht, I (MJB) talked again with the colleagues who initially nominated him and who knew him well during the activist period of his life. From those conversations, the last of Colby and Damon's[2] criteria emerged: Dr Echternacht embodies a sense of realistic humility about his own importance relative to the world at large, implying a relative lack of concern for his own ego. One colleague remarked, "I knew it would make a good story, but in retrospect, I'm surprised he agreed to be interviewed. When we tried over the years to honor him for his achievements, either at the local or state dental societies, he would decline, declaring that he was merely doing what was expected." Such "effacement of self-interest" is undoubtedly a reason why the nomination of Dr Echternacht as a moral exemplar was so enthusiastically supported by his peers.

References

1. Pellegrino ED, Thomasma DC. The Virtues in Medical Practice. New York: Oxford University Press, 1983.
2. Colby A, Damon W. Some Do Care: Contemporary Lives of Moral Commitment. New York: Free Press, 1992.

obligations for honesty, helping others, community involvement, and commitment. The fluoridation struggle illustrates all four values, but is a paradigm lesson in commitment. Jack thinks those four characteristics are his essence, personally as much as professionally.

Jack thinks the requirements of honesty assume an expanded meaning in practice. "There are so many opportunities you have where you could take advantage of a person. Patients don't know what is going on most of the time, even though you explain it to them. And there are so many times you could take a short cut or not do something the way it should be done. You just have to do things the proper way. When there's money involved, you can easily take advantage of patients. It is just a terrible thing when a professional man takes advantage of a patient."

Another essential value pertained to helping others. One of Jack's joys in practice was the thrill of helping people out of difficult situations. "You know," Jack said, "dentists and physicians are servants of the people. We really are. We provide a service that should be beneficial to people. There's a great deal of satisfaction derived from that, in addition to the monetary return." Sometimes he thought it would be wonderful if he could just concentrate on the treatment and not have to worry about charging his patients. In fact, Jack felt that the details of ordinary business life were sometimes beyond him. Without the help of his staff, there is no telling how much free dentistry he would have provided.

A value that emerges with special conviction is the obligation to pay back the community for what it has provided. "I believe that if one lives in the community and makes his livelihood from it, he should return that benefit by participating in the activities of the community to better it in any way that he can." Although Jack speaks quietly, in everything he says there is a rocklike grounding of force, sincerity, and often humor. Nowhere does he show more force and less humor than when he talks about obligations to the community. This energy comes from his frustration that many others do not share his commitment. The majority of people go through their lives without even a glimmer of what Jack considers to be so vital. "I've been on so many fund drives in my community, I get so disappointed with what people do, when I know what they could do. And that just bothers the life out of me. If all the professional people would do something, all these projects and things that you'd like to better the community with would be so much easier to accomplish. I just don't understand how you can take but not give."

Jack's beliefs about community service are an outgrowth of his practice. They are demonstrations of how the profession has enlarged his values. He had never thought about community involvement before he entered dental school, nor when he started his practice. He had received no prior encouragement in that direction from his family. Jack merely felt gratitude to his community and his patients for the good living that his family enjoyed. The satisfaction he gets from community projects is parallel to that which he gets from dentistry. In both, the benefits are tangible. "Like putting a filling in a tooth," Jack says.

Jack specialized in megaprojects. He found that he had a special talent for fundraising and used it to create a golf course at the Brainerd Golf and Country Club and to transform a floundering Young Men's Christian Association (YMCA) with few useful functions and no building into a vital organization with a new activity center. He later became president of the Brainerd YMCA and also served for a time as its national director.

The project that pleases Jack the most is the Brainerd Civic Center. It is an imposing building on the edge of town, big enough to hold a regulation ice hockey rink, locker rooms, a balcony, and concession stands. The Civic Center enabled the high school to field a hockey team. It is also used for ice shows, countywide ice hockey lessons, automobile shows, and other trade shows. Jack conceived the idea, organized the corporation that would own the building, and raised more than $1,000,000. It was a private effort, with Jack as part owner of the Civic Center and president of the corporation. From his own funds, he bought enough trees to beautify the building. Neither Jack nor any other directors received monetary compensation. After a few years, when income exceeded operating expenses, the corporation donated the Civic Center to the city.

Dr Echternacht has been involved in many other community efforts. Using his skill in taxidermy, which was a legacy of his childhood mentor, Dr Portman, he provided and still updates a six-cabinet display of about 120 birds and examples of their habitats at the Brainerd High School. (With regret, Jack states that the display includes a golden eagle that he shot approximately 20 years ago.) Besides donating mounted birds to the high school and to the vocational technology school, he taught taxidermy at the high school at no cost. He has also donated teaching time in the local dental assistant program. He is past president of the Brainerd Civic Music Association and has participated in various Boy Scout activities. In 1982 he was named Brainerd Citizen of the Year, after modestly declining the honor for several years previously.

An activity that Jack feels was his most outstanding professional accomplishment, apart from the promotion of fluoridation, was taking groups of dentists on an annual autumn hunting trip at the game farm at Little Falls. The close companionship in game hunting all day and enjoying the evening feasts was largely instrumental in making the Crow Wing County dentists the most cohesive group in the state.

Currently

These days Jack feels as idle as he has ever been in his life. He semi-retired at the age of 70 when Flo, his wife of 50 years, became terminally ill and died after a 5-year battle with cancer. During that time he cut back his practice to 3 days a week so that he could spend more time with her. Two years later he stopped practicing altogether. Today he takes care of his house on Gull Lake and enjoys golfing again. At present he is upgrading the display of birds at Brainerd High School.

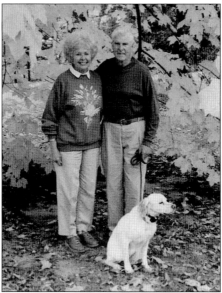

Dr Echternacht with his wife, Faye, and dog, Jill.

In 1994 Jack married again, to Faye Hickerson, an old friend. He and Flo had known Faye and her husband 30 years ago, when they all lived in Brainerd and belonged to the same social group. Faye and her husband were among those who moved away. Four years after Faye's husband died, she married Jack in Portland, Oregon, then moved back to Brainerd. Getting together worked out well for both Faye and Jack. She is an unabashed fan of Jack's, and sometimes provides details that Jack omits, such as being first in his class.

Jack feels slightly guilty that he has not been involved in any community activity since he retired. "For instance," Jack says, "in the paper last night, there was a call for bell ringers for the Salvation Army Christmas fundraiser. I said, 'Faye, how about that? Don't you think I ought to do that?' She said, 'Yeah, sure.' I said, 'No, really. Don't you think I should? I've got time. I could go over and spend a few hours.' Faye said, 'I think you've done enough for three lifetimes.'"

"But it does bother me a little bit that I don't do something like that."

Questions for Discussion

1. Dr Echternacht discovers important role models for himself as he reflects upon his life and the particular actions for which he was nominated as an exemplar. Who were his models, and what important lessons did they impart? Think about your own life. Are there individuals who influenced you to act in particular ways?

2. The commentary directs attention to several of the virtues of professional practice. Choose one or two of these and discuss them. Assess yourself and the professionals closest to you in terms of these qualities.

3. At the end of the commentary, Dr Echternacht is described as a virtuous person, yet the authors suggest that it is not his actions that contribute to such a judgment. What, then, makes him a virtuous person?

4. What lessons about collegiality does this story contain?

5. Persistence seems to have been an important virtue in Dr Echternacht's 30-year struggle over water fluoridation. As he reflects on that battle, however, what does he see as his personal shortcomings? What role do these shortcomings play in his effectiveness as a moral exemplar?

6. Discuss Dr Echternacht's views about gratitude to his community. Is his attitude an essential one for all practitioners?

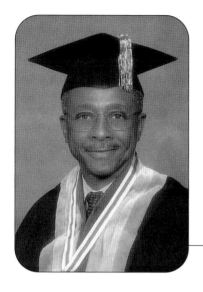

3

Hugo A. Owens

Dentist, Civil Rights Leader, Politician

For 44 years Dr Hugo A. Owens was a distinguished practitioner and community leader in Portsmouth and Chesapeake, Virginia, and also served for a time as president of the National Dental Association. Besides his proclivity for dentistry, he was driven by two other passions: politics and civil rights. In 1970 he was one of the first African Americans ever elected to the Chesapeake City Council. He was re-elected for the next term and appointed vice mayor, a position he held for 8 years. His political successes were preceded by his activities as a civil rights leader, which began in 1950 and lasted through the 1960s. In a remarkable series of negotiations and litigations, Dr Owens was the prime mover in the desegregation of the city of Portsmouth. In all three "careers," Dr Owens used dentistry as a home base for the expression of his activist philosophy of providing help for others when they were unable to help themselves.

Influential Early Years

Hugo Armstrong Owens was born on January 21, 1916. His name was the result of a negotiated parental settlement. His father wanted to name him Samuel Armstrong Owens, after Samuel Armstrong, the founder and president of Hampton Institute when Hugo's father attended college there. His mother liked Armstrong, but balked at Samuel. She said that no one would call her son "Sambo"—or any other nickname or caricature that would undermine his self-esteem and identity. Both parents, however, liked the symbolic reference to academe conveyed by the name Armstrong. In fact, his mother had dreams that a son of hers would one day be a university president. So they compromised and named him Hugo, after James Hugo Johnston, president of Virginia State University, which was his mother's alma mater.

The pursuit of higher education was a tradition in Hugo's family. His maternal grandparents had sent all their children through college, and his uncle, George Melvin, had become a lawyer. There was no question that Hugo also would go to college. In fact, with George Melvin living across the street, Hugo could not have survived comfortably with lesser goals.

With his imposing stature, fiercely intense eyes, and booming voice, George was a powerful influence on the aspirations of Hugo and the other four Owens children. Uncle George was a hard man to satisfy. If the children asked a careless question, he would shout at them, "You are asking a dumb question!" His frequent prognostications were considered declarations of how things ought to be. Uncle George said Hugo's older brother was going to be a minister, and so he was. Uncle George announced that Hugo's second brother should be a musician; he became one. Although George offered no specific career path for Hugo, he predicted that greatness lay ahead. He told Hugo, "If you were a white man, you would be governor of Virginia." Even today, after all these years, Dr Owens perceives his uncle's influence. "He helped shape my character, forced me to set goals, and inspired me to excel in everything I did."

Especially unforgettable is a memory of Uncle George from when Hugo was only 5 or 6 years old. To get to work, Uncle George took the streetcar every day from his village to downtown Portsmouth. Hugo said, "Many a night he came home bloodied because he refused to move to the back of the streetcar or get up to give whites a seat. I can still see him come in the house bloody, and my mother would say, 'What in the world happened to you?' And he would curse like a sailor and tell her. That's the kind of thing I grew up witnessing."

Dr Owens had been thinking about this story since he was first contacted about our interest in knowing the people and circumstances that had influenced his moral development. For his entire adult life he has looked back with pride at his uncle's courage under fire. It remains his paradigm for courageous, vigorous, and principled action. Dr Owens said, "When I did civil rights, I was my Uncle George."

Although Uncle George's experiences on the streetcar have given the mature Hugo Owens much satisfaction over the years, they had a much different effect on him as a child. At that tender stage, his uncle's experiences fostered feelings of anxiety, fear, and trepidation of white people. Even now, he said, part of him is still afraid of white people.

Hugo's Uncle George was not the only means by which he learned about the uncertainties of being African American. His grandmother had been a slave and recounted stories about the cruelty of the masters. Moreover, she raised concerns about the hazards of modern-day life as well. Hugo said her core advice to him was, "Never steal; never lie. If you want something, ask for it; don't take it. And whatever you do, never even look at a white woman; they will string you up whether you did anything wrong or not."

Coupled with the memories of these important people in his childhood, Hugo had geographic reminders of his personal circumstances and those of his ancestors. His childhood home was on property that his great grandfather had purchased when he came out of slavery. And the home where Hugo lives today lies almost equidistant from where both parents' ancestors were enslaved: 30 minutes in one direction for his mother's people and 20 minutes in a different direction for his father's people. On one wall of Hugo's house hangs a framed receipt dated 1855 for $2,400, the price paid by an ancestor to a plantation owner to free six of his grandmother's relatives.

Another major influence in young Hugo's life was religion. His mother, Grace, was a Sunday school teacher. His father, James, was deeply religious. A charismatic man who loved to talk with people, James became a deacon while he was still a college student at Hampton. Later he became a lay minister (everyone loved his elegant, colorful sermons), and he was a Sunday school superintendent for as long as Hugo can remember. On Sunday mornings, while Hugo's mother was preparing breakfast, his father would gather all five children to quote scripture from the Bible, sing a hymn, and, while on their knees with their faces in their chairs, invoke the blessings of the deity. "That was every Sunday," Dr Owens said, "so you see why I'm such a nut." Almost everyone who nurtured young Hugo was religious. The exception was George Melvin, who claimed to be an atheist.

The family emphasis on religion also provided an introduction to poetry. James Owens enjoyed the poetry of the Bible and started training Hugo to memorize the Psalms at the age of 4. More than 75 years later, Dr Owens can still quote the first Psalm. His mother quoted poetry to her children and often wrote poetry herself. Everyone connected with the Owens family learned to enjoy poetry, including George Melvin, who took pleasure in reciting the dramatic poems of Edgar Allen Poe. Hugo especially likes poetry. He used to quote poetry to his patients. Sometimes he opened meetings with poems. It seemed impossible to be with him for more than a few minutes without hearing a poem. He has also published a small volume of poems he has written. During our first meeting, he fortified the conversation with two or three selections from his favorite poets, Langston Hughes and Paul Laurence Dunbar, and one of his own that he had written for his son.

Hugo was bombarded with the relevance of religion to everyday affairs and the need to maintain high standards of personal conduct. The lessons were well learned. Religion continues to be a vital part of Hugo's life. He brought the values that he learned at home and at church—which were identical—to his professional life, his political life, and his involvement in civil rights. From the standpoint of how others should be treated, he believes that the Golden Rule should be the guideline. He believes that those who live by that principle have a peace of mind that others do not.

Heading Toward a Profession

By the time Hugo graduated from high school, he had some definite ideas about his future career. In his sophomore year, his biology teacher had presented information on the endocrine system that, he said, "was like a search light coming on in my brain." As a result, he read everything he could get his hands on about the endocrine system and decided he wanted to be an endocrinologist. However, Hugo also considered teaching as a career alternative, because he had no funds for graduate school.

Both of his parents had been teachers. His father's teaching career had not lasted long, however, primarily because of the low salaries for teachers, especially black teachers at that time. So with a growing family to support, his father became a letter carrier. This offered a salary that was more than twice as high as his teacher's pay. In a laboring community, it meant that Hugo was looked upon as a rich man's son. To add to the family income, Hugo's father eventually bought several acres of land and worked it as a farm.

When Hugo graduated from high school, he did not go directly to college as he had expected. His mother was ill, and it was up to him to take care of her. His siblings, all of whom were older, had already moved away from home. His father was extremely busy as a mail carrier, not to mention his activities in the church and on the farm. Hugo therefore delayed his entry into Virginia State University for a year, by which time his mother had recovered. During that year, besides caring for his mother, he did the housekeeping, learned to cook, read the classics, read poetry, wrote poetry, read more science, memorized all sorts of things, listened to radio broadcasts of the Metropolitan Opera, and courted Helen West, whom he would eventually marry. All told, he says, that year was "one of the finer periods" of his life.

At Virginia State, Hugo immediately entered student politics and ran for president of the freshman class. That

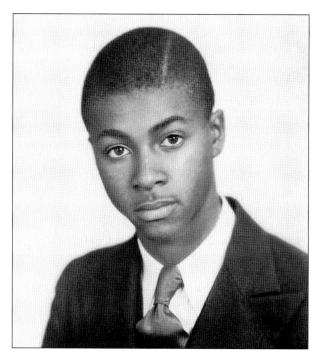

Hugo A. Owens, while attending Virginia State University (1938).

and his first attempt to run for Portsmouth City Council were the only elections he ever lost. Three years later, as a senior, he was elected president of the student body. It was in that office that he discovered something about himself that has been his hallmark ever since. It gave him great satisfaction to do things that other people needed to have done but could not do for themselves. In addition, he began to judge himself according to his success in making things happen and found that he was good at it. Hugo said, "When people say something ought to be done, I say let's do it."

Hugo received a bachelor of science degree from Virginia State University in 1939 at the age of 23. Although he had done well in all of his courses and still had dreams of becoming an endocrinologist, he did not apply to medical school. He knew that blacks were not being accepted in the Virginia schools, and he was not aware of opportunities for blacks in universities outside his home state. Even if he had known about those prospects, he lacked the money to attend medical school elsewhere.

He therefore decided to be a teacher, at least for the time being. For 3 years he taught chemistry and physics in Crisfield, and by the time he left to join the US Army in 1942, he had married Helen West and risen to the rank of assistant principal. He had even enrolled in a master's program in guidance counseling as the first step in becoming the son who fulfilled his mother's dream of a college presidency. As Hugo said, "That's what I was going for."

Reflecting on his young adulthood, Hugo said he was inspired by people he called "The Giants." These were orators who had messages of both practicality and great depth. He listened to their speeches as often as he could and contemplated their messages. The "Giants" included Mordecai W. Johnson, president of Howard University; Carter G. Woodson, historian and founder of the Negro History Month; Benjamin Mayes, president of Morehouse College; Howard Thurman, dean of the chapel at Howard University; and C. C. Spalding, a founder of the North Carolina Mutual Life Insurance Company. All of these men were African Americans who had achieved success and retained a sense of obligation to their roots. Hugo said that, distilled, their message was this: "First excel, then help others."

Hugo's enlistment in the Army started the process by which his inspiration took focus. He achieved the rank of corporal and became a personnel clerk because he knew how to type. Thanks to the opportunity provided by the Army Specialist Training Program, he had the opportunity to acquire further education. Even though he continued to lean toward medicine, he was uncertain about his future. He applied to medical schools, but also to dental schools, law schools, and meteorology schools. His first acceptance letter came from Howard University's College of Dentistry. Having absorbed the Army maxim of never turning down a chance to improve one's situation, he accepted Howard's offer. A week later, acceptances started to roll in from Harvard, the University of Chicago, Meharry, and other universities in all the disciplines he applied for. He entered dental school in the fall of 1943 and has never regretted his choice.

Hugo's life as a dental student was extremely busy, but not only with his studies. Although he was supported by the GI (government issue) bill, he still found it necessary to work. He took one job that kept him busy every weekday evening, and on weekends he worked as a dental assistant. Interestingly, his classmates elected him class president all 4 years. Hugo says, "They made me president for life; I was such a ham." In his yearbook he was referred to as "The Dean." Despite these diversions, he excelled in both classroom and clinic. At his graduation in 1947 at the age of 31, he received the award for excellence in preclinical studies, was elected to the Chi Lambda Kappa Honorary Society, and was made a member of Omicron Kappa Upsilon, a prestigious recognition of academic accomplishments.

Practice As Home Base

Enjoying His Practice

Dr Owens first practiced in Washington, DC, for a few months, filling in for a couple of dentists who were on vacation. He then accepted an offer to work with a dentist who was nearing retirement in Portsmouth, Virginia, not far from his childhood home. It was a good choice. Everyone knew his father and felt they could not go wrong with James' son. Hugo was well supplied with patients right from the beginning. He soon took over the practice and remained in Portsmouth for 44 years, not retiring until 1991 at the age of 75. He might not have retired then, but his nephew was available to succeed him.

Hugo enjoyed his practice immensely. Like his father, he loved to talk with people. He would joke with them, quote poems, and listen to their problems. He also enjoyed the technical aspects of dentistry and did most of his own laboratory work for bridges and inlays. Always a competitor, Hugo got special satisfaction from his conviction that he ". . . was delivering something to my patients that other patients weren't getting." He said dentistry taught him about the concept of perfection and the need to strive for it in whatever he did. The profession's concern for excellence was a good match with his personal philosophy.

In the early years of practice, Hugo saw another major advantage that dentistry had to offer: It permitted him to control his time. If he wanted to earn money in his office, he could do that. If he wanted to tend to a special project, he could do that instead. Usually his patients were willing to be rescheduled, and there was no one else whose permission he had to seek. As Hugo became familiar with the community and its problems, his activist tendencies reappeared and he came to appreciate the flexibility that a dental practice provided.

Listening to Patients

Hugo's awareness of his community's problems came sometimes from his own observations but often through the eyes of his patients. One such patient, Floyd Cooper,

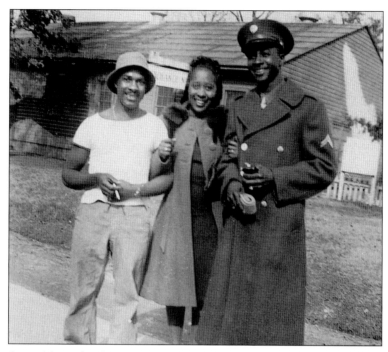

Corporal Owens *(right)* with his wife, Helen, and a sergeant at Fort Eustis, Virginia (circa 1942).

had had his fill of injustices and figured that Hugo was someone who might be able to change things. Floyd had never finished school past fourth grade, but Hugo said he was one of the most brilliant people he had ever met. He had been a caddie at the city golf course almost all of his life, but, being black, could not formally use the course for his own enjoyment. In 1950, 3 years after Dr Owens started his practice, Floyd spoke to him about this inequity, and together they devised a plan. Floyd assembled a group of five would-be golfers, including Dr Owens, who went to the Recreation Department and requested admittance to the Portsmouth Golf Course. Only one of the men, Floyd himself, had ever swung a golf club. The Recreation Department rejected their request. Led by Dr Owens, the group then embarked on a series of negotiations at progressively higher levels in city government. Everyone they met wanted to know if they could actually play golf, figuring that the probability was about zero. Dr Owens would respond, "How in the hell do we learn how to play golf? We don't own golf clubs. We don't have a place to play." The officials would then want to know why they wanted to play golf if they didn't know the game. Dr Owens pointed out, in logic that was to become the pattern for similar, future

negotiations, that their ability to play golf was not the issue. Their concern was that he and the others were paying taxes to the city treasurer. The city budgeted part of that money to operate the golf courses and the city park. However, even though he had contributed some of the tax money, he was prohibited from using the facilities it was supporting. Nevertheless, at each level of discussion, their attempts at negotiation failed. Dr Owens then switched to litigation. Using the same logic in court that he had in his negotiations, Dr Owens successfully led the first lawsuit against the city to open its parks and golf courses to African Americans.

A year later, Dr Owens had better luck with his negotiations. He successfully negotiated with the city of Portsmouth to have its first Alcoholic Beverage Control (ABC) store opened and managed by a black staff. Again it was Floyd Cooper who pointed out that every ABC store in Portsmouth that was located in a black neighborhood was manned by whites. This time Hugo worked through the existing political process at the state level, convincing a few key delegates that it would be in their long-term interest to support this change.

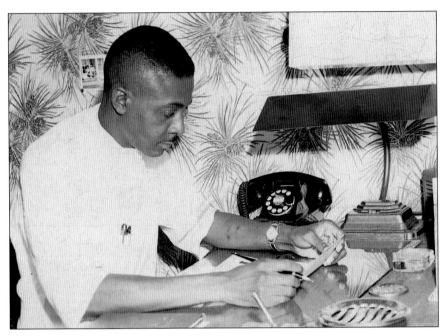

Dr Owens in his private practice (1950s).

Leadership in Dentistry

At precisely the same time that Hugo first became involved in civil rights, he was also making his presence known in the Portsmouth dental community. Hugo enjoyed working with people and appreciated what could be done when people work together in organizations. At that time the primarily white Virginia Dental Association was not admitting blacks. Therefore, African American Virginians formed their own state organization, called the Old Dominion Dental Society. Like the Virginia Dental Association, it was represented in the various communities by component societies. Portsmouth, however, had no component society. Hugo decided that it was time to create one and founded the McGriff Dental Society in 1953, in honor of a distinguished African American dentist who had practiced in the Portsmouth area. The McGriff Society is still thriving.

The year 1953 was busy for Hugo in many ways. He headed a group of citizens who put pressure on officials to upgrade streets and install curbs in the black part of town. Part of the pressure was the threat of litigation, and the city yielded. Also that year he won a lawsuit against Portsmouth that forced the city to stop its policy of maintaining white-only cemeteries.

Hugo paid for that lawsuit out of his own pocket, as he often did. However, he sometimes got help from other benefactors for these substantial expenditures, and people would come to his office unsolicited and donate a few dollars for the cause. Dr Owens was the point man in these activities, but not the only person by any means. Nevertheless, word was getting around that if you had a problem, Dr Owens was the man to see. Requests for help proliferated, and he was invited to speak all around the region. His civil rights activities expanded to the point that he was out of his office for about one third of his time.

In 1955 Dr Owens hired his first associate. The term "associate" by today's standards is appropriate in that it most often describes a business relationship between an established practitioner with a growing practice and a young dentist, usually fresh out of school. However, the term does not do justice to the relationships between Dr Owens and the 12 young dentists with whom he would work over the years. Dr Charles Sanders, dean of Howard University's dental school, who nominated Dr Owens as a moral exemplar, viewed him as a true mentor. Unlike the custom today, Dr Owens did not advertise for associates; he only responded to requests for help. Dr Owens not only offered support and guidance at the time the young graduates needed it the most, he also offered them as much flexibility as they could hope for. They could stay in his office as long as they wanted, until their own practice was established. Some stayed for 1 year, others for 2 or 3 years. All told, from Dean Sanders' standpoint, Dr Owens was the perfect alumnus: he mentored Howard graduates; he had the respect of his peers; he had a reputation for excellence; and he was a supporter of the college. At one time he had been on Howard's faculty as an extramural professor and had served as president of the university's dental alumni association.

Within the next few years, Dr Owens was elected president of the Old Dominion Dental Society and published a case report on the replantation of an avulsed tooth in the *Journal of Prosthetic Dentistry*. He also spearheaded a lawsuit that eliminated segregated housing, and organized a conference of leaders who recruited black students for formerly all-white schools. Dr Owens became president of the Portsmouth chapter of the National Association for the Advancement of Colored People (NAACP), as his father before him had been some 15 years earlier. During his tenure in office, he focused public attention on job discrimination at the Naval installations in Portsmouth, which resulted in a federal investigation and ultimate change. Here again, a lawsuit was avoided.

His Last Years in Civil Rights

In 1960 Dr Owens initiated a lawsuit against the city to desegregate the public library. It would prove to be his last litigation and his most satisfying experience. Emotions had been high on both sides, and he felt that he had been able to provide constructive leadership, avoiding the violence he had feared. Dr Owens had been trying to get blacks into the city library for 6 years. Finally, some small irritation that he can't remember set him off. He left his office, picked up his three children and the minister of his church, and drove to the library. He asked the head librarian how he could check out some books for his children. He suggested that parents at Rev. Wilson's 1,000-member church might also be interested. When the librarian said that they did not have any children's literature, at least for them, Dr Owens engaged in a series of escalating discussions with the library board, the city attorney, the mayor, and the city government. He initiated a lawsuit when it was

clear that the discussions were going nowhere. Once again the federal judge agreed with him, proclaiming, "The Portsmouth Library must admit Negroes or close up–lock, stock, and barrel."

After 10 years of intense activity, tensions began to subside. Whereas the decade of the 1960s was a time of civil rights conflict for the United States as a whole, many of Portsmouth's struggles were behind it. Nonetheless, some issues continued to surface. In 1964 Dr Owens headed a group of local medical and dental practitioners that successfully negotiated the desegregation of the city hospital. In the same year, he organized public demonstrations that led to the desegregation of other public facilities, including restaurants and department stores.

Finally, in 1965, when civil rights activists walked the 54 miles from Selma to Montgomery, Alabama, as a response to weeks of violence, Dr Owens organized and led the largest Selma sympathy demonstration in the country. They marched in silence through the city of Portsmouth to the waterfront and ended with the ceremonious reading of the names of those who had been killed. With each name, a red rose was cast into the water. When the names of the four girls who had been killed in a Birmingham church were read, a white rose was thrown instead. Telling this story affected Hugo as if it had happened today. Speaking increasingly softly and slowly, he seemed to be reliving the experience. At one point he stopped talking altogether.

Professional Disappointment

In the early 1960s Dr Owens joined the predominantly white Tidewater Dental Association. Shortly thereafter, he was nominated by two of his new colleagues for membership in the premier organization that recognizes leadership in the profession, the American College of Dentists. Based on the record he had already compiled, it would have been reasonable for him to be voted in. However, the regional chapter as a whole rejected his nomination, and it never went forward to the national organization. He was led to believe that he had been rejected because of his race, and perhaps because of his activities in civil rights. Although this incident happened a long time ago, it still had the power to affect him.

> "When people say something ought to be done, I say let's do it."
>
> *Dr Owens*

Expanded Leadership in Community and Profession

During the 1960s, Dr Owens began to turn his attention to more traditional sorts and greater variety of community involvement. Over a period of time, he became a director of the Tidewater United Fund and of the United Virginia Bank. He served as vice president of the Hampton Roads Public Broadcasting Corporation. Always present at the start of things, he was a founding member of the Southeastern Tidewater Opportunity Project, the new Eastern Virginia Medical School, the Portsmouth Chesapeake Council on Human Relations, and the Portsmouth chapter of the Congress of Racial Equality. He also had his first taste of city politics and his final electoral defeat. In 1965 he ran for the Portsmouth City Council and lost by 62 votes.

Late in that decade, Dr Owens became interested in preventive dentistry, a field that was just beginning to be recognized. Using that theme, he presented lectures to his Virginia colleagues and published two papers in state journals. One of the papers, appearing in the *Virginia Medical Monthly*, admonished his physician colleagues for indiscriminately recommending full-mouth extractions for patients whose teeth could be saved. His activities became known beyond Virginia, and he became a founding member and the first vice president of the American Society of Preventive Dentistry (ASPD), receiving a Founder's Award for his efforts. In typical form, Hugo began one of his national meetings with a poem, the opening lines of which were, "My dentist 'tis of thee, Member of ASPD." A few years later he published an article in the *Journal of the American Dental Association* in which he advocated that plaque control be added to prepayment insurance plans, an idea that was far ahead of its time.

By 1970, 23 years after starting his practice, Hugo was in full swing. Having moved to nearby Chesapeake, he ran for and this time was elected to the city council. He was one of the first two African Americans elected in that community. He was re-elected in 1972 and appointed vice mayor. He was re-elected three more times and served as vice mayor for 8 years before he retired undefeated in 1980. In that office, he brought minority representation to all the boards and commissions in the city and dramatically increased the employment of blacks in city government.

During this same period his community service expanded to higher education. In 1972 Dr Owens was appointed by the governor to serve on the Norfolk State University Board of Visitors, which in Virginia has broad governing responsibilities, ranging from selecting the president to keeping the mission of the institution on target. He served on the board as its secretary until 1980. He later served as rector, or chair, of the Board of Visitors at Virginia State University from 1982 to 1986 and at Old Dominion University from 1992 to 1996.

If, when Hugo "did civil rights," he was his Uncle George, when he did politics, he was his father. Functioning in civil rights and in politics was similar in some ways, but in other important aspects, it was quite differ-

Commentary

Dr Owens said, "[I was able] to do things that other people needed to have done but could not do for themselves." His willingness to identify moral problems and act on them seems to set him apart from many respected and accomplished practitioners and is an example of what Pellegrino and Thomasma[1] define as practical wisdom, or phronesis. Phronesis encompasses essential internal processes that give rise to morality.[2] These processes include sensitivity, judgment, motivation, character, and competence. Collectively they promote a practical kind of moral insight. Dr Owens displays this quality as he elicits the stories of racial injustices from his patients. He is able to discern moral choices that are justifiable and is motivated and committed to correct the injustices. More remarkable is his practicality. He consistently devises highly effective courses of action to achieve his goals. He displays this ability repeatedly, ever broadening the scope of problems he undertakes. By the time he is well into retirement, the "ethic of action" is so well honed that he is able, without preparation, to "lay out a plan for action" that results in a standing ovation. In the implementation of the action—throughout his lifetime—he habitually shows persistence, temperance, and prudence.

Like Jack Echternacht (chapter 2), when prompted to reflect on life events that shaped his moral actions, Hugo very quickly cited a paradigm example of courage in the face of injustice. He recalled with pride his Uncle George Melvin's drama on the streetcar in which he willingly risked physical harm to defy discriminatory policies. But, like Dr Echternacht, who recognized the downside of his father's courage in challenging the power structure in the community, Dr Owens understands the disadvantages of his uncle's confrontational style and is clearly influenced by the more temperate models demonstrated by his grandmother and parents.

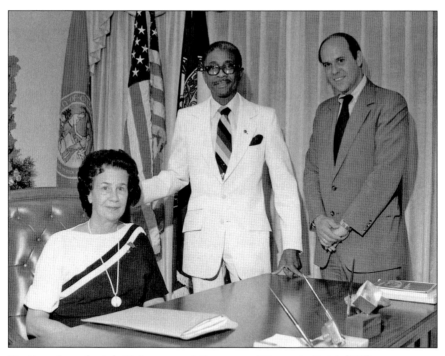

Vice Mayor Owens *(center)* with the mayor and city manager of Chesapeake, Virginia (1979).

ent. Similarly, his Uncle George and his father, James, were both principled men who acted on their beliefs, but in many ways they were quite different. Except when it came to religion, James was much less strict than George Melvin. More important, though, James was less rigid and less disposed to confront "the system." For example, while both men believed in teaching children how to defend themselves, his father would say, "A good run is better than a bad stand." James was much more willing than George to compromise. According to Hugo, his father's attitude would be, "You can't get all of the pie. Even if you want it all, you've got to share some." On the

Hugo was able to change discriminatory practices without inciting violence. In this respect, it appears that he learned the essential characteristic of temperance from his grandmother. She provided guides for living in a community where inequality is the norm. Her strategy went beyond basic integrity—the habitual disposition to personal honesty and truthfulness. In her view the only protection from bigotry was to conduct oneself in a way that did not draw attention to the biases of the white community. Temperance in righting racial inequalities in a community requires an exquisite awareness of the conditions of the community. A master of negotiation in the mold of his father, Dr Owens patiently worked through the community hierarchy using logic and reason to achieve his ends. Problems were called to the community's attention respectfully. The incidents at the golf course and the library are marvelous examples of respectful problem presentation. Demonstrating another hallmark of effective negotiation, he focused on interest, rather than positions. In the ABC liquor store example, he pointed to the long-term benefits of hiring black managers for stores in black neighborhoods. Only after negotiation failed did he turn to litigation. Even when pursuing litigation, he seemed to sense when there was sufficient external support to make the legal pursuit a good investment of time and resources. Leadership as modeled by his Uncle George Melvin is "standing up." Leadership as modeled by his father is "avoiding bad stands."

Reflecting on Dr Owens' accomplishments, we see an individual who led change to achieve social justice without negative notoriety. In all he did, he demonstrated both fortitude and a fine sense of prudential judgment. His fortitude is most easily understood in his expressions of courage, resilience, and staying power. Understanding where prudence fits in requires some comment. To be prudent is to discern the most appropriate means to achieve a particular end. Its essence is practicality, but it requires speculative wisdom as well. Certainly, Hugo Owens is intimately aware of the forces that shaped his intellectual maturity. He spoke of the expectations to achieve greatness and the expecta-

other hand, George Melvin's posture would be, "Look, you [expletive], you've done this to me; therefore I'm going to take it all." When Hugo became a politician, he came to fully accept his father's way. He realized that no matter how much power he had as an elected official, he still had to compromise.

When Hugo left city politics, he concentrated again on professional politics. He became increasingly active in the National Dental Association, which is primarily composed of African Americans. In 1982 he was elected Speaker of the House of Delegates, and in 1988, 3 years before his retirement from dental practice, he served as its president.

Hugo's contributions have earned him many awards. He received two Distinguished Alumni Awards, one from the College of Dentistry at Howard University in 1971 and another from Virginia State University in 1973. In 1989 Norfolk State University presented him with The President's Citation, and in 1992 Old Dominion University gave him its Martin Luther King Leadership Award. In 1996, not yet satisfied, Old Dominion again honored Dr Owens by renaming its African American Cultural Center the Hugo A. Owens Center. Over a period of some 30 years, Dr Owens was presented with "First Citizen" awards by the cities of Portsmouth and Chesapeake and two other organizations. In 1980 he was named "Citizen of the Decade" by Norfolk Newspapers, and May 23, 1986, was proclaimed "Dr Hugo A. Owens Day" by the city of Portsmouth. He has also received an array of local Founder's, Achievement, or Citizenship awards. In 1988

he was named an "Influential Black American" by *Ebony* magazine and received the Brotherhood Award by the National Conference of Christians and Jews. One of the things that pleased him the most was, in 1997, having a new school in Chesapeake named the Hugo A. Owens Middle School. Most recently, in 2000, Dr Owens was named by Dominion Resources and Virginia Power/North Carolina Power as one of ten people recognized for excellence in leadership in their "Strong Men & Women" series. He shares this award with such previous recipients as Colin Powell, Maya Angelou, and Douglas Wilder.

After Retirement

Dr Owens entered retirement with a great celebration. A group of his Virginia colleagues chartered a plane and took Hugo to Bermuda to celebrate his career. He said he felt like a hero. And he sailed for the first time at the age of 75. Hugo said he had never felt as liberated as he did then.

Since his retirement, he has continued to be active both in professional and community affairs, despite a heart bypass operation 2 years later. Although he does write an occasional poem, he prefers not to be sedentary. After our first interview in Chesapeake, he suggested that the next meeting start at 7:30 AM—he likes to start the day early. The morning meeting went as planned, then after lunch he drove me around the coun-

---

tions to pursue higher education. His family valued oratory and poetry. When describing the role of religion in the development of his character, he spoke not only about how the Golden Rule became his normative action guide, but also about the role of hymns and psalms in forging his interest in poetry. Interestingly, in the year he spent at home following high school, he engaged in activities relatively atypical for an adolescent. He read classic literature, read and wrote poetry, and listened to opera. At this early point in his life, the motivation for learning, promoted by his family, was internalized. A love of learning characterizes his lifelong personal and professional pursuits.

Turning to his professional achievements, we see a man who was, first and foremost, a technically competent dentist. Dr Owens took great pride in his ability to "give his patients a level of quality they couldn't get elsewhere." His assessment of his competence is not simply self-aggrandizement. His self-assessment was well validated by the dean of the Howard University dental school and by the extensive number of his

academic achievements and accolades. However, in today's view, a dentist is not only a technician but also a scientist. Dr Owens clearly stayed abreast of the evolving scientific basis for his profession and contributed to that body of knowledge through publications in scientific journals.

Another aspect of Dr Owens' perceptions and actions is noteworthy. When describing his conception of the caregiving partnership, he expressed a motto that was atypical in the paternalistic era in which he practiced. He spoke of "helping others help themselves." In his role as a professional, he recognized that the dentist's role as a nonjudgmental teacher and healer is critical to fostering the patient's cooperation in posttreatment maintenance and prevention of subsequent disease. In his roles as dentist and community leader, he illustrated the essential capacity, as described by Pellegrino and Thomasma,[1] to "co-suffer" with the patient: to create a bond through which the symptoms of the patient's condition and circumstances are filtered. Out of co-suffering comes the ability to use his competence—the cognitive

tryside of his childhood home until mid-afternoon. The next day, we started at the same hour. When asked about his evening, he said he had gone to two meetings, but confessed to having needed an afternoon nap.

Hugo's current activities still involve concerns over civil rights. A while back, he attended a meeting that was a spin-off of the Million Man March. The theme was a growing concern among Virginia's African Americans about their prospects for maintaining adequate influence in the state legislature. The general mood was one of increasing depression. Toward the end of the discussion, Hugo asked for the floor. Without any prior preparation, he laid out a plan for action that resulted in a standing ovation. As might be expected, he was asked to chair a new ad hoc committee whose mission was to get things done.

In May 2000 at the age of 84, Dr Owens attended a meeting of the American Association of Retired People. He wanted to see "how my peers are handling their aging. The most illuminating thing I documented is that they have a high regard for, and use, alternative health maintenance medications, treatment, and procedures." Dr Owens' response was to join with a few others to form a new organization, the Association for Integrative Health Care Practitioners. He says, "I am constantly reminded of my experiences when I joined with those who helped found the preventive dentistry movement in the late 1960s. You will be hearing of us very soon. We are planning our first convention here in Norfolk."

Dr Owens' decisive action at that meeting was characteristic of his approach to problems. He believes that failure to take advantage of an opportunity has unfavorable moral consequences. He attributes much of this belief to the influence of two men, Benjamin Mayes, one of the "Giants," and Paul Laurence Dunbar, his favorite poet. When Hugo was 18, he heard a speech by Benjamin Mayes that he has never forgotten. Mayes' message was that "the inevitable result of waste is want." For Hugo it means, "If you waste your moral upbringing, you will die corrupt. If you waste your time, you will suffer lost opportunity," and a few other admonitions as well. Of the various methods of wasting resources, the squandering of time bothers him most. Hugo quoted a poem by Dunbar that refines the consequences of lost opportunities and that helped direct his life (below).

Conscience and Remorse

"Good-bye," I said to my conscience—

"Good-bye for aye and aye,"
And I put her hands off harshly,
And turned my face away;
And conscience smitten sorely
Returned not from that day.

But a time came when my spirit
Grew weary of its pace;
And I cried: "Come back, my conscience;
I long to see thy face."
But conscience cried: "I cannot;
Remorse sits in my place."

and technical aspect of healing—to fit the unique predicament of the particular patient. He empowered the patient—or the community member—to participate in the activity to ameliorate the suffering.

Pellegrino and Thomasma[1] also affirmed that fidelity to trust, compassion, and self-effacement are indispensable traits of the "good professional." To trust, a patient must have confidence that the professional will not exploit his or her vulnerability, even when the professional has motives to do so. Nowhere is "fidelity to trust" better illustrated than by Dr Owens' relationship with his young associates. He supported the fledgling dentists and allowed them to remain in his practice as long as needed, until they were ready for their own practices to thrive. Rather than acting competitively toward the younger colleagues, he illustrated a cooperative and supportive role.

Finally, Dr Owens participated fully in the monitoring and self-regulation of his profession. He joined his local dental society and, based on his extensive community service, was nominated by his peers for membership in the American College of Dentists. However, membership in the larger organization was denied, a rejection that appears to have been more hurtful than the other discriminatory rejections he experienced. Much like Jack Echternacht, he maintained his relationships with peers, despite their lack of support, showing a remarkable disposition to move forward in the face of rejection. In fact, Dr Owens sees this ability as the essence of who he is. Moving forward—cheerfully, compassionately, and competently, with temperance and prudence—in service to others describes Hugo Owens. Like his own heroes, he has become a "giant" in our time.

References
1. Pellegrino ED, Thomasma DC. The Virtues in Medical Practice. New York: Oxford University Press, 1983.
2. Rest JR. Morality. In: Mussen PH (series ed). Flavell J, Markman E (volume eds). Handbook of Child Psychology: Cognitive Development, vol 3. New York: Wiley, 1983:556–629.

In all my discussions with Hugo Owens, he seemed a remarkably positive person. There was little evidence of resentment or negativity, attitudes one might expect to creep into the life of a man who had faced so many adversities for his race. When asked about this observation, he reflected on his views and experiences. Hugo thinks that the qualities that allow him to avoid the dangers of negativity are linked to the very essence of his makeup, which is his "ability to not be emotionally or physiologically bruised by the rough deals that life deals to one. I've seen people literally destroyed because things didn't come out the way that they wanted to. I've seen people miserably hurt by things that are hurtful. But you have to be tough enough to withstand them, and I think perhaps that is the one thing that has made it possible for me to be able to survive in some very hostile conditions. I get the greatest pleasure out of being able to help people overcome things that they couldn't deal with themselves. I think more than anything else that's why I got involved in civil rights and certainly why I got involved in politics." This kind of activity is Hugo Owens' trademark: helping others to help themselves.

In Closing

In the foyer of Hugo Owens' home hangs a picture of a man reaching down over a wall, stretching toward an arm that is desperately struggling to reach the helping hand. The hands of the two men are not yet joined together, but help is on the way. Hugo said that he perceives himself as the man reaching down to help his neighbor. The picture, however, misses another part of his philosophy. Hugo said that if he were an artist, he would paint a second picture that would place himself *below* the man in trouble. The revised painting would show Hugo pushing as hard as he could from beneath. Perhaps with his effort the man would rise above and surpass Hugo. Getting the man out of the pit is only the first step. Developing self-sufficiency so that the man can move beyond the mentor is the higher goal.

Questions for Discussion

1. Dr Owens describes contrasting role models that helped him forge a way of being and interacting that appears to be an important dimension of his success. Who were these role models, and what important lessons did they impart?

2. What special abilities seem to characterize Dr Owens' remarkable success? What implications does this have for your own life?

3. What basic philosophy does Dr Owens have about taking on a "fight"? What role, if any, does this philosophy play in his success in dealing with difficult issues?

4. What kind of disposition does Dr Owens display in the face of adversity?

5. Which of the expectations of a professional (listed in Appendix C) stand out in this story? Continuing learner? Service to society? Acquisition of knowledge?

6. What virtues of professional practice (see Appendix D) does this story illustrate? Assess yourself and the professionals closest to you in terms of these qualities.

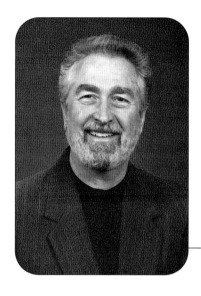

4

Brent L. Benkelman

The Good Practitioner

Dr Brent Benkelman has practiced oral surgery in Manhattan, Kansas, since 1971. Having grown up in a tiny farming town in western Kansas, he opted for the lifestyle of a smaller community after graduating from the University of Missouri at Kansas City School of Dentistry in 1966 and completing his training in oral and maxillofacial surgery in 1969. His experiences since then have revolved around family, practice, and community. With his family as his first priority, he has participated in various community activities, including a church-operated food pantry, an emergency shelter for the homeless, and Habitat for Humanity. He was nominated as a moral exemplar in dentistry for his dedicated commitment to his patients and because he understands and cares about the complexities of his patients as human beings, placing his own financial gain secondary to the interests of his patients.

Dr Benkelman's nominator, Nancy Habluetzel, has known him as a friend for 20 years and an employer for 7 years. The qualities she saw in him on a personal level were "deepened by my observations and interactions with him professionally." From her perspective, "His choice of Manhattan, a relatively small community, over more metropolitan areas exemplifies his commitment to people as opposed to his own financial gain." He is absolutely dedicated to his patients. "His firm rule is that we see people in pain, whether or not they are able to pay, and without concern for how busy our schedule is." He trains his staff to ask questions of patients who call with problems in order to determine which ones are truly emergencies. "If there is any rea-

son to suspect an emergency, Dr Benkelman will *always* see that person. His fees also reflect his concern for patients, as he strives to minimize their costs. [His] practice includes many people who are unable to make full payment at the time of service." Perhaps most revealing, Nancy said, "Brent prefers not to be apprised of those patients who have not paid him—an example of his desire to treat all people as worthwhile individuals deserving of respect."

Unlike the long-term relationships that many general practitioners enjoy with their patients, oral surgeons typically see their patients for more episodic care. Nancy Habluetzel thinks that Dr Benkelman's satisfactions come from doing his best to make a difficult surgical experience easier. "Dr Benkelman takes great pride in his ability to distract patients–he tells jokes and generally entertains as he attends to the serious business of their dental health. Many people even tell us they didn't know he had taken the tooth out. I consider these comments to be not only an indication of his surgical skills, but also of his genuine concern for the well-being–physical and emotional–of his patients."

Genuine concern for patients emerges as Brent Benkelman's trademark. Ms Habluetzel especially remembered one busy morning when, despite a full schedule, "four unscheduled people just came by to see Dr Benkelman. Not one was turned away; not one was made to feel intrusive." In particular, she recalled a woman in her early 80s for whom Dr Benkelman had extracted some teeth and placed an immediate denture, which another dentist had provided. Some months later the denture was giving her some trouble, and rather than go to her general dentist she came to see the oral surgeon. "Dr Benkelman patiently made the necessary adjustments [and] as is his custom, he also visited with her. As she was leaving, she asked him how much she owed him for his work, and he replied, 'How about a hug?' It brings tears to my eyes as I picture that lonely little lady giving and receiving a much-needed hug. Dr Brent Benkelman is a man who understands and cares about the complexities of his patients as human beings."

Nancy Habluetzel told me (JTR) that she thinks that one of Brent's important qualities is that "he understands what's really important in life, and I agree that what's important in life is people. I think that's what he puts first. I don't mean that he doesn't want to make a good living, because he does; but I don't think that's his prime concern. I just see him treat people with respect. Brent is perceptive about the emotions of others." He spends time with his patients, and he talks to them in the same way that he talks to his friends. Nancy said, "I think he's always open to that possibility [of friendship]. Brent is Brent. At a restaurant, if the food doesn't come right away, he will go around talking with people, whether he knows them or not." Furthermore, with respect to patients, she says he presents himself the same with the farmer as with the ophthalmologist. He is always the same. "He doesn't see–or he doesn't very much see–that he's the doctor, and you're the patient. He isn't perfect. Don't get me wrong. He doesn't always

> "Dr Brent Benkelman . . . understands and cares about the complexities of his patients as human beings."
>
> *Nancy Habluetzel*
> *Dr Benkelman's nominator*

live up to these [expectations], but I think that's his philosophy."

Sometimes Dr Benkelman's patients do become his friends. One such person, LeRoy Johnston, said that their friendship started on the operating table under general anesthesia on a snowy New Year's Day in 1980. That morning Mr Johnston had spread hay over the snow for the horses to eat. His favorite filly was being muscled away by the other horses, so he moved some alfalfa off to one side and tried to lead her there. The filly would not be led and stubbornly kicked sideways, catching him in the face. A couple of teeth hit the snow, but they were the least of his problems. Fortunately he remained conscious, walked to the house, and eventually made it to the hospital where Dr Benkelman treated him. Brent remembers it clearly. He said that LeRoy had fractures in both his midface area and his mandible, as well as lacerations of the lip and tongue. The surgery took about 6 hours and was followed by a life-threatening bleed a few days later. All LeRoy remembers is that there were 60 or 70 sutures.

Months later, completely healed, LeRoy was walking past Dr Benkelman's building to see an orthodontist for follow-up care when the window in Brent's office went up. LeRoy could see a patient sitting in the chair. Brent leaned out and said, "Hey, LeRoy, you don't talk to me anymore?" LeRoy said, "In my mind I was thinking, 'Well, he patched me up and kicked me out,' and that was it. It never occurred to me that this was something different than the doctor and a patient, right? So, I went in and we chatted, and from then on we started hunting together and fishing together and taking trips together and drinking beer together. It's been a 20-year deal. I always felt just like I was his older brother."

It was not only with LeRoy Johnston that Brent made friends. When LeRoy sold his ranch and moved 30 miles further north, Brent continued to join him for hunting and fishing. LeRoy said they would go into a little country restaurant, and everybody would say, 'Hey, Brent! Hey, Brent!' He knew more farmers up there than even I did, and I was living there. I think he told me he worked on everybody that was in the room." LeRoy suspected that Brent received this kind of response all around Manhattan.

Undoubtedly, much of the way that people respond to Brent is merely a reciprocation of Brent's views about them. Brent Benkelman is an outgoing, generous, and friendly person who is the same whether he is in the office or elsewhere. He also is an organizer. LeRoy said, "You come into a group and everybody is buzzing around Brent." After a hunt, he likes to process his own deer meat into steaks, sausage, and especially bratwurst. He then finishes off with a big party at his house. He also likes to organize New Year's Eve parties and kite-flying days on Easter. When he started to make beer, he created an association of like-minded connoisseurs. When LeRoy Johnston and his wife sold their second ranch and moved to their new condominium in Manhattan, Brent organized a surprise housewarming.

Quite apart from Brent's social skills, however, LeRoy appreciates his skills as an oral surgeon, even when LeRoy is awake. He had a wisdom tooth extracted by Brent under local anesthesia, which was "like having a fingernail cut." In addition, LeRoy said he is an "incredibly honest" man who is extremely serious about his profession. When a group of friends would go hunting, LeRoy recalled, "We'd be waiting with our guns, two or three guys, and there was always a chance that we'd get a call. Brent would have an accident or something [to take care of]. He'd just drop everything for his patients. He would never worry about his fun. He was very dedicated." LeRoy said that interruptions such as those happened quite frequently.

Through the eyes of others, Dr Brent Benkelman is seen as an oral surgeon who is both competent in his skills and dedicated to his patients. His dedication apparently stems from his egalitarian views of all people as "worthwhile individuals deserving of respect." He enhances and implements these moral qualities with a personality that is gregarious, friendly, and generous. A look at both his early years and his professional life give further insight into Dr Benkelman as a person and as a professional.

Growing up in Western Kansas

"Brent Layton Benkelman, born of humble origins, in a pitiful little county in western Kansas." This was a typical Benkelmanian response to a request for background demographics. Born December 23, 1941, he was the oldest and shortest of three boys. He said that he was the shortest "because being first born, they don't feed you enough." Being the oldest, though, he had the opportunity to be the ringleader, a position he has never relinquished.

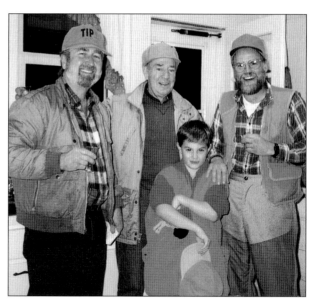

(From left) Dr Benkelman with LeRoy Johnston, Eric Turtle, and Jim Turtle after a day of hunting.

Small-Town Life

McDonald, Kansas, where Brent grew up, is positioned almost as far in the northwest corner of Kansas as it possibly could be; the Nebraska border is only 15 miles away. Just across the border is Benkelman, Nebraska, a town named after some of Brent's forebears. McDonald had approximately 300 people, and when Brent was in high school, they fielded a football team with only 18 players. Furthermore, Brent said, "It was people farming small farms when I grew up there." Now, farming in McDonald "is no longer a small land game"; it is for people with large holdings of land. As a result, there are fewer farmers and smaller towns, McDonald being one of them.

His father, Willie (Charles Wilmot), was a farmer whose experience was typical for the region. He lived in town but farmed small parcels of land both in McDonald and in outlying areas. He was definitely not a big landowner. Brent remembers that his father also sold casualty and crop insurance, "to keep his boys in beer and shoes." Unlike most people in McDonald, Willie had degrees in civil engineering and agriculture from Kansas State University.

In the years that Brent lived in McDonald, few farmers actually lived in town. Mainly, Brent said, "There were the teachers, the merchants, a few widows, and a handyman or two." There was one block in the community that contained Brent's house, a tractor store, a vacant lot, and a house for the blacksmith. His grandmother, his great-grandfather, his grandmother's sister, and his great uncle lived in the next block. Brent said, "All in the back of that were granaries, corn cribs, and Quonsets, and where we parked the tractors, and where the gardens were, and the chicken house."

Almost everyone in the community, except for a "few wicked people," as Brent said, went to church. Catholics and Protestants were about equally divided. Brent said that it was basically a religiously oriented farming community in which "everything pretty much goes back to nature." There was a certain philosophy about those people, a certain fatalism about weather. The whole year could stem on one little hailstorm just before harvest. The whole crop could be gone.

McDonald was full of frugal people who made ends meet, but only by the smallest of margins. They survived by working hard and helping each other. Children in McDonald were raised by the entire community. It was like an extended family that seemed to go on forever. They were available for him, concerned about him, kept an eye on him, and, Brent said, they would "tell on me when I did something wrong. Everybody kind of looked out for everybody else, and if you did something wrong, your parents found out about it. The only thing that got home sooner than you was the bad deed."

Family Life

Having his parents find out about his behavior was not a big problem. Brent has fond memories of his immediate family, especially of his father. Like Brent, Willie was the kind of person everyone in town knew. Adding to his sociability was his excellent singing voice, which brought him many invitations to sing at weddings and funerals, thus accounting for the majority of times he was ever seen in church. Willie was a fair-minded person who was full of encouragement and high expectations. Brent and his two brothers understood and accepted their father's expectations, which served as a substitute for heavy-handed discipline. Willie pushed his sons to achieve and readily supported everything they did. In fact, everyone in the family attended all the athletic events and stage productions in which the boys participated. Brent thinks they showed up not because they had to, but because they wanted to. It was a matter of love.

That sense of belonging was extended to people outside the Benkelman household. "Our place was always a haven. If anything was going on, everybody knew that if there was a light on in the kitchen, come on in. If it was after a ball game, or if there was a dance, or if we were out on a date, somehow there would always be cocoa on the stove. It was mainly our best male friends, mine and my brothers.' We'd come in, and Dad would sit there and talk with us about our games or our dates or whatever we wanted. All the kids would come in–he was available. He was not a father you didn't want to be around. It was welcoming. The whole experience was very formative." Brent's mother was an essential component of that experience as well. "I would always sit and talk to my mom while she was cooking or working in the kitchen. She imparted values and wisdom during those talks."

In fact, Brent's entire McDonald extended family left its mark. His great-grandfather lived with his grandmother, his grandfather having died when Brent was about 5. Brent does not remember his grandfather very much, but neighbors have described him as one of the kindest men they had ever known. This appealed to Brent as an aspiration for himself. His great-grandfather was a general store owner and farmer who accumulated farmland in an unusual way. "During the dust bowl years [drought] when people had to sell out, they gave him deeds to the land, because he had extended them [the kindness of] credit." Thus, like Brent's father's land, his grandfather's land was scattered about. Brent's grandmother taught piano and Sunday school and played piano at the church. His great-aunt also was a Sunday school teacher. Through eighth grade, Brent spent every Sunday with those two women. Their collective influence on him was great.

Brent remembers going to church even in his earliest days. Church camp provided more intense experiences later on. Adding to the impact of the church was the fact that almost the only social event available for Protestants was the Wednesday night church youth group. He said that religion became especially meaningful to him during his adolescence when "thoughts of being the right sort of person were really important to me. [I realized that] I needed to do things that I learned in the Bible by example."

College and Dental School

Brent graduated from high school in 1959 after lettering four times each year in band, football, track, and basketball. He had always assumed that he would go to college. In his class of 12 he was the salutatorian and proved to be the only one to earn a college degree. He said, "I thought I was above average until I got to college."

Brent attended Kansas University, and even though he enjoyed 1½ years as a sprinter and long jumper on the track team, he said that college was "no fun for me. It was psychologically difficult. It was too large." His academic background from McDonald was limited, and in terms of relationships, it was "hard to go from a town of 300 to a class of 300. . . . You have to remember that I was going to a big liberal arts school, coming from a small farming community. Most of the people from the large towns didn't think very highly of anybody that came from the 'outlands.' We were pretty much [hickish] people." It wasn't that Brent was not able to make friends; it was only that he had to put up with the snobbishness of the eastern Kansas urbanites toward the farm boys. This was a deterrent to the development of his characteristic participation in community affairs, the only exception being a brief membership in the Young Republican Club. Brent said, "When I got back to a fairly intimate learning relationship, like dental school [with classes of 116], that was much better for me. It took me 1 year in dental school to find my niche. After that I liked it. You knew everybody in your class."

Before Brent left home for college, he had mainly thought he wanted to be a farmer like his father. However, he had no idea how he could ever accumulate the huge acreage that was increasingly required in modern farming. In addition, his father had not particularly encouraged his sons toward farming. Then there were his father's brothers. Uncle Ward was a physician in Montana, and Uncle Bob was a dentist in Denver. Brent's grandfather also had a brother who was a dentist. The idea of professional school pleased his father. With these influences, Brent said he began to think about dentistry early in his college career. "It seemed like a good thing to do, because I really liked Uncle Bob." If Brent ever were to have considered anything else, it would have been the life sciences: human biology or wildlife biology.

The other reason Brent gives for turning toward dentistry was the liberal arts curriculum at Kansas University, which perversely forced him to take some language classes. After a semester of Latin and a week of French, he decided it was not for him. The idea of

> "We all have a certain amount of dues that we need to pay. It's not like I'm going to suffer if I give a few things away."
>
> *Dr Benkelman on providing free care*

speaking a foreign language appealed to Brent, if only he could have avoided learning the grammar. Thus, he took the final step toward dentistry. His grades were good enough for dental school after 3 years of college, and so, encouraged by his two dentist uncles, he took the dental aptitude test and did well. Whatever the influences that led to dental school, Brent said that his decision to apply was a turning point. Before that "I was sort of a wandering generality. We all do better when we have a focus."

Although the predominant focus of dental school was learning the techniques of patient care, he began to learn about the philosophy of caring for people. Brent said, "We were coached to think of people as an entity, rather than just a tooth. We were reminded of that a lot by the instructors that I had. But that's difficult to do. When you are trying to learn specific talents, it is difficult to associate what you are doing to an entire situation." Brent said that it was not until he became more experienced in oral surgery that his sense of caring developed more. "I'm a better listener now than I used to [be]. I try to perceive those things that patients need rather than the things that I need. If I could go back and be as skillful then as I am now, I'd have been a lot better off. Experience is wonderful."

Brent entered the Univerisity of Missouri at Kansas City (UMKC) School of Dentistry in 1962, spent 4 years doing not much more than studying, and graduated in 1966 at the age of 25, as he said, "just a pipsqueak." His dream during most of his years in school was to practice general dentistry in Denver with his Uncle Bob. However, he had begun to think about surgery early in his senior year, and Bob had said now was the time to apply. After he was accepted, he debated whether to accept, and Bob said now was the time. So he did.

Choice of Lifestyle

Brent stayed at the UMKC for his training in surgery, which he completed in 1969. In the last year of his training he married Virginia Owings, and when he finished his program, he joined the Air Force as a way of having more time to decide where they wanted to live. Missoula, Montana, and Ft Collins, Colorado, were

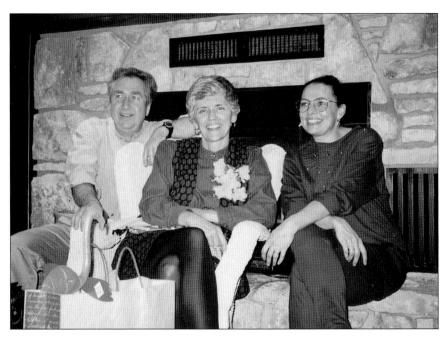

Brent and his wife, Virginia, host a birthday celebration for Nancy Habluetzel *(center)*.

possibilities. They liked Kansas City as well, but Brent said, "I needed to be closer to the country. There were too many cars, too many people." Being stationed at an Air Force base in Florida had made them realize that they did not want to be too far from their extended families. So they settled in Manhattan, Kansas, a university town of 25,000, which, as it happened, was only 305 miles from both families. Brent said, "Manhattan was about as small a town as an oral surgeon could have ever been supported in."

When asked what he thought about Nancy Habluetzel's opinion that his choice of Manhattan was a sign that his primary interest was people as opposed to financial gain, Brent answered by referring to his childhood. Both he and Virginia had grown up in a frugal environment. While Brent doesn't remember going hungry, there were some years when the crops were bad and life was tough. However, regardless of how good or bad the weather, the work of farmers never changed. That was what life was all about. He said, "You worked six days a week. Sunday you got off. And that was just routine. Money was something that just happened." He feels the same about his own life today. "What I do is I work, and I have a certain amount of money to spend. I have to work. That's just a given. If you can imagine

yourself inside that concept, that's sort of my thinking about money. I don't think of my job as earning me so much an hour. I think of work as work. I work and then I have so much money. That's sort of the way I grew up. . . . My philosophy is that if you make up your mind to go ahead and do something and be diligent about it, you can do it." He said that while he was considering dentistry as a career option, he does not remember ever associating the idea of dentistry with money. "It was just something to do. A good way to get along."

Reverting to his discussion of why he settled in Manhattan, Brent said, "Probably I came here as much to be close to the lakes and hunting, and to be able to get out to the country quicker, and to be closer to parents, and to be away from big cities, as I did thinking about the money." In fact, making money was difficult at first. In his first year of practice he had to take out a loan to cover his expenses, and it took 7 or 8 years before he was financially comfortable. Now things are different. His practice is thriving. Manhattan has grown to 40,000, and Kansas State University has about 20,000 students. Now that general dentists are referring extractions to surgeons, third molar removals alone could probably keep him going.

The Practice

When Brent was trained, the scope of oral surgery was considerably narrower than it is now. Extractions and management of fractures were the primary foci. More advanced surgical procedures had either not yet been fully developed or were left to physician-trained surgeons. For example, oral surgeons did no orthognathic procedures and placed no implants. When these procedures became popular, Brent enjoyed learning the skills. He has been placing implants since 1984, virtually since the day they were approved by the Food and Drug Administration. The same is true for other state-of-the-art practices in oral surgery, including sinus grafting and bone grafting. Brent and his partner, who joined him in 1991, also do a lot of biopsies, third molar extractions, and canine exposures.

Brent performed orthognathic procedures for 10 or 15 years, but when his partner wanted to do more, Brent was happy to let him handle all the orthognathic cases. "I'd worry about them a week before, and then I'd worry about them for a week afterwards. Two weeks of worrying about one case is too much. Trauma you don't have to worry about as much. You just have to get right to it." Brent does wish, however, that trauma cases could be timed better. "I just hate to work in the middle of the night anymore. It's easier during the day." Nevertheless, fractures are a fact of life. Within the weeks before the interview, he had treated two trauma cases: facial fractures in a boy who ran a motor bike into a truck and a displaced fracture in the edentulous mandible of a man who was hit by a steel pipe. On the first day of the interview, a Sunday, he had visited the hospital to check on another man whose fracture he treated.

Regarding his approach to his profession, Brent said, "One of the things that I've always done is . . . set my limits on what I will do, and then I try not to ever compromise. [For example] I say I'm never going to take out a tooth on somebody whose systolic blood pressure is over 190 or their diastolic is over 110. You compromise that, and you start having problems. Just little things like that. Decide on the things that you know are going to be right, and you never have to change your mind about it."

Dr Ken Lyle, a Manhattan general practitioner and longtime friend of Dr Benkelman's, thinks that Brent uses general anesthesia and sedation much less than most oral surgeons. In doing so, it is necessary to expend significant effort in communication. Perhaps, Dr

Lyle said, "It's the 'Life on the Prairie' syndrome, in that he wants to be able to be resourceful and handle anything that comes along. . . . He is [also] very perceptive and he wants to be tapped into that pipeline, the psyche of that patient that is under his care, and he wants to read those vibes that are coming through. Whatever it is he picks up on, he can't have it squashed out, because it limits his ability to deliver the type of care that he wants for this person. We all realize that the physical aspect of care is only one small wedge of the pie. We do a lot of other things for our patients."

Working with Patients

Humor and Persistence

In general, Brent said, "I guess my basic philosophy of practice has always been to do things as easily for people as I possibly can, so that they don't feel like they've ever had to endure anything. So that it's more an, well, an enjoyable experience." He laughed at that prospect. "When you're having oral surgery, it's difficult to say that, but that's been my basic goal. People are usually nervous when they come to see me, so I think my use of humor allows them to [relax]." His humor comes out in various ways, usually as "corny jokes and puns," as Ken Lyle said. For example, Nancy Habluetzel said that in discussing upcoming surgery with a woman and her spouse, he might say, "You are not allowed to do housework for 3 weeks." Or he might admonish an adolescent awaiting removal of a third molar to remember that there should be "no kissing for a month." Corny or not, the patients love it. Brent said he also uses humor to try to get patients to take better care of themselves. Sometimes he tells them, "'You know, you have not been standing close enough to your toothbrush, and you're a dirty dog for not doing it.' I'm honest about things like that, and they understand that, but I'm not going to berate people, because it doesn't help."

Working with patients who do not seem willing to take care of themselves is one of Brent's biggest frustrations. Nevertheless, he persistently encourages patients to get general care if they are not currently doing so. No matter how hard he tries, though, some patients "will be back and back over a 10-year period until you've got every one of their teeth out. They won't brush, they won't see a dentist. That's frustrating to me. But still, you've got to do something with them. I probably don't care as much about them as a whole as I do somebody who's going to be compliant, but I try not to allow that to temper the kind of treatment that I'm going to give them. I'm going to treat them just as gently as anybody else, be as nice to them, not scold them."

In addition, when he disagrees with the judgments of referring practitioners, Brent chooses to deal with them directly. His typical approach, as Dr Lyle attests, is to let the patient know about the difference of opinion and call the practitioner. When asked if this annoys Brent's colleagues, Dr Lyle said with a little smile, "Yeah! It's an annoyance, but it's the right thing. I can live with that. I see it that Brent and I are sharing a common frustration. He is frustrated with the fact that I don't see things clearly enough to know what the correct answer is, and I feel the same way about his view. We just professionally coexist and work it out somehow." In the most complex cases, usually involving combinations of restorative dentistry and prosthodontics, Brent stops by Dr Lyle's office and they do work it out.

> "I guess my basic philosophy of practice has always been to do things as easily for people as I possibly can, so that they don't feel like they've ever had to endure anything."
>
> *Dr Benkelman*

Generosity and Respect

As Nancy Habluetzel said, Brent does not like to know whether his patients are able to pay for treatment. One reason is so that financial status does not influence the treatment options he offers. "What I would like to do is to present them the best possible treatment plan and give them the alternatives and let them make the choice. I think that's what everybody should do. I don't think you should exclude a procedure because you think somebody can't afford it. I don't think you should omit something [that is less than ideal] because they have a lot of money. People should know what they can do and make up their own mind."

More than that, though, Brent said, "If they're having pain, I say get them in. If they don't have any money, I just do it. I don't care. That's been basically my philosophy." He doesn't even want his staff to inquire about the method of payment when patients call in. "It doesn't matter to me. If they're having a problem, they need to be seen." Sometimes patients refuse necessary treatment because they cannot afford it. Rather than turn them away, Brent has said, "'This just needs to be done. Let's do it.' I put the bill away, and I say 'This is what you owe me. I'm not going to send you any bills. If you ever want to pay me, you can.' I've had a few people pay me 2 or 3 or 4 years down the road." Occasionally, someone takes advantage of him,

Commentary

Brent Benkelman was nominated as a moral exemplar for the compassionate and caring way he treats his patients. We admired him and selected him for this remarkably developed capacity. As his story unfolded, however, our esteem deepened. His narrative illustrated his careful concerns about executing each of the roles and responsibilities of the health care professional,[1] and doing so with an uncommon balance between personal and professional commitments.

For the young person aspiring to become a professional, there are important lessons to learn from Dr Benkelman's views of his professional obligations and how they relate to his personal life. More importantly, he models a professional who is not only successful but very happy. He pursues competence as he expands his skills in oral surgery. He values learning and builds opportunity for learning into daily living, eg, reading journals as he rides his exercise bike. He habitually and actively serves his association through both leadership and the lowlier tasks of mundane committee work. He engages in self-regulation—setting for himself standards for professional practice. He is willing to speak to his peers about professional standards that he questions. He unequivocally puts the interests of his patients above his own as he enters into the caregiving partnership, and he readily treats anyone in need. To assure that everyone is treated respectfully, he maintains a blind eye to the patient's personal resources so as not to compromise the patient's right to know the full range of options. The inability to pay is not allowed to interfere when a real need presents. Yet even in the giving, he allows the person to maintain dignity by saying, "I'm not going to send you any bills. If you ever want to pay me, you can." Fulfilling the essential professional obligation for some measure of pro bono work, he is moved to engage in other forms of service to his community. He attributes his disposition for giving to his roots in religion and community.

Much of Brent Benkelman's perspectives on work, on personal worth and achievement, and on competence, caring, self-regulation, professional monitoring, and service to patients, profession, and community stem from his experience of grow-

but it doesn't seem to bother him. "We all have a certain amount of dues that we need to pay, you know. It's not like I'm going to suffer if I give a few things away."

Giving away services and money to the community is part of what characterizes both Brent and Virginia. They both say that it is basic to their lives that if someone calls, you help them. It just spills over into dentistry. If you have a skill, you utilize it. "Maybe it goes back to that basic old Christian attitude [that] you do better [in caring for other people] if you give everything away. Could it be possible that I actually feel a little bit guilty about being as successful as I am and having everything that we have, so that it doesn't bother me to give away the services that I have to give away?" Aside from professional services, Brent and Virginia donate money in other ways as well. "A gift given in secret is the most fun. We give a lot of things anonymously, because I don't care to have my name on all those lists." It also prevents him from getting a lot of plaques of recognition that he does not want.

From Ken Lyle's perspective, Brent's sense of community pervades his concept of dental practice as well. As he perceives it, "[Brent] thinks of his dental patients as being the community, as an extension of growing up in western Kansas, and that part of our job as dental practitioners here is to take care of people before we take care of ourselves."

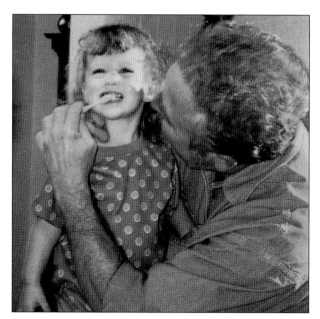

Dr Benkelman teaches a granddaughter to brush her teeth.

Investment in the Community

What goes on outside Brent's office reflects what goes on within. He said that from "time to time" in the roughly 30 years he has been in practice he has been

ing up in the heartland of America. Hard-pressed by the Great Depression and the great drought of the 1930s, people in the heartland developed respectful perspectives toward natural resources and work. The land is important for survival, but people are custodians of something they cannot control. Work requires careful planning and cooperation, but its outcome is often uncertain. People in the heartland have come to view work as having an intrinsic value regardless of its outcome. If the outcome is a bountiful harvest, the success is attributed to the goodness of God rather than to the skills of the farmer, though skillful effort is both expected and required.

The heartland conception of work is present in Brent's story. For Brent, work is not a means to an end, but a way of life. Further, work is not all-consuming; it is balanced with other roles—those of father, husband, friend, and community leader. Although one engages in all these roles, there is a certain priority to work, especially when one is committed to put the interests of others above the self, as is the health professional. For Brent, leaving a planned recreational activity to handle an emergency was common. The possibility of interruption did not

deter him from planning and engaging in recreation. Yet he did not express anger or disappointment at having to abort his plans in order to care for a patient. The experiences of farming prepare one to continue in the face of disappointment and spawn a sense of parsimony and frugality as one learns to live with uncertainty. It teaches one to practice the adage "waste not, want not," which is part of Brent's internal value system.

The heartland perspectives on self-worth and the worth of others are also visible through Brent's narrative. Anyone who grew up in the heartland of America knows that what Garrison Keillor regularly asserts on "Prairie Home Companion"[2]—that all the children are above average—is, in a profound sense, essentially true. They also know that, while everyone is above average, no one is superior. Are all children truly above average? Clearly not; but the maxim represents an attitude: Everyone should be treated with respect, and no one should consider himself or herself superior. This worldview promotes a sense of equality: While individuals may be respected for personal qualities or achievement, no one is superior. This view tempers tendencies toward self-aggrandizement, just as it tempers

active in various dental societies and medical groups: the Manhattan Medical Center (twice as president), the Medical Staff at the Mercy Health Center, the local dental society, the Kansas Society of Oral and Maxillofacial Surgeons, and the Midwestern Society of Oral and Maxillofacial Surgeons. He served the American Dental Association as a consultant on hospital and institutional dental services for 4 years, was on the Kansas Dental Association's Council on Dental Care Programs for 5 years, and has been treasurer of the Kansas Society of Dentistry for Children for 4 years. Along with a number of surgery talks to local groups, he has also presented on "The Treacherous Molar and the Maxillary Sinus" at an international conference in Belize, which, Brent was quick to say, was organized by a friend. His friend also convinced Brent to make a few volunteer service trips to Belize. Locally, he participates in the Donated Dental Services program and sees patients that the local health agency refers.

In the larger community, almost all of Brent's many activities, and Virginia's too, involve service to others. Often they revolve around their church. For example, Brent said that when he was serving as a deacon, he helped to organize a local food pantry network, which is now distributing 400,000 pounds of food each year. Since his role was only to help set up the pantry, Brent said that for the last 10 years he has "done nothing more than donate money." Within the church itself, he

is now an elder: in Brent's words, "the ruling clan." Presbyterians love meetings intensely, and he said that he hasn't worked so hard since he organized the first joint meeting with the Southwest Society of Oral Surgeons, when he was president of the Midwest oral surgery group.

Other community activities include the Optimist Club, which named him Man of the Year in 1974. Brent said this honor was bestowed "because I ran the tee-ball program that summer, and it took a real man to do that." According to him, this consisted of mowing the baseball diamonds every weekend so the youngest children had a place to play. He said he doesn't do very much for the Optimist Club now, although he does help out with three or four projects, including the sale of Christmas trees. Apart from Optimist Club activities, Brent has worked on an emergency shelter for the homeless, participated in a local program in which people both donate household items and provide home-oriented services for people who need assistance, and helped with Habitat for Humanity projects. He said his involvement with Habitat was minimal. "I went down and helped a couple of times to build on one house, but now I just donate." This comment is typical of his view toward all his current community activities. His phrasing reveals his intent to view his accomplishments honestly and without exaggeration.

When their children's activities started to reach beyond their home, the adult Benkelmans changed their

intolerance toward those who are disadvantaged. With his characteristic "me second" midwestern modesty, Brent attributed his "Man of the Year" award from the Optimist Club to the fact that he mowed the lawns for the tee-ball tournament. Clearly, he has internalized the heartland views on self-worth.

Through Brent's story, we see a person who absorbed the values of his community during childhood, then grew to model those values to others. The community unambiguously communicated its central ideas of helping one another and caring enough about others, including the children, to participate actively in raising those children. This included "tattling" on unacceptable behavior when necessary. For Brent, additional values were instilled by a grandfather who had a reputation for being "one of the kindest men [people] had ever known," by a father who was so welcoming that teens stopped by "just to talk," by a family that attended and celebrated each child's events, and by a community where church was a central focus and everyone attended—except for "a few wicked people," as Brent jokingly put it. These conditions helped to shape the hall-

mark values of generosity and other-centeredness in our current exemplar. The lessons of childhood were well learned, and they are reflected in Dr Benkelman's views both about patients and about relationships with friends, family, and colleagues.

Growing up in McDonald, Kansas, set the stage for Brent's acceptance of the concepts of caring and community. However, Brent perceives that his sense of caring and his concept of dentistry as a caring profession have evolved. As he reflected on the model of caring his dental faculty tried to instill, he observed that it is difficult to be concerned about the whole person while focusing on perfecting the skills necessary to treat a single tooth. It takes time to be able to see the person and his or her particular need as primary and the tooth as secondary. Dr Benkelman now considers himself a listener, one who needs to connect to the lived experience of the person, to understand the illness and the meaning of that illness to the person. Only with this understanding can the professional heal the person, not just fix the tooth. The fact that Dr Benkelman uses less general anesthesia and sedation than is typical of his peers is

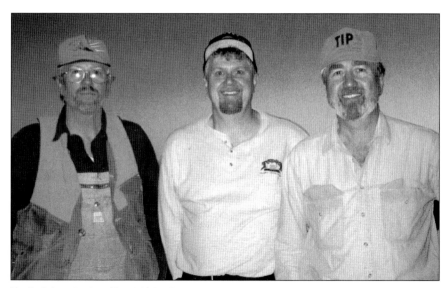

The Benkelman brothers *(from left)*: Bill, Paul, and Brent.

focus of projects. At church Brent and Virginia taught Sunday School for the junior high group for a time, and they chaperoned the church youth group on a ski trip to Colorado. They also volunteered many hours for school events. For the 8 years that their daughter Jami was in track, Brent officiated at events from the long jump in high school to the triple jump at the Big 8 college championships. When Jami graduated from high school, he stopped officiating. Melissa was interested in music and plays. When she was in the concert chamber choir, they sponsored 49 students to travel and sing in Florida. Virginia said she just viewed it as her responsibility. "If you are in a community, you need to give back to the community. The community is supporting you, then you need to support it." Brent agreed and added with a smile, "Virginia would have killed me if I didn't. The more you involve yourself, and the more things that you do, the more you benefit from those things."

evidence of his remarkable ability to reduce anxiety and instill confidence, enabling the patient to undergo procedures without trauma. He achieves this relaxed atmosphere with corny jokes and puns and with a level of acceptance that helps people see him as friend and helper—even someone who needs a hug—rather than as doctor.

Brent's profound respect for persons of all walks of life and his tendencies to minimize achievements are further evidence that he possesses each of the indispensable traits of the authentic professional. Growing up in western Kansas, he learned a way of being that involved modeling himself after those admired in the community and setting standards as a guide to action. As a result, he does not endlessly reflect on his actions, nor does he spend time arguing with himself when temptation presents. Instead, he simply follows the guideline he established for himself. This is not to suggest that he does not evaluate his guidelines, especially those that are based on scientific evidence, but it does suggest that he does not endlessly reflect. Action, rather than reflection, characterizes Dr Benkelman's life. In some cases,

actions are the results of habit. In others, they result from thoughtfully considered judgment, as in the case of the conditions for treating a patient with high blood pressure. Finally, Dr Benkelman seems to have achieved the kind of optimism Seligman[3] describes as a quality that distinguishes effective people. "Optimism works not through unjustifiable positivity about the world, but through the power of non-negative thinking."[3p211] Dr Benkelman does not ignore his faults; but on the other hand, he chooses not to focus on them, perhaps recognizing that to do so is debilitating. He would prefer small nudges, as he perfects a way of being that is consistent with his heartland values.

References

1. Bebeau MN, Kahn J. Ethical issues in community dental health. In: Gluck GM, Morganstein WM (eds). Jong's Community Dental Health, ed 4. St Louis: Mosby, 1997:287-306.
2. Keillor G. Lake Wobegon Days. New York: Viking Penguin, 1985.
3. Seligman M. Learned Optimism: How to Change Your Mind and Your Life. New York: Simon & Schuster, 1998.

Currently

The word that best describes Brent Benkelman's life and practice, he said, is "busy." He had taken a partner in 1991 to reduce his workload, but in the past 6 years or so he has become excessively busy again. For the first time in his life, he now resorts to making lists of things to do so as not to forget anything. "When you get to be a certain age, you have so many things that interest you, that it's difficult to get them done."

Brent presently works 4 days a week, 10 hours a day, a schedule he adopted after his father died. At that time, the Benkelman brothers sat down to go over his papers. They saw that Brent's father and his two brothers had written to each other year after year about getting together, but they had never done it. As a result, Brent and his brothers, Bill and Paul, try to get together frequently and do things they all enjoy. Additionally, each of them also makes a deliberate effort to take off one day a week as an "advance" on their retirement while they are still active and able. "I take Tuesdays off. I consider that part of my ultimate retirement, while I am able to do the things physically, maybe not always financially, that we wanted to do. But I can get out and walk and hunt all day now. I might not be able to do that, because of my knee, 4 or 5 years from now. So I at least have 45 days a year of retirement that I wouldn't have had otherwise."

One of Brent's goals is to become a better person. He wants to read more and become "more well-rounded" and less preoccupied by things that aren't worth worrying about. Brent also said he thinks that he is not very good at expressing his feelings about things. He joked, "I try not to be too introspective, because I'm afraid of what I'll find. I'd just as soon improve without knowing that I was bad to start with. Sneak up on it! Let's head off these bad tendencies before I notice they're there!" Above all, Brent said, "I am evolving . . . [and trying] to become a more positive, bigger person."

One would think that Brent is already positive enough. He is usually the personification of the Optimist's creed: "To look at the sunny side of everything." Given his generally positive outlook, a good friend who is a general surgeon gave Brent the nickname "Dr Happy Tooth." For better or worse, that is now his designation by the Manhattan medical community.

Nevertheless, Brent said he needs to "learn how to listen a little bit better," an aspiration that pertains less to his patients than to other people around him. "I'm really patient with [my patients]. You know, you can spend so much time being patient, you use it all up." At times Brent thinks that his relationship with his employees is wanting. Sometimes he is too abrupt with his staff, and he gets upset over small things, such as when someone makes an unnecessary photocopy of a document. Harking back to his frugal upbringing, he said that he might be "a little overboard about not wasting money." He may also overlook the effect of his decisions on his staff. For instance, on a busy day, if asked to see an extra patient, Brent will gladly make room in his schedule. He doesn't mind staying late, but he forgets that his staff has to stay, too. Generally speaking, though, Nancy Habluetzel thinks Brent's flaws are nothing more than the opposite side of the coin of his virtues.

Considering his perceptive observations and concerns about his patients, it is difficult to know whether to believe Brent's deprecatory assessment of his introspective capacity. It is easy to see, however, that action rather than reflection continues to characterize his life. He is as busy at home as he is during his 10-hour workdays. His evenings and weekends are filled with church, community, and professional activities. His role as a church elder alone consumes many evenings each month. Whenever possible, his "retirement Tuesdays" are occupied by hunting, fishing, or taking his dog, Sunny, for a run. Time has to be set aside for on-call responsibilities and continuing education courses, and he reads his surgery journals at home on an exercise bicycle in front of a large window overlooking reddish-brown prairie grass. Over the years, Brent has also found time to finish and restore antique furniture, which is displayed throughout his house. His energy level is not deficient, to say the least. He also tends to be restless and impatient. However, he commented that compared with his younger years, he is now the model of placidity. Hours into the interview he said, "You would have never gotten me to sit still this long 20 years ago." However, he said that he still does not like to sit still at a movie theater, and continuing education courses are torture to sit through. He doesn't even sit down for very long while he works.

So Dr Benkelman continues to keep busy doing the things that he has always done. He does not philosophize about his egalitarian approach to professional and personal relationships, nor does he think about how others judge him as exemplary for his dedication, generosity, and concern for his patients. Instead, with his roots in the understated, caring fellowship of the western Kansas plains, he just works steadily, and if someone calls, he helps them.

Questions for Discussion

1. What virtues does Dr Benkelman's story best illustrate? Assess yourself and the professionals closest to you in terms of these qualities.

2. Which of the expectations of the professional (listed in Appendix C) are illustrated by Dr Benkelman's activities? How does he manage the responsibility for lifelong learning? How do you (or will you) manage yours?

3. What is the heartland concept of work that shaped Dr Benkelman's life? How does this compare or contrast with the ideas you grew up with? What perspective helps him balance the demands of work and play? How does the heartland perspective on self-worth as described in the commentary mesh with Pellegrino and Thomasma's perspective on humility?

4. Dr Benkelman speaks about a sense of caring that develops over time. He contrasts his sense of caring now with that which he felt as a professional student. How do you characterize the challenges to the development of caring during dental school and as a practitioner?

5. What lessons does Dr Benkelman's story contain about dealing with people? With fearful patients?

6. Professionals sometimes worry about being taken advantage of if they are "too giving." How does Dr Benkelman manage that concern? Do you agree with his approach?

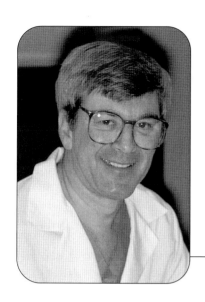

5

Jack A. Whittaker

Activism for Access to Care

Dr Jack Whittaker grew up in Bowling Green, Ohio, in a family atmosphere that was dominated by sports and nurtured by sportsmanship. Planning on a career in dentistry since high school, Jack graduated from The Ohio State University College of Dentistry and in 1965 opened a general dentistry practice in Bowling Green. After 3 years of facing his deficiencies in providing competent care for children, he entered the pediatric dentistry program at Columbus Children's Hospital. In 1970, he returned to Bowling Green to establish his specialty practice and remains there still. From the earliest days of his practice, Jack has treated low-reimbursement Medicaid patients. Eventually realizing that most of his colleagues were not doing likewise, he became concerned that children who needed care were not getting it. As a result, he began a long process to effect change. Within the profession, he campaigned to encourage both generalists and specialists to accept Medicaid patients. Simultaneously, he forged a successful relationship with an influential elected official in state government that brought about a significant and much-needed increase in the rate of Medicaid reimbursement to dentists. Apart from his practice, Jack has expressed his concern for children through coaching and off-the-field leadership in baseball, football, and ice hockey.

Dr Whittaker was nominated as a moral exemplar in dentistry by Dr Ann Griffen, an Ohio colleague in pediatric dentistry. In a 1996 letter, she wrote, "The story begins with Jack showing up at an Ohio Academy of Pediatric Dentistry meeting [in 1992] to speak his mind about an issue that was bothering him. He was concerned about the lack of access to dental care for Medicaid- [welfare-] funded children in Ohio, and he said so in a slightly shaky voice. He wanted some other practitioners to see these kids. He didn't point any fingers, but rather talked in generalities about the difficulty

that patients had in finding care. He told us that he couldn't turn the patients away, but that they were coming from long distances to see him and they were filling his available practice time. He told us that they were an astounding 50% of his practice."

Dr Griffen continued, "Now, we all knew that you lost money seeing Medicaid kids, and the high-volume Medicaid-dependent practices we were familiar with were either academic centers or substandard 'mills.' But this guy looked like any other competent, successful private practitioner. He went on to tell us that he had been audited by Medicaid investigators [for what turned out to be] minor billing errors. . . . My guess is that they were suspicious of him because of his high volume. The amazing thing was that despite financial penalties, and the humiliation and hurt of being accused of fraud, Jack went right on seeing these kids because he considered it his moral responsibility. I don't think the rest of us would have done it. Most refused because of the low fees, some because of the difficulties in filing claims, and some because of the general unattractiveness of the families. I don't believe very many of us would have persisted in the face of harassment."

Commenting on his activities after the Ohio academy meeting, Dr Griffen said, "Not only did Jack keep seeing these kids, he spent the next few years figuring out how to improve access for kids all over the state. He started by trying to negotiate with the bureaucrats in the Medicaid system. When promises didn't lead to any change, he started visiting legislators. Other members of the academy helped in these efforts, but it was really Jack's energy and persistence that kept it going. The result was action by a powerful state representative with an interest in kids that led to substantial increases in Medicaid fees. The legislator became the attorney general, and she attended our last Ohio Academy Meeting to receive a special award and watch while we recognized Jack for his efforts."

Dr Griffen concluded her letter: "Throughout, Jack was very modest, always wanting to credit others with the work. He obviously felt good about being recognized, but it was clear that that was not his motivation for doing what he did. In my estimation he's a genuine moral hero: He did what he thought was the right thing for no reason other than it was right; he suffered for doing it; and he persisted until what he saw as a wrong was righted."

When I (JTR) asked Jack Whittaker to comment on Ann Griffen's account of his activities, he said that it was fairly accurate, including the part about his shaky voice. "I was very emotional, and my voice was cracking, I guess. I talked for about three minutes, and I sat down. You could have heard a pin drop." The reason for the silence was that Jack had just described the current status of access to dental care for Medicaid children in Ohio, especially with respect to pediatric dentists. He had told them "that I had called every pediatric dental office in Ohio, some 110 guys maybe, and only 23 would take the welfare card."

Experiences with Medicaid

To appreciate what happened at that 1992 meeting, one must go back to the first days of Jack's pediatric practice, which began in 1970. In those days, the Medicaid record system was primitive, and it took 6 months to get paid. Even so, Jack said, "I've always taken welfare. I saw all the kids. The poor kids have been around forever."

Why did he choose to treat Medicaid patients? "They are *kids*, and I didn't think it made any difference. I didn't get paid as much—that was the first thing you noticed. But there was money there, and it didn't bother me. We just worked them in. I was in practice probably 5 years before I finally figured out that about one third of my patients were welfare." Jack said he was not alone in seeing Medicaid patients in those years. "Everybody was seeing them, but there weren't that many [Medicaid patients] when we first started. In the late '70s and then in the '80s, it started to build."

By the end of the 1980s, his practice had grown to 40% to 50% Medicaid. Jack said, "I noticed we were starting to get kids from farther away. We were getting them from 30 miles, 40 miles away, because no one would see them anymore . . . I had kids coming [all the way] from Van Wert, Ohio. In order for them to get here, they had to go by 260 dental offices, [including] four pediatric dental offices, to get to me with toothaches. Their faces were swollen; they were in pain. Now there's something wrong about that! And that's what got me going—that's what got me mad." Jack said, "It was kind of a gradual thing, but I started getting on my soapbox. And for 2 or 3 years I just got mad at everybody because they weren't seeing welfare."

It is not that Jack doesn't understand dentists' reasons for not wanting to see Medicaid patients. Young practitioners, for example, have major financial obligations. Every Friday, Jack teaches in a general practice residency program at the Medical College of Ohio in Toledo. He said, "When my residents finish dental school, they are $85,000 to $100,000 in debt, and their biggest worry is making their monthly payments starting next July." Taking on patients that don't provide much income is not high on their priority list. Money is not the only issue, however. When onerous Medicaid paperwork yields financial penalty, it is difficult to be enthusiastic. For many years, the Medicaid reimbursement rate was in the range of 25% to 35% of usual and customary fees. In addition, Jack said that when he asks dentists why they don't see Medicaid patients, they tell him about the frequent problem of broken appointments and the occasional breach of personal hygiene. They say they are afraid the Medicaid patients will drive their private patients away. Although Jack thinks the fear of losing private patients is nonsense, he admits that the dentists are sometimes right about the hygiene issue. "Sometimes we sit back there and cut fingernails and wash their faces."

Despite the acknowledged negatives of Medicaid, Jack said, "I'm frustrated because I really care about the kids. When there's an injustice done, or when people are in need of help, you've got to do it. If you're in the 'kids' business, I think you should take care of kids. It's just too bad that I can't help them all."

Occasionally Jack gets as upset with the dentists who treat Medicaid patients as he does with those who don't. He said there are a few dentists who abuse the system by providing the quick preventive procedures but refusing to perform the more time-consuming restorative procedures, often without telling the parents. Jack said, "Then they see them 6 months later and tell them the same thing. You get tired of seeing these little kids being pushed all over the place."

One of Jack's major sources of irritation is the tendency of segments of the profession to overstate or misrepresent the degree to which dentistry provides care to the disadvantaged. For example, there are claims of reduced-fee programs for children that actually render little treatment; humanitarian awards for treating underserved populations in distant countries given to people who refuse to treat Medicaid patients in their own communities; and leaders of organizations who do not treat Medicaid patients themselves, but who praise the profession for its goals of caring for all.

Working for Change

Jack converted his frustrations to actions designed to increase the number of dentists who treat Medicaid patients. His extemporaneous 3-minute plea to the Ohio Academy of Pediatric Dentistry was the first in a series of efforts to improve access to care. He also served on the access committee of the Ohio Dental Association and, for a time, wrote letters for its monthly newsletter urging participation in the Medicaid program. Whenever he gives a continuing education course, he urges the participants to get involved. He encourages mothers who cannot get dental care for

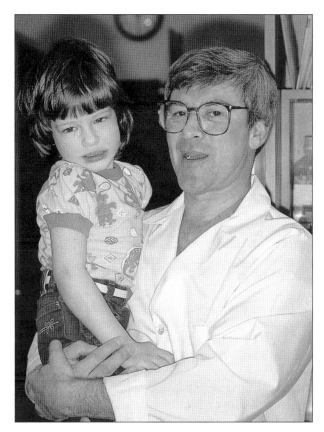

Dr Whittaker finds satisfaction in the hugs he gets from Medicaid children. "They're so happy you'll take care of them."

their children to write letters to appropriate organizations. He writes letters about the issue to officials of the US government. He writes letters to the *ADA News* and sends e-mail messages to leaders of the American Academy of Pediatric Dentistry and the American Dental Association when they make what he feels are self-serving statements about how well the profession meets its responsibility to care for all children.

Besides encouraging Ohio dentists to see Medicaid patients—which, incidentally, he feels has had little effect except to incite criticism—Jack launched a much more successful campaign to increase the rate of Medicaid reimbursement for dental services in Ohio. He reasoned that if reimbursements were higher, then more dentists would enroll as Medicaid providers.

Jack's efforts started in 1991, a few months before the Ohio academy meeting. He had obtained some information from the state that showed that of the 6,000 dentists in Ohio, 1,790 (roughly 30%) were signed up as

Medicaid providers. While this number was not large, it was respectable and suggested that the problem may not be severe. Since his impression was that there were fewer providers than the number suggested, Jack and Dr Bill Fye, a pediatric dentist from Cincinnati, decided to look further into the issue. Jack started by calling several individuals who had submitted rather modest requests for reimbursement. At that point, his strategy was that he would call their offices, state his name, and announce that he was doing a survey on Medicaid providers. From their responses, Jack said, "I thought they were seeing welfare patients 18 hours a day." It seemed to Dr Whittaker and Dr Fye that the enthusiasm they were hearing for treating Medicaid patients did not match the information provided by the state. They needed to get better information.

At about the same time, a dental hygienist at a clinic for poor children in Toledo who knew of Jack's concern arranged a meeting between Jack and Betty Montgomery, an influential state senator. The agenda was to discuss the difficulties of providing dental care for Medicaid children. His need for better data that delineated the problem became more imperative, but he was not sure how to get it. He said, "So one day," he said, "I was working away, and I had a brainstorm. I got out our association telephone directory, and I called all the pediatric dentists in the state of Ohio. I would pretend I was a father, and I gave different scenarios at different times." The circumstances of "his child" ranged from needing a checkup to suffering severe pain, orbital swelling, and fever. "[My staff wasn't] happy with me because I was making too many phone calls and had patients lined up out the front door. There were times they walked up and unhooked my phones. [Overall] I probably called 7 or 8 offices a day, so it didn't take me very long. In less than a month I had pretty good statistics."

He used these data for his meeting with Betty Montgomery in February 1992. Jack beefed up the data with several pages of color photographs that he had taken of small children with advanced dental caries, lopsided faces, and eyes swollen shut. He hoped the vivid pictures would help compensate for the limited data. These were also the data that Jack presented to the Ohio Academy of Pediatric Dentistry just a few weeks later. Firmly committed by that time, he was happy that, "They asked Bill Fye, myself, [and two oth-

> "Dr Whittaker did what he thought was the right thing for no reason other than it was right."
>
> Dr Ann Griffen
> Dr Whittaker's nominator

ers] to work on this thing. Whenever you go some place and [complain], they put you on a committee. Am I right?"

His meeting with Senator Montgomery was successful, even though he had no valid information on general dentists. They talked for almost 3 hours. Jack said, "Betty Montgomery told me what to do and how to do it." Jack was so encouraged that he arranged a meeting with Representative Randy Gardner, the Republican majority whip, whose children were patients of Jack's.

Of primary importance was the production of additional and reliable data about the participation of general dentists in the Medicaid program. Jack therefore decided that his next action would be to make random calls to at least 500 other dentists in Ohio. Jack said, "I hit every corner of the state. I called Cincinnati. I called Youngstown, Dayton, Akron. I called Cleveland. I called Bellefountain. You name it, I called it. I found that less than 5% would see my welfare child. So I really had some backing there." These data paved the way for subsequent legislative action.

In his first meeting with Senator Montgomery, she had made it clear that it was also necessary to write to legislators and talk to them personally. Additionally, he needed to talk to the people in charge of policy making for dentistry. Jack followed her instructions faithfully. Furthermore, the senator said it was necessary to never let them forget it. Jack said, "Every time she saw me, she said, 'Keep going. Keep going.' Her point was to keep their attention focused."

With respect to the composition of letters, especially to the legislators, Senator Montgomery told him to keep it simple, and so he did. He said, "If you put it in 18,000 words and 24 pages, single spaced, they're not going to read it. They could care less. But if you can say, 'Dentistry–Kids–Welfare–No money,' now they've heard that." Furthermore, he handwrote every letter on yellow paper in big script just so they would be sure to notice it. His strategy seemed to work. Jack said the majority whip told him, "There wasn't one senator in Ohio that did not know me, because I was persistent. I sent letter after letter after letter, and I got replies. I made phone calls. If you're smart, the first thing you want to do is get to their main aide. Once you get there and you can convince them, you'll get to the legislator. You do not accomplish one single thing unless you see the actual legislator. I'll guarantee you that."

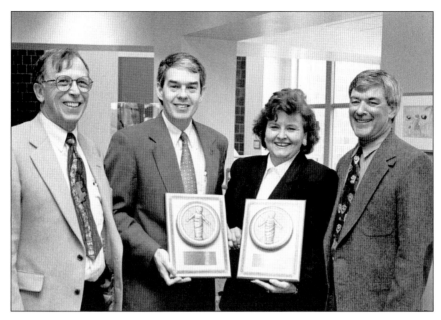

Dr Whittaker *(far right)* and Dr Bill Fye *(far left)* with Majority Whip Randy Gardner and Attorney General Betty Montgomery after the Ohio Academy of Pediatric Dentistry presented them with awards in 1995 for their efforts to improve access to care.

Jack did not limit his letters to Ohio. His committee decided to present their problems to the federal government. Jack wrote to the Secretary of Health and Human Services, using the same handwritten letter on yellow, lined paper and the same photographs he had shown Betty Montgomery. Shortly thereafter, the Secretary's office called to thank him for what he was doing. Later, after some Ohio dental public health officers went to Washington, DC, for a meeting, Jack said they told him that some federal officials "talked about a dentist from Ohio who sent some pictures. It was me."

In Ohio, with Jack's persistence and Senator Montgomery's generous help, the prospects for increasing dental Medicaid fees were improving. The time for voting was drawing closer, and she had arranged for Jack and Bill Fye to see the budget director and the director of human services, in order to ensure the acceptance of change at those levels. Additionally, Jack felt it was necessary to see Governor Voinovich, who was running for a second term in 1994 on the Republican ticket. He called Senator Montgomery, who herself was running (successfully) for attorney general. She was having a campaign party in Toledo and arranged for Jack to attend. Jack estimates that there were 35 corporate chief executive officers and himself. The governor moved

around the room shaking hands with everyone; Jack said, "He stepped up in front of me, read my name tag, and said, 'Dr Whittaker.' I said, 'Hi, I'm Jack Whittaker, one of your Medicaid providers.'" The governor laughed and told Jack what he wanted to hear: Governor Voinovich's administration would give him the backing if they could get it through the legislature. Jack said, "My feet didn't even touch the ground when I walked out of that place."

In 1995 the legislature approved the increased fees; they took effect on January 1, 1996. Instead of being paid roughly only 35% of their customary fees for children, dentists would be paid 50% to 60%, depending on the procedure. The fees for procedures on adults were lower, but still much better than they had been. Jack said, "The nicest part about the whole thing was that dentistry sat down with government, and we made decisions as to where the money was to be spent and how much we should pay for [certain procedures] and where we should put the most emphasis." There was a group of 12, including Jack, Bill Fye, and other representatives of the Ohio Dental Association, that did the work for dentistry.

Although Jack's motivation through the entire process was to improve access for low-income children, he is somewhat embarrassed that the outcome has almost doubled the part of his income that comes from Medicaid. He is concerned that someone will say, "Well here, Whittaker, you've just lined your pockets."

Jack has not received criticism for lining his pockets, but his use of fictitious fathers has received considerable disapproval. Immediately after the Ohio Academy meeting, Jack said a colleague told him, "What the hell are you doing things like that for?" He has had similar responses from others too, Jack thinks, not only for what he did, but also for being so confrontational with his colleagues. He said some members of the Ohio Dental Association "would not even look at me."

Referring to the criticisms, Jack said, "I've put some burrs under people's saddles, and maybe I've been unfair to a lot of people, but I don't really care. What I mean by 'I don't really care' is that I was determined that something had to be done. I was tired of people saying they were doing all these wonderful things when they weren't really doing much."

Many of his colleagues approve of what Jack is doing. At meetings, people say to him, "Way to go, Whitt. Take care of those kids." "I think you're doing a wonderful job." "We're glad you're doing it." "Then I say to them, 'Would you help me?' That's the way I look at it." Jack thinks there is not much evidence that his approving colleagues do, in fact, help. They cannot quite take the final, committed step. Jack said, "I don't mean to make everybody sound bad. I think there are some very good people, and I would say that 90% of them act professionally. It just happens to be that the Medicaid thing is a big issue with me. I think, overall, we're okay [as a profession]. I think it's there. But I'm still not going to say we are a really, tremendously caring profession."

Jack is optimistic for the future, though, especially because of the new dentists, despite their burdens of debt. "In the last 6 or 7 years, the younger dentists coming up have a completely different look at things. I just feel a difference there; I don't know why. And whether they are seeing welfare, I have no idea. I'll probably be calling them all up some day to find out."

Whatever ambivalence exists within the profession about treating Medicaid patients, it is clear that dentistry appreciates what Jack and his collaborators in state government have accomplished. In 1995, the Ohio Academy of Pediatric Dentistry gave a luncheon to honor Jack and Bill Fye and present Betty Montgomery

and others in state government with a special award. A year later, the Ohio Department of Health awarded Jack for his efforts in advancing the health of children.

Understanding Jack's Actions

"Whittaker University"

In order to make sense of Dr Whittaker's concerns for the disadvantaged, his willingness to act, his anger, and his impetuous behavior, it is necessary to take a look at the circumstances of his childhood. Jack Allen Whittaker was born on February 22, 1936, and has been a Bowling Green resident for most of his life. His father, Ray, had grown up in Sandusky, Ohio, as a 5-foot–8-inch star football and basketball player. After high school, Ray worked briefly as a fireman, then joined the Marines during World War II. It was not until his late 20s that Ray considered college and moved to Bowling Green. Bowling Green State University (BGSU) was an easy choice for Ray because his brother Bob was head football coach there. Another brother, Jim, followed shortly thereafter. Jim starred in track and worked as an assistant football coach while he went to college. Ray served as equipment manager for the football team, starred on the basketball team, and, when he graduated, got a job as the BGSU freshman basketball coach. At the same time, Jack's mother, Betty, along with both of his aunts, also worked at BGSU in the president's office or the dean of students' office. Jack said, "They used to call it 'Whittaker University' in the '40s and early '50s, there were so many of them around." There are pictures all over the athletic department of Bob, Jim, and Ray, especially Ray, since he had been voted into the BSGU Athletic Hall of Fame. Ray made a lifetime career for himself at BGSU. After a few years as assistant basketball coach, he served as director of housing and progressed thereafter to dean of men, then dean of students.

Jack's mother became secretary to the president and then ran the financial aid office for many years, despite not having a college degree. This office provided her with extensive contact with the athletes. Her efficiency and unruffled manner earned her the distinction of being the first woman to be given a BGSU Athletic Award. Despite her prominence in the university community, Jack said that at home, "She was a quiet little

> Jack looks at the problems of access to dental care for low-income children with intense emotion.

thing. She was kind of a one-step-behind [her husband], two-steps-to-the-left type of person." Jack said that this relationship did not seem to bother her at all, but his personal opinion was that "my mom was squelched." At work, whatever she did, she did it quietly. Jack said, "She would do things for you, and that's the last you knew of it. You never heard of it again. Another thing about my mother: There's only been two names ever spelled by the band on the BGSU football field, and my mother's was one of them."

Sportsmanship

Considering this background, not to mention that his house was next to the baseball field, it is not surprising that, "Athletics was a big part of my growing up." Ever since he was 4 years old and doing well in sports, he was used to someone saying, "Hey, good job!" and giving him a pat on the bottom. He said, "It always meant something." In fact, at the very beginning of this interview, Jack used the same words to speak about his nomination as a moral exemplar. "You can't imagine how it makes you feel when someone else in your profession gives you a pat on the bottom and says, 'Hey, good job!' That's probably the most rewarding thing you get out of the whole experience."

Jack said, "Athletics teaches you a lot." He grew up with his Uncle Bob preaching, "'Look, if you want to be an athlete, you've got to take good care of yourself.' So, I knew I had to do those things, because I wanted to do good. [Athletics] teaches you to get along with other people. And there is the camaraderie that goes along with being on a team, and you're all going toward the same goal at that particular time. I enjoyed the closeness." He said that athletics taught him "to respect others. If I played against you, I respected your trying. If a guy played really good, I would tell him about it after the game."

Much of his affinity for sports was his love of competition. "I'll compete anytime, anyplace. If you want to throw pennies, we'll throw pennies. I don't care if I get beat if I just try hard. I want to do the best I can. My dad's philosophy was, 'Work hard, but have fun doing what you're doing.' That's what I try to tell little kids [in my coaching]. I don't want the superstars. Just give me the 10 kids that really want to try hard. You can't win every time. When you win it's fun; when you lose you feel bad, but so what! You could always win next time. Does that make sense? My Uncle Bob was the same way as a football coach, and my dad was the same way in basketball. They wanted to win, but you weren't going to die if you lost. You just work harder the next time."

Jack believes that what is most important is that each child on the team gets a chance to play in every game. Jack said his Uncle Bob was the same way. "I think the biggest thing about him was his fairness. [He] used to have some 50, 60 kids on his football team, and just about every game they all played. I'm not saying they played evenly, but they all played."

Bob Whittaker had other principled ideas that now appear unorthodox. He had started coaching at BGSU in the late 1940s, a time when BGSU offered no football scholarships. This was a state of affairs that Bob liked. When he went to high schools to recruit players, he preached the need for a good education. Players were expected to take paid jobs around the university, but nothing more. In the early 1950s when the university started the move toward scholarships, Bob balked because he disapproved of the emphasis of athletics over academics. When the university first awarded football scholarships, Bob quit. To be precise, he quit as football coach and took a job as track coach. No scholarships were offered for track. Life was very different then.

The Athlete and His Father

Jack was not only immersed in the culture of sports and sportsmanship, he was also a very good athlete. In high school, he played baseball, basketball, football, and track, lettering twice in each sport. He excelled at football, where he starred as quarterback. The memories he carries of those days are primarily feelings of encouragement. "No accolades, just a pat on the bottom. And when my dad would watch us play a football game, he wouldn't say, 'Now, you should have done this, and you should have done that.' He would just say, 'Hey, good job!' That's all he'd say, and walk away. As long as he said that, I felt good."

There were many times, however, when Jack wished his father had been more demonstrative. "My father never said 'I love you.' I tell my kids that every day that I see them, and I think the reason I do is because my dad never said it to me. . . . My mom didn't say she loved us too many times either. They were not affectionate people." In addition, his father's university position was extremely demanding, and his father, in Jack's words, was "a kind of a self-centered person. . . . My sister and I always felt we weren't first, and I think that carried over. That influenced me to make sure that my kids were first in most cases." This does not mean that Jack thinks his father did not love him. He said, "There's no question. He was so proud the day I graduated from dental school, you can't believe it. That was just the greatest thing. He was just as proud as he could possibly be. And I wanted him to hug me, but he didn't."

Ray Whittaker expressed his feelings for his son in other ways. He never missed a sports event that Jack was involved in, whether it was football, baseball, or track. Jack said, "He was a chaperone for the high school dances, college dances, too. I was always proud of him and proud of my mom, too. And my mom more so later in life, because I never realized what she actually did, since my father was kind of the centerpiece of our family."

His father attracted attention in whatever he did. Jack said, "He worked hard. He worked too many hours. He was an 8:00-in-the-morning-to-8:00-in-the-morning type of person. He was in the university when a lot of the Vietnam riots were going on in Ohio. And so, being the dean of students, he was in the thick of it." Unlike some universities, BGSU stayed open despite the riots, and Jack thinks it was because of his father. He related a story some friends had told him: "There was this kid from Cleveland [who] was leading the riot. He was standing

> "Work is so rewarding to me. I take care of some of the most seriously ill children. I affect their lives. I make them feel better. I keep them healthy."
>
> *Dr Whittaker*

out in front screaming and yelling, 'Let's go!' And they were starting to charge the ROTC building. My father just took off, ran down this little incline, and tackled him. The crowd dispersed, and that was it." His act somehow dissipated the tension, and campus life continued undisturbed. Jack said, "They told me that story; I just died laughing. I could just see my dad doing it."

The student from Cleveland was expelled from school, but was readmitted in the next semester. Jack said, "I guess he told the kid, 'When you think you want to come back here, you give us a call,' and when the kid called, my dad got him back in the school. I saw him do that on different occasions. He felt it wasn't his job to kick the kid out of school. It was his job to try and keep a kid in school. There were students he had to kick out of school that would afterward come back and thank him for straightening them out. There's lots of stories like that."

There were also stories about his father writing letters to people whom he thought had committed an injustice. Occasionally, such confrontations occurred face-to-face. Late in his career, while at a university party, his father publicly berated the president for some official acts that he thought were wrong and harmful. Although his father's behavior seemed to lack propriety, Jack said, "He did not want to embarrass [the pres-

Commentary

Jack Whittaker's story addresses one of the more perplexing challenges for the profession: meeting the responsibility of service to society. Like Jack, we interpret this responsibility as an obligation that goes beyond providing care for those who can pay. The generally accepted viewpoint is that one ought to give back to society a part of what one has been given—partly because the privilege of practicing a profession is ultimately granted by society, partly because the general public heavily subsidizes the training of heath professionals. Jack Whittaker's rationale is less theoretical. He treats low-income children because they need his help and because he cares about them.

Most professionals are involved in some form of giving to others. Dr Echternacht, our first exemplar, believed giving back to the community to be obligatory, and his actions went far beyond minimal expectations, sometimes to his detriment. Many people find that giving is a rewarding experience; and if

one has something to give, the process can be rather painless. Giving money is probably the most painless thing to do, especially when it's accompanied by a tax break. Generosity becomes harder when effort is required day after day, one's income shrinks, and one's sensitivities are challenged, as with Dr Whittaker. It may be distasteful to provide care to people who rely on government resources and are said to make no effort to acquire honest work. It may be unpleasant to treat patients with physical or mental disabilities, and when patients are dirty, self-destructive, abusive, or demanding, the unpleasantness becomes repugnance.

Jack Whittaker sees himself as a person whose sense of caring has been enlarged by a lifetime of experiences working with children—primarily as a pediatric dentist, but also as an athletic coach for young children. He enjoys what he does and expresses a profound sense of gratitude for the skills he possesses and for the opportunity to serve others. He has always thought of himself as a caring person. However, in reflecting on his earlier years as a dentist, he now feels that the depth of his

ident], but [the president] had refused to meet with him. So, when my father came eyeball to eyeball with him, he just ripped him apart. He was using four-letter words and everything, this old man yelling at [the president]."

Jack admits that his father "was a cantankerous old man. I have a lot of his traits, and I find myself saying things like he did or writing letters like he did. I told you that he wasn't around very much. When he was around, he wasn't that pleasant to be with. He was kind of a grumpy guy, kind of ornery, 10 times more opinionated than I ever thought of being, and I'm damn opinionated." Later in life, especially after he experienced a heart attack, Ray Whittaker became even more curmudgeonly. Jack said he hopes that when he gets old he will avoid that label, though family members aren't so sure he'll be able to.

Into Dentistry

When Jack was a junior in high school and obliged to make a career choice for vocational day, he decided he wanted to be a dentist. This was a switch from his previous inclination to be a coach, but not surprising to anyone. His father had always talked about the advantages of a profession, and there were many things Jack liked about his own dentist, Dr Norm Huffman. Dr Huffman, Jack said, "was just such a nice guy, nice and easy, and he took good care of me. . . . He [also] had a nice house and

a nice car." However, Jack said, "I was scared to death to go to college. My father was at the university, my mother was at the university, and I thought if I go there I have to do good, and I didn't know if I could." His grades in high school were average, he said. "Some Cs and Bs, an occasional A in chorus or gym or something like that."

His academic performance turned around after high school. He spent the 1954 to 1955 academic year at Manlius, a prep school in New York. He went there on a baseball and football scholarship. "If I hadn't been in athletics, I probably would not have been able to go there." The Manlius experience gave his academic confidence a great boost. "I studied hard, worked very hard, and did well."

His performance at Manlius also gained him football and baseball exposure at San Diego State University. Jack recalled, "I went out there, and my dad decided that because I was going to the west coast, that he'd leave his job here, and he and my mom moved the entire family to California." What actually happened was that his father, who was 10 years into his job as dean of students, had negotiated a leave of absence. To support his family, Jack said his father "taught high school and coached basketball. He got back into coaching again." Jack stayed at San Diego for only one semester. He injured his knee, had to quit playing football, and returned to Ohio to complete his college education at BGSU. After having to wait an additional year in California, his father reacquired his deanship, and the Whittakers moved back to Bowling Green.

---

caring at that time was superficial. His experiences in treating disadvantaged children and his encounters with an unresponsive system that discriminates against these children has fueled his sense of caring and precipitated a passion for addressing the injustice. His success, at least with respect to raising Medicaid reimbursement rates, has only intensified his sense of caring and his inclination to challenge his peers to take up the cause.

Jack believes that much of who he is stems from growing up in a family that was dominated by sports, with special lessons on teamwork and fairness from his Uncle Bob and his father. Under their guidance he learned to work cooperatively in an environment that respects and develops each individual. He seems to have applied these concepts in his dental practice and works in an atmosphere of support from loyal employees who are treated respectfully and fairly. In fact, he thinks that the collaborative environment in his office is a major reason why he loves his work so much. For Jack, work, like athletics, is fun and brings an intense sense of enjoyment. Furthermore, in

parallel with his concept of what athletics ought to be, the fun comes not so much from winning, but from developing and maintaining an effective, caring team.

Based on his experiences with Medicaid, Dr Whittaker does not see dentistry as an especially caring profession. Certainly, there are many caring professionals who, like Jack, provide exceptional service to individual patients and their families. But Jack is talking about a larger conception of caring. He does not see the dental profession as a cohesive group who work together for a larger goal—the promotion of oral health for society. In Dr Whittaker's efforts to provide more care for Medicaid children, he confronts some of the same issues faced by dental ethics educators. Helping well-intended dental students develop and articulate a broad understanding of the roles and responsibilities of a professional is a special challenge. While dentists, lawyers, and physicians convene with camaraderie in professional organizations and study clubs to promote their professional and technical interests, there is seldom a clearly articulated sense of their larger purpose.

Jack graduated in 1959 with a dual major in biology and chemistry.

Jack married immediately after college. He then entered dental school at The Ohio State University under a draft deferment. Dental school kept him extremely busy. In addition to classes, for the first 3 years, he worked 20 hours a week in a blood lab doing cross matching. This almost paid for his dental education and helped support his family, which included three children by the time he graduated.

Clinically speaking, his skill developed moderately easily, but, as Jack said, "I think I'm a lot better now than I was in dental school. I'd better be." In his first experience with operative dentistry techniques—which he refers to as "the pits"—he drove his high-speed handpiece through his mirror. However, overall his experience was a good one. "I was lucky," he said. "I had great patients. They always showed up—pure luck. I had good friends who were way better students than I was, but their patients wouldn't show up half the time. I got all my requirements done with time to spare." Focusing on something that had a purpose for his future was very satisfying.

Jack Whittaker received his DDS in 1963 and then fulfilled his obligation to the Army, where he had two very different experiences. One was the exhilaration of beginning a new life, receiving his first meaningful paycheck, and having time left over to play flag football and baseball. The other was being depressed by the Vietnam war. "It just didn't make sense to me. I thought, 'God, if my kids ever grow up and they have to go to this war—boy, this is crazy.' I became somewhat unpatriotic."

Working with Children

Jack's time in the Army also reinforced his interest in working with children. He had liked it in dental school, and he enjoyed it even more in the Army. He said that he wanted to treat children more but he was not very good at it. Acting on those interests, however, was out of the question. He was married with a family and needed an income.

Jack left the Army in 1965 and set up a general practice in Bowling Green. He said, "I was the new young dentist in town, and the old guys didn't want kids, so they sent them to me." Before long half of his patients were children, which only served to increase his frustrations of not being able to manage them. Jack said, "They're a challenge. I mean, think about what we do. We take a little 3 year old, and we stick needles in his mouth. We put a raincoat [rubber dam] over his mouth and drill holes in his teeth. They're a challenge, but how could you not like kids?" To make matters worse, he knew everyone in town. Jack said, "These people were sending me their children, and too often I couldn't work on them. . . . I could not sufficiently and efficiently take care of children." A precipitating event in his decision to pursue his

When Dr Whittaker, in a shaky voice, first stood up in a professional meeting to speak about the problems of access to care for Medicaid children, he was not speaking to a community of peers who had the consciously articulated mission of promoting the oral health and welfare of their community. The professional association was not engaging proactively to see that the needs of the community were being met. They were not even actively engaged with their state system to work together for fair Medicaid reimbursement rates. If the association had had a mission that was more in line with the larger societal expectations of professions, Dr Whittaker would not have been so reticent to discuss what he had noticed about the access problems. Perhaps because he believed that the reason for practitioners' reluctance to provide care was truly the unfair reimbursement rates, he did not challenge his colleagues with the same level of moral indignation he seems to show today.

At present Jack looks at the problem of access to dental care for low-income children with intense emotion, sometimes with outrage at his colleagues' shortcomings. He is more willing than most to confront them and reveal their excuses and misrepresentations. He is an outspoken activist who engages in contentious methods that expose his profession's reluctance to take care of the disadvantaged. Through enormous persistence, he engages in activities that effectively raise legislators' consciousness about the issue and ensure that the public shoulders its fair share in the finance of care for those who cannot care for themselves.

For Jack Whittaker, the victory turns out to be hollow. He learns that low Medicaid reimbursement is not the primary reason that many practitioners refuse to treat disadvantaged children. Their reasons range from concern about broken appointments and the fear that their paying patients will be alienated through distaste for low-income patients' personal hygiene. As far as Jack is concerned, the concerns are insufficient and self-serving. The more excuses he hears, the more incensed he becomes. He feels especially annoyed when the caring characteristics of the profession are publicly exaggerated

interest in treating children was his defeat by a frightened 5-year-old child with Down syndrome. Jack said, "I went out to the waiting room to get him, and he turned around and ran right through the screen door." His father caught the child in the parking lot and brought him back. However, Jack said, "I never even got to see if he had teeth or not. And that night I went home and said [to my wife], 'I don't know what I'm going to do.'" In the following year, 1967, Jack sold his practice and, with his wife and their three children, moved to Columbus to enter the pediatric dentistry program at Children's Hospital.

Jack finished the program in 1969, spent another year at a center for children with developmental disabilities, and returned to Bowling Green to establish his specialty practice, which he runs today. His professional life is extremely busy. He spends the first 4 days of each week at his office, which is located in the town hospital's professional building, and sees 30 to 50 patients each day, depending on the trauma cases that come from the hospital. He is on call at the hospital for trauma for both adults and children. His practice includes many children with physical and mental disabilities, and he takes care of mentally disabled adults as well. The last day of the week he teaches in the general practice residency programs at two hospitals in Toledo. This is one of the days he values most. He is pleased that the residents seem to value it, too.

The atmosphere in his office is friendly, and his employees tend to stay with him for years. Jack said he follows his father's advice to take good care of your

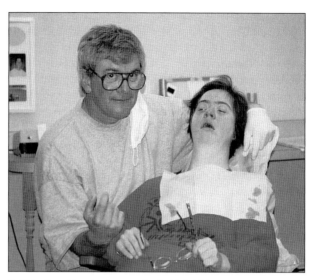
Dr Whittaker with a developmentally disabled child.

employees: "People don't work for you; they work with you." Employee benefits include a profit-sharing plan and a shared decision-making process both for purchasing and for hiring. Jack said, "That's what keeps people working, and that's what keeps people happy. That's the reason I go to work. They provide comfort for me at that office. I'm so lucky. I have tremendous people I work with, and things just run nice and smoothly every single day. It's a nice, calm, relaxing atmosphere, and that's the reason I can practice the way I do."

or misrepresented. Indeed, when practitioners who fail to treat Medicaid patients at home are honored for their humanitarian efforts abroad, usually in some exotic place, he feels especially indignant.

What are the basic issues? How do they arise? How can they be addressed so that we promote a more cohesive profession, focused on the long-term purposes of the profession? There seem to be two fundamental problems. One is the nature of service to society and what that might mean. The second is the responsibility of the professional to cooperate with peers to promote the oral health of the community.

Many young people enter dentistry with an idealistic and perhaps altruistic view of themselves as future professionals. Yet for most, the exact nature of the roles and responsibilities of the professional are not well understood.[1] In fact, some are quite surprised to learn that the expectation of service to society extends beyond providing services to those who can pay. A few have such an expansive conception of responsibility toward others that if their actions matched their beliefs they would

not be able to maintain a viable practice. Many are surprised at the expectations related to professional self-regulation and self-monitoring. When responsibilities to participate in organized dentistry are introduced, they often are quick to point out that one is not legally required to join a professional association. Distinctions between what is legally required (the minimum standard) and ethically required (the aspirational standard) are not understood. Even if students accept that they have a responsibility for service to society, they are subject to the same intervening financial and cultural factors that Jack Whittaker heard from his colleagues.

Other reasons for the reluctance to respond to the needs of the disadvantaged are forms of self-deception. Of importance from this standpoint is Goleman's[2] reminder that effective human functioning requires a certain amount of positive self-affirmation. The challenge is to differentiate positive self-affirmation from self-deception. Each of us has a capacity for developing elaborate and internally persuasive rationalizations for prioritizing nonmoral values over moral ones. Also, we tend

Jack presents the same concepts of practice management to his residents at the Medical College of Ohio. He also tells them his personal experiences with the risks of practice. About 3 or 4 years into his pediatric practice, Jack was working about 80 hours a week. No one else was available to cover night call at the hospital emergency room. He would sometimes get called in four or five times a week, and was often up until 2:00 in the morning. In addition, he was in debt from starting his practice and from buying a house. He said, "I loved what I was doing, but it was killing me, and I didn't know it. I got pretty heavy into drinking, Demerol, and Percodan, and a few other things, just to stay awake or to go to sleep. The drugs were so easy to get. I'd come home at night, after everyone was in bed, and I'd sit down and drink four beers and a half bottle of Schnapps so I could sleep." This went on for about a year, the first half of which Jack was unaware that he had a problem. It ended abruptly late one night when he experienced acute anxiety and skin pain over his entire body. Even his hair hurt. He was hospitalized and sedated for 9 days and away from work for 2 weeks. Since then, his life has been essentially normal. He has had no interest in drugs, and he drinks a glass of wine a couple of times a week. He considers himself extremely fortunate.

> "My caring has been more intense in the last 7 or 8 years. When I saw changes take place, that's when I realized how important [caring] was."
>
> *Dr Whittaker*

Jack's crisis was a shaping experience. He saw how easy it was to become trapped in self-destructive behavior, even when you thoroughly enjoy what you do. The experience taught him to be less self-centered and helped him to realistically differentiate between the important and the trivial in his life. It helped him to view his financial concerns with the perspective of time. He appreciated dentistry even more. He tells the residents what happened to him and hopes that they listen.

Jack also tells his residents, "I hope that you have as much fun in this profession as I have had in the last 25 years, because I love it. I actually love it." In fact, he said he wishes he could practice 30 more years. "I have a beautiful practice. I have people coming to me from hundreds of miles away [who value my services]. I can't think of anything neater than that. These are selfish things, but you have to feel good about yourself. And feeling good about yourself—that to me is being successful."

Jack reiterates emphatically, "I love to come to work. I'm 60 years old, and I've been doing it since 1963. [I do it] because I want to do something nice. I feel like I want to take care of these kids, and nobody else around here can do it except me. And nobody wants to do it, and that's the sad part about it. But it's so rewarding to me. . . . I take care of some of the most

---

to shield ourselves from anxiety by avoiding painful truths or pretending not to notice them. Goleman points out that when we fail to realize that we did not notice the distress of others, "there is little we can do until we notice that we failed to notice how failing to notice has shaped our thoughts and deeds."[2p24] Thus the mind protects itself against anxiety either by rationalizations and self-deceptions or by diminished awareness. The challenge then for Dr Whittaker and for ethics education in general is to (1) sensitize professionals to the needs of others, especially those unlike themselves, (2) foster a reasonable sense of personal responsibility for others, and (3) help professionals see that if they collaborate to serve the needs of the less fortunate, no one will be unduly burdened.

It is pretty clear that many, if not most, practitioners recognize their responsibility to provide care for the disadvantaged. Take, for example, the formal recognition that Jack received from the dental profession in Ohio and the informal praise from individual colleagues, even those who were not treating Medicaid patients in their own practices. Another example is

seen in the responses of the practitioners Dr Whittaker called in his first attempt to survey Medicaid participation by dentists; many exaggerated their involvement to the point that the information was useless. There are also stories about dentists who abuse the system. An example cited in Jong's[3] textbook on community dental health shows dentists who use the Medicaid funding allotment of money to provide diagnostic assessments to low-income children in school settings, then send a note to the parents indicating the child's need for services and the name and address of the nearest dentist who could provide the care. The needed care, of course, is not covered because funds have been exhausted.

Stories such as the last example above are what drives Jack Whittaker to say and do things that anger his colleagues. Such actions detract from the fact that Dr Whittaker is a professional of extraordinary compassion. He is able to look beyond what many find as objectionable and to care about each child. His moral imagination is stimulated to extend his concern to the parents and their unique predicaments in life. His reward is the

seriously ill children. I affect their lives. I make them feel better. I keep them healthy. I prevent children who have had open-heart surgery from having serious illness due to their bad teeth. I don't think they can get along without me. Not very many people can do what I can do. How does that sound? Doesn't that sound wonderful?"

Day-by-day Jack's biggest sources of satisfaction are the thanks he gets from the mothers and the hugs he gets from the children. Furthermore, he said, "Ninety percent of that comes from Medicaid kids. They're so happy you'll take care of them."

Other Activities

Almost all of Jack's other satisfactions relate to children and to sports. In 1970, the year he opened his pediatric practice, he started coaching: baseball in the spring, ice hockey in the winter, and always with "the little kids." He continued his active coaching for more than 20 years, finally stopping in the mid-1990s to allow more personal time. Until recently, Jack himself was a regular participant in softball and ice hockey. He slowed down noticeably in his mid-50s after an ice hockey game with 20 year olds in which he received three broken ribs from a blow by a hockey stick.

Over the years, Jack has served on Bowling Green's recreation committee, been a founder and president of a youth hockey program, and served as commissioner of

the baseball league that has the youngest children—a position he still holds. He and two others were responsible for persuading Bowling Green High School to accept ice hockey as a varsity sport. Jack said, "Everything pertained to kids. I can't think of anything nicer to do."

As a coach, he said, "I'll teach them a lot of baseball and a lot of hockey, and they'll have fun. And that's the most important thing—to have fun. Certainly not to win every single time we go out there, or to play all the time. I tell the parents that everybody's going to play equally. Everybody gets a chance." Jack is his Uncle Bob recycled. And it might have been Ray Whittaker who said, as Jack does, "I don't want the superstars. Just give me the 10 kids who really want to try hard. That's what's fun."

Coaching children has its frustrations, too. Primarily, they relate to the single-minded desires of parents for their children to excel, to play every moment of every game, and to win. Jack thinks that these views about sports are destructive to children and detract from the most meaningful lessons in living that sports can offer. All he could do was to present his concept of coaching at the beginning of each season so that parents would understand—and hopefully accept—what their children would be experiencing. Even so, Jack is full of stories about how parents try to enhance their child's opportunities at the expense of others. Some parental manipulations were quite innovative, if not grossly excessive. All abrogations of fair play, both the routine and the extreme, were frustrating to Jack.

gratitude expressed by his patients and their parents. What further sets Jack apart from most is that he also feels moved to act on behalf of all children and parents who are disadvantaged. It is interesting to reflect on his development as a health care professional. In his earliest years he cared about doing things well, but now he thinks his perspective was superficial. As he learned to do things well, his focus on caring shifted from techniques to people, particularly children. It is clear that being a part of a profession has furthered his moral development.

As passionate as he is about his responsibility to care for others, he is equally passionate about addressing injustice. His persistent political efforts to improve access by raising Medicaid reimbursement have earned him the praise and recognition of his colleagues. During the process he became exquisitely aware of the ways that some professionals deceive themselves into believing they are good and caring practitioners. Challenging his colleagues in his father's impetuous manner, as he feels compelled to do, has earned him the criticism of

many of his colleagues. This is difficult for him because he much prefers, and even needs, personal affirmation and endorsement. He thinks that his lifelong uncertainty about his father's love and affection has created that need for affirmation. However, when it comes to his profession, even though he pays a price, he cannot help but call attention to self-serving behavior and claims of altruism that promote the image of caring but do not require personal sacrifice.

References

1. Bebeau MJ. Influencing the moral dimensions of dental practice. In: Rest JR, Narváez DF (eds). Moral Development in the Professions: Psychology and Applied Ethics. Hillsdale, NJ: Lawrence Erlbaum, 1994:121–146.
2. Goleman D. Vital Lies, Simple Truths: The Psychology of Self-Deception. New York: Simon & Schuster, 1985.
3. Bebeau MJ, Kahn J. Ethical issues in community dental health. In: Gluck GM, Morganstein WM (eds). Jong's Community Dental Health, ed 4. St Louis: Mosby, 1997:287–306.

The frustrations Jack felt in coaching are linked to those he experiences in dentistry. His second wife, Cindy, whom he married in 1984, puts it this way: "There is always something he is striving for. He's always been setting injustices straight. If it weren't in dentistry, it would be about kids not being treated fairly in being put on baseball teams, or that they wouldn't be treated fairly in hockey. I think he's always defending the underdog." Jack agreed. He said, "I don't like to see people being taken advantage of. That bothers me. I don't like it at all. I don't care who it is—if it's my family, or your family, or somebody I don't even know."

Views of Himself

In trying to understand Jack's perspective of himself, I asked him what is so important about himself from a moral standpoint that he wouldn't be himself without it. He responded, "I think I honestly care about other people. Not just about dentistry, but about all phases of life." As he views it, "The end result of caring is all the rest of the stuff. That's the reason I worked with the welfare system. That's the reason I coached and why I work with my residents the way I do."

Jack said he had always viewed himself as a caring person, but that his perspective of caring has broadened considerably since dental school. At that time his concerns were more about learning the skills necessary to perform good quality treatment on a consistent basis. He said he cared about his patients but that the depth of his concern was superficial. In those days, treatment to him "was something that you had to get done. To a dental student, I don't think your patient comes first in your mind. When I first got out of dental school, [caring] was one one-thousandth of what was on my mind." It was not until his stint in the Army that he began to understand what it means to have the responsibility to take care of people and to appreciate the value of what he did.

Even after the Army, the pressures of debt from starting a practice kept Jack from fully realizing the value of his work. "You can't put a value on something that you're doing, because you don't know the end result. Is it going to turn out good? Is it going to turn out bad? Am I doing the right thing?" It is only with the perspective of time that Jack feels especially good about the practice he created.

Jack added, "I'm not just talking about dentistry. A lot of things have changed in the way I feel about life in general. Maybe that's just growing older. But my caring, I think, is now more intense in the last 7 or 8 years than it was prior to all this." He relates much of this change to his attempts to improve access to care. Jack said, "A lot of it is related to my work, and who I take care of, and realizing that when you do care, something can get done. I cared about things, and I wanted things to get done and wanted things to change. When I saw changes take place, that's when I realized how important [caring] was. It's like I was given a whole new life. It's too bad I couldn't have learned that about 25 years ago. I've missed a lot. I'm serious. There's been a change."

Jack's umbrella of caring extends to religion. "Religion, to me, is just caring for another person. A good religious person ought to care about everything, all the people, every person." Jack said that he is religious, though not outwardly. Formerly Episcopalian, he developed a friendship with a Catholic priest in the Army who led him to convert to Catholicism while in the Army. He had previously attended Catholic services with his first wife and their four children, but conversion had never entered his mind. Needless to say, his status as a Catholic does not immunize the church from his criticism. "I get so upset when I see churches being built when they should be taking care of poor people. I know I'm narrow-minded, but I keep thinking, churches are to take care of people."

The same juxtaposition of Jack's criticism and endorsement pertains to human beings as well as to institutions such as dentistry and Catholicism. Jack said, "I won't hesitate to say if I think you're wrong. But I don't do it because I dislike you. I just do it because, at that particular time, I think you are wrong." He hopes that the same consideration is extended to him, but fears that it is not. In fact, Jack has a great interest in having people like him, which he thinks stems from his youthful concerns about his parents' love for him. As Cindy said, "He likes everything to be rose colored. He likes everybody, and he likes everybody to be happy and get along. And he goes out of his way to make sure a lot of people get that." Nevertheless, despite the conflict, if he sees a problem, he has to speak up.

Currently

At present, except for his abrupt reduction of direct participation in sports, not much has changed in Jack's life. His practice is as busy as ever. He continues to be involved in the affairs of Bowling Green University, where he established The Ray and Betty Whittaker Scholarship for a graduate of Bowling Green High School who wants to go to BGSU and major in some aspect of music. (His parents had enjoyed lasting friendships with members of the music department, and Jack thought that at least one nonathletic connection with the Whittaker name ought to be made.) He continues to write letters to the university as well as to his colleagues. Recently, when the new president of BGSU spoke about the problem of poor student attendance at football games, Jack wrote him a handwritten letter, on yellow paper, offering the top 10 reasons why attendance was poor, beginning with the preferential parking enjoyed by the administration at the expense of the students. Jack continues in his efforts to sensitize his colleagues, both in Ohio and nationally, to the issue of dental care for low-income children.

Recently Jack was appointed by the Ohio Director of Health and Human Services to serve on its Medical Advisory Committee. This is a group of 15 people of diverse backgrounds whose function is to advise the state on how to spend its health care dollars. Jack is the first dentist to sit on this committee in more than 15 years. Even Jack's participation in sports is scheduled to get a boost. Jack has started to get in shape to participate in the New York Yankees baseball "Fantasy Camp."

Jack is also reflecting on whether the climate for increased care for Medicaid children is improving. He tries not to be discouraged, even though the rise in Medicaid fees did not result in more Ohio dentists treating Medicaid patients. However, Jack knows that the issue is complicated and intimately connected with the economy of the country and the culture of the profession. Over the past few years, there have been some national conferences addressing this issue. Furthermore, most recently, the newly elected president of the American Dental Association placed access to care at the top of the profession's priority list. In his home state, the invitation to sit on Ohio's medical advisory committee is a good sign. The frequent pats on the back he gets from his colleagues about the good job he is doing are also encouraging. Jack just wishes their good will would translate into action.

Fundamentally, Jack is confident that action will take place soon. He expresses his optimism in this poem:

> For the little Medicaid kid with acute lymphatic leukemia,
> For the little Medicaid kid with hemophilia,
> For the little Medicaid kid with cerebral palsy,
> For the little Medicaid kid with a seizure disorder,
> For the little Medicaid kid with only a foster mom,
> For the little Medicaid kid with a swollen face,
> For the little Medicaid kid who is deaf and cannot speak,
> For the little Medicaid kid . . .
> It's been very tough. We keep trying, and I honestly believe, very, very soon, many will care for the little Medicaid kid.

Questions for Discussion

1. Dr Whittaker feels a sense of righteous indignation over the failure of his colleagues to treat medical-assistance patients. Is his indignation justified? What might he have done to encourage his peers to share the burden?

2. Has this story enlarged your sense of responsibility to serve? Does the profession collectively have a responsibility to provide service to the disadvantaged? How can you and your colleagues address the access to care issue in your community?

3. Dr Whittaker believes that being a part of the dental profession has enhanced his moral development. What is it that so affected him?

4. Dr Whittaker treats many patients in his practice who have significant dental needs. He feels that he cares about his patients and enjoys dentistry so thoroughly in part because he is able to make a valuable impact on their lives through the treatment he provides. How do you feel about these observations in terms of your current or future practice?

5. Was Dr Whittaker overzealous in his attempts to obtain adequate data on Medicaid activity among his state's dentists, or did the importance of his goal justify his actions?

6. How would you react to Dr Whittaker's realization that after his long but successful fight to increase Medicaid reimbursement, there was no significant increase in the number of providers? What would be your next step?

7. What virtues of professional practice does this story illustrate? Assess yourself and the professionals closest to you in terms of these qualities.

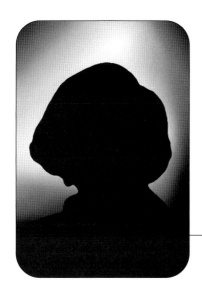

Janet Johnson

Am I My Brother's Keeper?

Authors' Note: This is a story about a whistle-blower, or, in accordance with recent literature, one who engaged in "positive deviance."* Unlike the others in this book, Janet Johnson's story is presented anonymously. The detailed circumstances of her life and the particulars of the original case have been changed because of Dr Johnson's concern that the use of actual names and circumstances would cause her and other key people in the case—including not only the dental assistants who lived through the story with her, but also the offending dentist—to relive the painful experiences that resulted from the incident. Although the facts of the case have been changed, we have attempted to present it so as to preserve the level of gravity of the original incidents. All quotes used are the original interviewee's actual words, and they pertain to comparable and representative situations in the original story.

Dr Janet Johnson graduated from a West Coast university in 1991. After 5 years with the US Public Health Service, she took a job in a general practice residency program at a Northwest hospital. Within a few months, she realized that her supervisor was flagrantly disregarding basic requirements for the safe administration of sedation for his anxious and uncooperative patients. After unproductive discussions with her supervisor and then the hospital administration, Dr Johnson took action that culminated in the filing of a complaint with the state board of dental examiners. The board's investigations uncovered more evidence of misconduct, and the offending dentist's license was eventually revoked for 2 years. Dr Johnson was widely criticized, even physically threatened, for what was falsely perceived as the unjustified reporting of a peer and a misplaced attack on the use of sedation. She was nominated as a moral exemplar in dentistry as someone who placed the interests of her patients, and ultimately her profession, above her own.

*Spreitzer and Sonenshein[1] define *positive deviance* as intentional behaviors that depart from the norms of a particular group in honorable ways. They suggest that whistle-blowing is a very specific form of positive deviance from ethically questionable organizational norms. The whistle-blower refuses to follow an illicit organizational norm and also departs from an organizational norm of silence. The authors also suggest that whistle-blowing behavior must be intentional and voluntary and relate to what one ought to do, that is, be "honorable."

Setting the Stage

Dr Janet Johnson graduated from a West Coast dental school in 1991 at the age of 26. Feeling the need for additional experience before entering practice, she joined the US Public Health Service for what turned out to be a 5-year term. Much of her assignment was with Native Americans in Arizona and New Mexico. During that period, she acquired considerable experience in the use of sedation and general anesthesia—enough, in fact, to make her wary and respectful of both their benefits and their hazards. Wanting even more experience in these areas, she decided on a career in hospital dentistry. When she left the Public Health Service, she took a job in a general practice residency program at a hospital in the northwestern United States. Married within the previous year, she immersed herself in the challenges of being on her own as a new professional. However, events soon occurred that were to change her life for the foreseeable future.

Besides Dr Johnson, the hospital dental clinic employed one other full-time dentist: her supervisor and the general practice residency program director, Dr Edward Cross, a man of approximately 45 years. It also supported four general practice residents, five part-time dentists, and five dental assistants, two of whom were extremely competent and had worked at the clinic for a long time. The continued existence of the general practice residency program depended on each person's ability to contribute to the generation of income, and everyone felt the pressure to produce. Dr Johnson spent practically all of her days either supervising residents or treating patients. If she had any spare hours, they were spent in committee meetings. She barely had time to reflect on how well she was meeting her own responsibilities, let alone on anyone else's job peformance.

Nevertheless, within months, Dr Johnson began to have misgivings about her supervisor, especially the way he administered sedation, a technique that he employed frequently—too frequently, she thought. Her initial cause for concern was that he sometimes did not use the help of dental assistants during his sedation cases. Dr Johnson said that this was something she would never even consider doing, given the inherent complexities of the situation—checking nitrous oxide/oxygen percentages, assessing patient responsiveness and airway patency, evaluating blood pressure, heart rate, and respiratory rate, and monitoring oxygen saturation and expired carbon dioxide concentration, not to mention performing the dental treatment itself. Not only did using qualified assistants make sense, it was also required by the professional sedation guidelines. Furthermore, when he did use dental assistants, which in fairness to Dr Cross was the greater part of the time, it seemed like he chose the least experienced of the five. This seemed odd to Dr Johnson; if it were her, she would want the most competent help she could get.

As the months passed, Dr Johnson became a careful observer of Dr Cross and his sedation cases but saw

Commentary

Am I my brother's keeper? Janet Johnson's response is an emphatic "Yes!" She says, "When you see real harm, you just have to do something."

This case dramatically illustrates the professional's fundamental roles with respect to self-regulation and monitoring of the profession. For the professional who observes questionable conduct, a responsible course is to look carefully at the evidence, consider whether colleagues would agree with the judgment of misconduct, and then speak to the professional whose conduct is troublesome. This was the course taken by Janet Johnson. For the professional whose conduct is being challenged, a responsible course is to listen carefully to the critique, reflect on standards of practice, and, if necessary, consult with respected experts—all in order to judge whether one's conduct is within the bounds of acceptable practice—and then take appropriate steps for the future. To do otherwise is to suggest that one lacks not only competence but also character. Dr Cross took none of these actions. It is not a virtue to stand one's ground in the face of evidence that one's practices or procedures are below the standards for professional practice. Nor is it a virtue to berate, belittle, or retaliate against a colleague or subordinate who has the temerity to question one's actions or judgments.

Think how differently this case would have ended had Dr Cross adopted a professional stance with respect to questions about his professional judgment. Consider also how differently this case might have ended if the hospital administration had taken seriously their responsibility to investigate charges of questionable practices and then helped these dentists to seek expertise in setting standards for sedation use.

As this case unfortunately illustrates, professionals may act defensively rather than look at the evidence. They may attack subordinates for challenging their authority rather than participate in reflections on the standards for professional practice. They may brand the accuser as a troublemaker rather than

nothing new and unusual. But when she looked at the charts of some of Dr Cross's patients, many of whom were children, her concerns deepened. To begin with, his record keeping was sloppy. Although data entries occasionally appeared for heart rate or blood pressure, they were sporadic and unaccompanied by any of the more sophisticated techniques of pulse oximetry or capnography. These deficiencies were disturbing but not surprising. It would be difficult to adequately monitor vital signs without the help of well-trained assistants, and impossible if there were no assistants at all.

To compound matters, the sedative doses Dr Cross was using were large enough to induce deep sedation, a state in which the risks are substantially increased. However, he had never acquired the training required to perform deep sedation.

The use of deep sedation can be very alluring to the clinician. Unlike conscious sedation, its consequences are much more predictable and effective. Difficult-to-manage patients become relaxed and unresponsive, and their treatment becomes much easier. One might even be tempted to undertake some kinds of treatment without an assistant.

However, under deep sedation patients whose airways become compromised due to the head being inadvertently flexed forward are at risk for losing reflexes that permit self-correction of the head position. If such an event occurs and the clinician is not trained to handle it, oxygen deficit, brain damage, or even death can result. Furthermore, if a trained assistant is not present,

the position of the head can all too easily be overlooked while the operator concentrates intently on the technical aspects of the care.

After a few more months, the two most competent dental assistants, who had been observing Dr Johnson closely for her reaction to Dr Cross's use of sedation, came to speak with her. They had sensed her concerns about Dr Cross and wanted to talk about their own experiences with him. They told her that their relationships with Dr Cross had deteriorated significantly over the 15 years he had worked at the hospital and had reached a low point over the issue of sedation.

The assistants voiced several concerns. They thought he did not monitor his sedation patients properly: His doses of sedative agents were large, and the way he managed difficult patients—often with excessive physical force—was often objectionable. They felt that at the heart of the problem was the fact that Dr Cross lacked skill in managing anxious and uncooperative patients. In their view, it was this shortcoming, more than anything else, that drew him to sedation and then to its excessive use.

As the assistants told the story, during Dr Cross's early years at the hospital, he hardly used sedation at all. But because so many of his patients presented management problems, he decided to try a chemical approach, beginning with light sedative doses that produced only conscious sedation. Over time he used sedation more, even though he was never very successful with it. One of the important problems with conscious sedation is that

---

work to resolve professional disagreements. And they may reveal only part of the story in order to shift attention from their incompetent use of a procedure. When accused professionals act in these ways, the consequences for the accuser can be profound, as we saw with Dr Johnson.

Dr Johnson had expected that once the facts were known, her colleagues would support her. Instead they viewed her as a pariah. Whereas she had been popular and respected in dental school, she was denounced and shunned for having the temerity to attack a popular and well-connected professional. When asked if she would do it all over again, she seems somewhat ambivalent, not because she questions the rightness of her action, but because of the far-reaching and clearly unanticipated personal attacks that she endured as a result. What should have been a professional discussion about whether certain practices met standards of practice turned into a contest of wills. Reflecting on the drawn-out process, including her own role as an instrument of the board, Dr Johnson observes, "It became a contest—winning rather than looking at what you did."

Reading a story of this sort is disturbing. We wonder how often dentists fail to discuss problems with their colleagues, as well as how often dentists are unwilling to consider criticisms responsibly when confronted. Is a story of this sort an anomaly or a common occurrence? In this case, both staff dentists and residents had noticed the questionable practices but demurred from taking action. Is the reluctance of Dr Johnson's peers to report the misconduct of a colleague that unusual? Even if the educational system stresses the affirmative duty to report incompetence or misconduct, it may be particularly difficult to overcome early socialization that labels and condemns informants as "snitches" and "tattletales." A 2002 study[1] of medical students' perceptions of the affirmative duty to report misconduct indicate that less than 40% feel they *should* report and only 13% said that they *would*. Furthermore, the number of students who thought they should report declined during their years in medical school. In focus group interviews that followed the survey, students indicated that misconduct should be addressed—but that perhaps someone else should do it—not

sometimes it works and sometimes it doesn't, and prediction either way is difficult. When sedation is ineffective, it is much harder to provide good treatment. Therefore, in order to better control his pediatric patients, he began to rely heavily on the hand-over-mouth (HOM) technique.[†] The assistants were particularly outraged to see that his version of HOM sometimes included clamping the children's nostrils shut. In any case, the HOM technique and its variations seemed to upset his pediatric patients even more. Eventually, Dr Cross took the next step and increased the dosage of the sedative agents. Predictably, it worked, and eventually it became his approach of choice for any patient who appeared to be at all troublesome. Since he was now working in the realm of deep sedation, his patients' behavior improved, but they also tended to become unresponsive and unable to respond to stimuli.

The assistants also said that they were shocked at the number of patients Dr Cross treated who had significant medical conditions–either inpatients or those who had recently been discharged from the hospital. The last straw was when they discovered that Dr Cross rarely consulted with the medical staff about these patients.

At this point they requested a meeting with him in order to voice their concerns. Dr Cross responded in no uncertain terms that they were there to follow his orders. If they didn't like it, he would find other people to do the sedations with him. And that is what happened. The two assistants refused to work with him on sedation cases. The assistants with whom he did work

were never trained properly, and he often chose not to use an assistant at all.

The two dental assistants also told Dr Johnson that they had spoken to her predecessor about the issue. He had acknowledged the problem but had chosen not to become involved.

A few weeks after this disturbing conversation, Dr Johnson was moved to action by a story that spread rapidly around the clinic. This time it came from one of the other dental assistants who was still helping Dr Cross with his sedations. Reportedly, during the sedation of a pediatric patient, the child thrashed about during the early phases of treatment. Eventually, the child calmed down and treatment progressed satisfactorily until, near the end of the visit, the assistant noticed that the child's face was blue. At that point, Dr Cross belatedly started to attach the pulse oximeter to the child when he noticed that the child's head had slipped off the neck support and was bent forward. No one had any idea how long the child's head had been in this compromised position. Dr Cross replaced the neck support and the child's skin gradually returned to its nor-

---

[†]The HOM technique is a patient management approach employed for uncooperative children. In its least controversial application, in which the clinician places a hand over the child's mouth and quietly talks with the child, it is a way of arresting adverse behavior and helping the child concentrate on the operator's requests. However, its image is often associated with the abusive, even angry use of power as the operator's hand covers the child's mouth and forcibly moves the head into the headrest. Because of this association with abuse, HOM is now considered controversial and has been the source of litigation against its users. When HOM extends to covering the nose along with the mouth, its use is especially onerous. At present, most practitioners who use HOM acquire parental consent first.

---

them. Feelings of trust and camaraderie that develop during professional school contribute to the reluctance to report. In a related study,[2] as many as 65% of students from a prominent US medical school reported some degree of discomfort at challenging other members of the medical team over perceived wrongdoing. Apparently, the drive for self preservation, coupled with this general discomfort of reporting and the real or perceived fear of retaliation, work against professional self-regulation—at least at these early stages of identity formation.

What is it that distinguishes Dr Johnson from her peers who declined to address the issue? In our view, Dr Johnson demonstrates a level of moral maturity (identity formation) that is uncommon for someone in her early thirties.[*] She appears to have internalized the values of the profession—for example, to put the interests of others before the self and to engage in regulation and monitoring of the professions—and made them part of her "self system." Thus, unlike novices and students who reportedly are unsure of their responsibility to report or, if they do see it as a responsibility, see it as someone else's, not theirs,

Janet sees this responsibility not as something for others to do, but rather as something she must do. For her, to not act is to violate the self. To fail to act also violates what the assistants should rightfully be able to expect of her. She expects support from the hospital administration, and thus is disappointed when it is not given.

Let's examine this stage 4 identity.[†] Dr Johnson is self-assured. She takes action when action is warranted. Furthermore, she has a keen sense of her responsibility to those the profession serves, particularly the disadvantaged—the "underdog," as she

---

[*]A recent cross-sectional study of identity development of military professionals[3] supports Kegan's observations that advanced levels of identity are rarely achieved before midlife (see Appendix E). Because Dr Johnson elected not to reveal her true identity, we are not able to portray the factors that shaped her identity as we were for other exemplars. For a more complete description of psychologists' view of the development of the moral self, see the commentary in chapter 8 (Donna Rumberger). In it, we draw examples from Dr Rumberger's life story to illustrate the stages and transition phases on her journey to moral maturity.

mal color. It was a dramatic treatment session that left everyone shaken.

Dr Johnson checked the patient's chart and saw that, as she had suspected, the child had been given sedative doses that were sufficiently large to be compatible with deep sedation. The chart made no reference to the anoxic incident, but indicated—falsely—that the pulse oximeter had been used to monitor the patient's response. The chart also revealed that the child, age 7, had been a longstanding patient of the hospital and was being treated for pulmonary stenosis. There had been no medical consultation for this patient.

Based on this alarming information, Dr Johnson decided to survey more of Dr Cross's patients. She examined the charts of all the patients he had seen over the previous 3 months. She discovered that her concerns and those of the assistants were completely justified. His doses of sedative agents were dangerously high. He was assisted by inappropriately trained personnel— or no personnel at all. He rarely used the standard electronic monitoring techniques. His documentation of treatment was shoddy but, surprisingly, included incriminating information. For example, he recorded the excessive dosage of sedative agents and the absence of monitoring. Worst of all, he had administered deep sedation to several children with systemic diseases with-

out consulting a physician. Janet quickly reviewed the medical component of the charts for the latter group of patients but saw no obvious changes in their conditions following dental treatment.

In addition to the disturbing evidence from the charts, Dr Johnson was beginning to form impressions about how the residency program was being managed. Dr Cross's cavalier attitudes about sedation had obviously spread to the residents, who, she thought, were employing it far too often. Although it was true that they were becoming experienced and confident with its use, Janet felt that their self-assurance and skills were without intellectual foundation, full of misinformation, and devoid of adequate concerns for safety. They were proceeding through their program with a false sense of security that could lead to major problems in the future.

Janet Johnson said that the whole situation with Dr Cross was extremely upsetting. At first, even after what she had heard from others, she "always gave him the benefit of the doubt and said that everybody does things their own way." Now, however, with indisputable evidence of her supervisor's inappropriate treatment practices, and despite an acute awareness both of her own junior status and of the fact that Dr Cross had vastly more clinical experience than she did, she nonetheless knew that some sort of action was required of her.

often referred to them during the interview. She also has a keen sense of responsibility to her professional colleagues and to staff. She supported her subordinates, the assistants who were troubled by actions they thought were harmful. She didn't turn the problem back to them, claiming that she couldn't judge because she wasn't there. Instead, she investigated. When she had satisfied herself that the problems were significant, she used appropriate procedures—direct communication—

for addressing her superior. When this didn't work, she went to the hospital administration. When this, too, proved ineffectual, she tried to work within the system rather than go directly to the state board of dentistry or the guardians of the children who had been harmed. She wanted to have questions of professional competence addressed by those who were most likely to resolve them without escalating the situation or enraging the public. Ultimately, the hospital's patient advocate, not Janet, involved the state board of dentistry.†

†A stage 4 identity is marked by psychological independence and by an integration of personal and professional values. Describing a stage 4 military professional, Forsythe et al[3p367] point out that, unlike earlier stages, where tangible rewards (stage 2) or how others feel about or judge the professional are defining to the sense of self (stage 3), the stage 4 professional has "an internal compass for proceeding even when he (or she) is receiving ambiguous or conflicting signals from others. In short, he can function as an independent decision-maker, one who shapes the environment in which he operates instead of merely reacting to it." These dimensions of the moral self are at least prerequisites to what Colby and Damon[4] refer to as the uniting of self with moral concerns, a defining feature of their exemplars. Moral maturity is described as an integration between moral reflection and habitual moral action that goes to the heart of the capacity to live out one's moral commitments.

†It is interesting to note that the patient advocate's action addressed issues for future patients who might come under Dr Cross's care rather than issues of harm to former patients. It seems that reporting to the board foreclosed the possibility of reparation for those who had been harmed.

Another effect of reporting to the board was that it eliminated the possibility of holding the institution accountable not only for the harms to patients, but also for an organizational climate that supported the wrongdoer and discouraged accountability. In fact, addressing the hospital's organizational climate became all but impossible. The fact that prior residents and staff dentists had observed the issues but had not had the courage to address them suggests a prevailing organizational climate that ultimately worked against Dr Johnson.

Making the Charges

The first thing Dr Johnson did was to discuss her concerns with Dr Cross. During an unpleasant meeting, Janet said, "He refused to do anything." Over the course of the next few months, they had several more discussions, which, in retrospect, Janet thought served only to antagonize him. His position was that his experience in dentistry was far superior to Janet's, and he felt fully justified in what he was doing. He would make no changes. He accused her of unfairly attacking his use of sedation when it was clear that it was by far the best way to manage the troubled patients in their institution. He countercharged that she was endangering her patients by not using enough sedation. Janet said that the more they talked, the more determined he was to do it his way: "He was going to do it come hell or high water." In fact, he insisted that she follow his lead in the use of sedation as often as he did. Ultimately, she said, he told her, "You either do it my way or you leave."

Unfortunately for the two dental assistants, Dr Johnson had told Dr Cross about their role in making her aware of the problem. She said that as soon as she had finished talking with him, he had called them in and denounced them harshly. Janet said she could hear it all through the thin wall that separated their adjacent offices. He screamed at them and told them how unprofessional it was for them to criticize him—he was the doctor! "I mean it was knock down, drag out. Not the kind of thing you would expect happening in a workplace," she said.

The work environment was getting worse every day. Janet said she thought about quitting the hospital, but even if she did, "There was no way I could leave the situation the way it was." Dr Cross's mismanagement of patients should not continue. Her next step was to go to the hospital administrator, which proved to be a disappointing experience. Janet felt that he viewed the situation as nothing more than a dispute between a green employee and an experienced supervisor. Perhaps, he suggested, she would be happier with employment elsewhere. From there, she went to the hospital's patient advocate, who was uncertain about how to proceed, given his lack of experience with dentistry. Because of this, he called the state board of dentistry for guidance. The board indicated that it would be an appropriate case for them to look into. Acting on this advice, the patient advocate submitted the necessary documentation to the board.

> "There was no way I could leave the situation the way it was."
>
> *Dr Johnson*

Could Dr Johnson have developed a better plan of action? It is hard to know. Regardless of whether she could have responded more effectively and Dr Cross could have responded with less defensiveness and more maturity, the issue remains as to whether and under what circumstances a professional should report. Janet's belief is that you don't report the small things, but you do report circumstances where there is real harm. Certainly, the American Dental Association Code of Ethics supports the duty to report.[5] Interestingly, the whistle-blower literature[6] suggests a somewhat different orientation, however. It indicates that whistle-blowing is more effective when the issues are less serious, are infrequent, and have been occurring for a shorter duration. It also suggests that the legitimacy of the whistle-blower is an important factor. From that standpoint, Janet, not the assistants, was certainly the one to do the reporting.

The challenge for anyone who contemplates whistle-blowing—besides considering the seriousness of the offense, its frequency, and the strength of supporting evidence—is to assess two things: the wrongdoer's potential reaction to the challenge and the moral climate of the institution, when, as in Janet Johnson's situation, there is one. However, in many ways, the questions below apply as much to organized dentistry as they do to a hospital or other employers; even if a solo practitioner is the wrongdoer, there are the various relationships within the dental community to consider.

With respect to the wrongdoer: Does it seem likely that raising questions about competence will trigger retaliation rather than openness to the concern? It may be possible to garner clues from reflecting on how the wrongdoer has reacted to more minor challenges to judgments. If the reaction has been generally positive, the whistle-blower may consider direct com-

[5]Section 4C of the American Dental Association's Principles of Ethics and Code of Professional Conduct,[5] Justifiable Criticism, states that "Dentists shall be obliged to report to the appropriate reviewing agency as determined by the local component or constituent society instances of gross or continual faulty treatment by other dentists."

Action by the Board

The board took the charges very seriously and spent almost 2 years exploring them. It hired an investigator and took depositions from Dr Johnson, Dr Cross, the two dental assistants, and other current and former hospital employees. It heard Dr Johnson's descriptions of the cases that she had witnessed and requested more documentation. The board also asked her to write up past cases that she had never even heard of, some from as many as 10 years back. Altogether she reviewed the charts of some 45 patients, from which representative charges were developed pertaining to 12 patients.

The board also needed to confirm that Dr Johnson was telling the truth. To this end it interviewed the dentists who previously had worked at the hospital under Dr Cross, including the dentist mentioned by Dr Johnson's two dental assistants. They all gave the same information: What Dr Johnson said was correct. When asked if they ever considered reporting Dr Cross, they said no—there were too many factors that worked against such an action. They felt their only option was to leave, and that is what they did.

Dr Johnson's life was in turmoil. She said that she worked each day from 8:00 AM to 5:00 PM and returned home to work some more: "I would finish doing the housework, and then I would start working on the board case. I would be up until 2:00 or 3:00 in the morning, and then I had to be up [early to get] to work

by 8:00." At the hospital, Dr Cross was still her supervisor, although he spent much of his time at work preparing for the hearings. Their relationship was extremely tense.

The board's investigation verified everything that Dr Johnson had presented, and more. During interviews of parents whose children had clearly received high dosages of sedative agents, the board discovered that four of the children had recently developed symptoms of intellectual dysfunction. Furthermore, their medical records showed that the onset of the dysfunction was compatible with the dates of the deep sedations. As a result, the board expanded its scope to include not only possible transgressions of the dental practice act but also whether Dr Cross's actions had caused physical harm to his patients and created risks that were serious and potentially lethal.

For example, the board cited the use of deep sedation three times on a 7-year-old girl with Down syndrome who had a mild respiratory infection and heart disease that was scheduled for corrective surgery. No medical consultation had been obtained prior to the dental care. The dental treatment consisted of scaling and polishing plus the placement of occlusal restorations on all four first molars. None of the caries lesions were extensive. The board stated that the standard of care for general dentists practicing in their state prohibited the use of deep sedation on a patient with the child's degree of dental disease and physical condition without appropriate medical consultation and the

munication. If the reaction seems negative, it may be better to involve a third party at the outset.**

With respect to the institution, it is important to assess the general climate of the organization. Is there evidence that the organization is responsive to challenges? On less serious matters, does it listen to employees and take appropriate action where indicated? If advice is not taken, does the organization offer defensible reasons for not addressing the perceived wrongdoer or wrongdoing? These assessments would help the potential whistle-blower decide whether to address the issue internally or to move immediately to channels of reporting external to the organization. External reporting is more effective when the wrongdoing is of a serious nature.[6] For nonserious matters, external groups may be inclined to attribute the

complaint to organizational infighting and be less inclined to support either party.

Despite legal protections for whistle-blowers, most experience some form of retaliation. Whereas retaliation is usually an effort to control the whistle-blower through fear, its effectiveness depends in part on the strength of the real or perceived threats. The net result of the potential whistle-blower's analysis may well be that the consequences are too great to continue pursing the concern. However, when wrongdoers retaliate, they run the risk of harming their own case. For the whistle-blower, the retaliation itself may serve to confirm an important suspicion: that the initial act was not a mere mistake or professional disagreement, but an intentional act of wrongdoing.[8]

One last consideration with respect to reporting: Whereas it may be tempting to try to report anonymously—presumably to avoid retaliation—there are real risks to doing so.[9] First, the concerns may be dismissed because the organization concludes that the anonymous accuser either has a weak position or isn't giving the accused a chance to confront the accuser. Second, if

---

**Parker and Holloway[7] point out that whereas personal interventions may seem more collegial, they not only are more personally demanding but also present the greatest risk of personal damage and professional disintegration.

required training. Further, it said that Dr Cross's treatment of the patient was inhumane and risked injury to the patient, including cerebral anoxia.

Although the abovementioned patient was one of those who had suffered cerebral dysfunction, the board decided not to charge Dr Cross with actually causing the brain damage for that patient or any of the others. Its rationale was that it was easier to determine that inappropriate and risky professional behavior had occurred than to determine a cause-and-effect relationship between the behavior and its outcome.

Instead, the board chose to make its charges based on thorough documentation of the risks to the child with Down syndrome and the three other patients—all children—with intellectual impairment. Medical consultations had been requested for none of them, and none of their charts showed evidence of adequate monitoring of vital signs or oxygen/carbon dioxide physiology.

One of these cases was a 4-year-old boy with cerebral palsy and extensive dental caries who underwent deep sedation four times. A dental assistant who was present gave deposed evidence that she thought the child's respirations were slowing and at one point had stopped altogether. When she told Dr Cross about her concerns he briefly continued treatment before stopping to check the child's airway.

The second case was a 9-year-old girl with severe asthma and moderate caries who underwent deep sedation twice. Based on his own documentation, during one visit Dr Cross had difficulty establishing adequate local anesthesia. As a result, he administered multiple carpules of the anesthetic agent—the total dosage exceeding that which was known to be safe. No dental assistant was present at that appointment. During another visit, when a dental assistant was present, Dr Cross reported that he covered the child's mouth and nose in an attempt to control her behavior.

The third case was that of a 4-year-old boy with nephrotic syndrome and extensive caries who had undergone deep sedation four times. A dental assistant was present and, during a deposition, said that the child appeared to be experiencing seizure activity. Dr Cross continued treatment during the seizures.

In addition to these cases involving medically compromised children, there were scores of others with clear evidence of inappropriate doses of sedative agents. There were also several instances that had no apparent link to issues of behavior. For example, the board's investigator uncovered several instances of missed diagnoses of obvious oral pathology such as large periapical lesions and dentigerous cysts and of much-documented failure on Dr Cross's part to provide adequate supervision for his residents.

After 5 days of hearings, the board found Dr Cross guilty of both negligence and malpractice and ordered him to surrender his license for 2 years. During that time he was required to obtain psychiatric evaluation and counseling and participate in designated continuing education courses. Dr Johnson said that this was "the most severe punishment that this board has ever laid on anyone."

---

the whistle-blower doesn't provide sufficient evidence of wrongdoing, the recipient of the complaint has no way of seeking additional information. Third, if the whistle-blower is highly credible, remaining anonymous weakens that credibility.

For the whistle-blower who has less credibility based on education, training, or position in a hierarchical organization—as was the case for the dental assistants in the Johnson story—revealing one's identity only to the complaint recipient may be an appealing option, as it at least facilitates the investigation. Doing so, however, surrenders power to the complaint recipient. Should the complaint recipient wish to influence the whistle-blower, it would be possible to threaten the whistle-blower with betrayal of confidence.

One of the best aspects of the socialization of professionals is a sense of collective identity and collegiality. Also important, however, is the development of a professional stance toward self-regulation and self-monitoring. Although these attitudes can be cultivated during every aspect in the life of a professional, most important is what happens in professional schools.

What steps can educational institutions take to overcome the early socialization that results in distrust and dislike for professionals who responsibly deal with the misconduct of their colleagues? How can the early socialization that labels and condemns such individuals as snitches and tattletales be reframed as young professionals take on the affirmative duty of self-regulation and self-monitoring?

First, the dean of the professional school, along with senior members of the profession, must make clear to entering students, perhaps through didactic instruction, the expectations for professional self-regulation and self monitoring. The responsible management of fellow colleagues with problems is an affirmative duty for all people within the profession, whether students or practicing professionals. In addition to introducing students to procedures for addressing misconduct, schools should promote student governance and peer review to enable students to experience this affirmative duty. In doing so, the construction of effective methods of instruction is essential. We think students need opportunities to practice these duties with hypo-

The Price Paid

Janet felt that the board's decrees fully justified her reporting of Dr Cross, but hardly anyone else agreed. Despite his pervasive clinical irresponsibility, Dr Cross had a friendly and outgoing personality and with few exceptions was well liked by colleagues. In addition, his family had money and was well known in the state's most populated area. Furthermore, almost every dentist in the state knew him personally, or knew of him, largely because he had been president of his local dental society and was very active in the state dental association. In a few years he probably would have been its president, were it not for Janet's actions. As a result, the immediate reactions of his colleagues were disbelief that the board had acted with such stupidity and outrage that Dr Johnson—a virtual newcomer to the profession—had the gall to accuse such an obviously innocent person. In the eyes of these dental professionals, Dr Cross's reputation was ruined, and the blame fell on Janet Johnson.

The primary problem was that most of the dentists in the state never really understood what the case truly embodied. This was true even after the board issued its decree and its findings of fact—the latter being either ignored or omitted from discussion. Perhaps the most plausible explanation was that because of their allegiance to a trusted colleague, most of the profession didn't *want* to understand what had happened. In addition, the most visible issue was the use of sedation, especially for children with medical problems. For many dentists, the case represented a dangerous attack on their right to use sedation—any sedation whatsoever—rather than its abusive use by an unqualified person. One commentary in the state dental association's journal considered the board's action to be the end of humane dental care for patients with medical problems. Some members of the hospital dental staff complained that the board's ruling kept them from adequately treating their patients. Others expressed concern that the board's actions would set a stifling precedent that would affect the autonomy of dental practice.

Unheard in conversations among professionals, however, were comments about the board's findings that Dr Cross often administered deep sedation without consent of any kind or had denied a child's pretreatment request to use the bathroom or that there were several documented failures to provide required antibiotic prophylaxes. Also ignored was that when his attempts at deep sedation didn't work and the patient's behavior continued to be unruly, he frequently administered extra doses of sedative agents in the middle of treatment.

The negative reaction of members of the profession to the action of the board was extremely disturbing to Janet, but the personal repercussions were even worse. In the hospital, tensions were high. Although Janet was a hero in the dental clinic, in the top echelons of the administration, they viewed her as a troublemaker.

---

thetical cases that provide opportunities for coaching that would help them to confront a problem effectively and respond to a confrontation appropriately. Such instruction must go beyond the simple judgment that something should be done and that the professional, not some generalized "other" like the state board of dentistry or the dental school administration, must actually do something. A very effective form of instruction utilizes role playing in which students not only have to confront a colleague with evidence of wrongdoing but also have to assume an appropriate stance when feedback directed toward them suggests they are the wrongdoer. Students must have the opportunity to practice the professional stance whether feedback is given in a supportive or a hostile manner.

If the development of a professional stance is cultivated, it should be possible for professionals to engage in more productive dialogue about a wide range of professional judgments, including the various levels of adverse outcomes that signal the potentially impaired or incompetent professional. Morreim[10p19] provides guidance for identifying levels of adverse outcomes in order to distinguish "ordinary mishaps and sad stories from real mistakes indicating incompetence."

Level 1 is nothing more than a complete accident, such as an unusual equipment malfunction. At *Level 2*, a well-justified decision unexpectedly turns out badly. *Level 3* describes instances in which competent professionals disagree. These are common in the professions. When professional disagreement occurs and there is also an adverse outcome, what counts is not the outcome, but whether the decision was well founded. *Level 4* describes poor judgment or skill. Every professional makes such errors, even if only rarely. Someone misses a caries lesion on a radiograph that, in retrospect, is painfully obvious. Or, someone forgets to ask a patient about aspects of his or her health history. The judgment of incompetence in such cases can be made not for a single error alone, but instead when the practitioner shows a pattern of errors. At *Level 5* are egregious violations of the standard of care. An example is the practitioner who claims he can cure multiple sclerosis by removing amalgam fillings or makes other unfounded health claims.

Among her colleagues, dentists she thought were her friends began to ignore her. Most withdrew silently, but some told her to her face that she should be ashamed of herself for reporting and ruining her boss. Perhaps, they thought, she was looking to take over his job. Worst of all, she received a number of threats, some of which made her fear for her life. One such threat was tucked under her car's windshield wiper while she was at work. The physical intimidation did not last long, but the denunciation by her peers went on relentlessly for several years. In addition, the criticism by members of the profession extended to the two dental assistants who had helped her.

Rejection by friends and colleagues was something new for Janet, and being labeled a troublemaker was almost unimaginable. Previously, acceptance and endorsement had been the hallmarks of her life. In high school, college, and dental school, Janet had always been popular. She had been elected to one office or another at each level, and in dental school she was twice elected a class officer. She obviously had been looked upon as a leader and, by all accounts, one who could be depended upon for constructive ideas.

Janet felt that the negative reactions of colleagues occurred because "they only knew a little bit, and they didn't check things out for themselves before they jumped on the bandwagon." She said, "It wasn't because they agreed with what [Dr Cross] was doing. It wasn't even that they knew what he was being charged with. It was only that they had been told a portion of the story."

Part of the problem was that Dr Cross was able to influence the way that the story was told. When he received the board's charges, he was also given the depositions made by Janet and all the others who gave evidence against him. As part of his strategy for preparing for the hearings, Dr Cross actually distributed parts of the depositions to selected colleagues around the state. Each dentist was given a section and asked to research the topic of that section and to help develop positions that Dr Cross could use in his hearing. Dr Cross also attempted to ensure that the recipients of his request were properly motivated. In a letter that accompanied the depositions, he disclosed that it was Dr Johnson who had reported him, that she was spreading her false accusations across the state, and that the hospital administration and the medical staff were unequivocally on his side and had admonished her for unethically spreading her gossip across the state. Except for the fact that she had reported him, nothing else was true. Janet learned about Dr Cross's letter from one of the dentists who had received it.

Janet felt isolated and beleaguered by the series of adverse consequences that she had unwittingly unleashed by her actions. She said, "It was a tremendous nightmare! There were so many things going on at the same time, there was no way you could solve all of them. And there was no support anywhere. I was by myself doing this."

For Level 4 or 5 adverse outcomes, the observer also assesses whether the act violates a fundamental norm of professional practice and, secondarily, whether the action was intentional. First it is necessary to determine how clearly the action violates the norm or ethical standard, then one must consider the seriousness of the violation. As Morreim[10p23] points out, some acts are intrinsically wrong regardless of whether they cause anyone physical or psychological harm. Other deeds are both intrinsically wrong and serious violations of the norms of practice because the harm is "virtually certain, not speculative." With respect to ethical duties, there are also differences of opinion—instances where good practitioners with good intentions can disagree.

Whether an act violates ethical duties is also a matter of judgment. However, when a professional retaliates against a colleague who raises questions about competence, he or she may be unknowingly undermining the whistle-blower's assessment of the colleague's intentions. In other words, the retalia-

tion confirms that the actions are not mere incompetence, which could be corrected, but something more diabolical.

As important as the skills of professionals is the atmosphere of the organization. One study in the organizational literature[6] indicates that when whistle-blower claims require great change or are of long duration, the issue is less likely to be resolved. The more serious the allegation and the more entrenched the practice, the more likely that the whistle-blower will experience retaliation. Whereas whistle-blowing is usually more effective when internal channels are used—especially when the wrongdoing is less severe or of shorter duration—reporting channels that are external to the organization should sometimes be considered. External routes may be particularly effective when the whistle-blower has little power and the wrongdoing is very serious. On the other hand, in instances where outside forces become involved, the whistle-blower is more likely to experience a wide range of retaliation.[6]

Upon Reflection

Years have passed since this life-changing event occurred. Dr Cross has been reinstated as a practitioner. Dr Johnson's life has slowly returned to normal, or at least close to it. A few of the former friends who had condemned her actions have visited her personally and expressed regret for their unwarranted criticisms. One of the dentists who had publicly denounced the board wrote the board a formal letter of apology.

Still, the events of this story have had a profound effect on Janet Johnson's life. Her marriage did not survive the stress of the charges, the preparation for the hearing, and its aftermath. She experienced a series of stress-related health problems. Her plans for a career in hospital dentistry have changed. She has left the hospital and is now practicing dentistry in other circumstances.

When asked if she would do it all again, Janet's thoughts remain conflicted. Her first response was, "Yes, I would have done the same thing again." This is what emerges when she remembers her outrage for the way that patients were being harmed and for Dr Cross's systematic mistreatment of society's lowest income groups. She says, "The major thing that runs through my life is, I can't stand a bully!"

But on the other hand, Janet said, "I was frightened the whole way through—actually scared to death." Although she knew that she was doing the right thing, "if I'd known how it was going to affect my family, . . . [that]

> "The major thing that runs through my life is, I can't stand a bully!"
>
> *Dr Johnson*

there would have been so much sadness, I wouldn't have been able to do it. It was good I didn't know."

Overall, Janet says that reporting a colleague to the state board "doesn't ruin you. It was difficult personally, but I got lots of respect." For example, some of the dentists and residents who had worked at the hospital and quit rather than do something later confessed they were ashamed of their lack of courage. One said, "I should have done something—prevented something."

Basically, she feels proud of what she did and says that the further she gets from the situation, the more she sees its positive effects. Having remarried and begun a family, one such effect is the conviction of having "set a good example for my children."

The experience has also made her more confident in herself and her own authority; on the other hand; she says, perhaps too confident. She tells a story about her conviction that a policy of the state department of dental health was causing adverse effects. Dr Johnson met with the state director to discuss it. When she didn't exactly get the reception she had hoped for, she became angry, and "flaunted my power and success." In effect, she threatened that she had been successful before in dealing with problems and that they would do well to pay attention to her now.

Looking back on that embarrassing conversation, Janet isn't proud of her use of a "bully tactic" to draw attention to her issues. The main result was negative. She concluded, "Even if you are working out of respect for patients, people can come to fear you."

Thus, if one wants to ensure an organizational climate that supports reflection upon one's practices and appropriate responses to challenges of wrongdoing, it would be important to create a culture of response. To do so, the organization would start with less significant cases of practice in order to create a culture of self-assessment and reflection. For example, a group practice might begin by asking dentists to reflect on new record-keeping standards and then to evaluate their own behavior about applying the standards consistently. Such a self-assessment might be followed by a periodic audit in which professionals assess each other. Establishing a culture of peer review, the organization could move on to more challenging record audits for a variety of diagnostic categories, such as endodontic care, placement of sealants, or general improvements in periodontal health of patients diagnosed with periodontal disease. Even in practices with only a few employees, it is important to establish a culture of self-reflection and self-assessment. We cannot expect individuals to act at the leading edge of their ethical abilities if the institution does not support them.

References

1. Rennie SC, Crosby JR. Students' perceptions of whistle blowing: Implications for self-regulation. A questionnaire and focus group study. Med Educ 2002;36:173–179.
2. Feudtner C, Christakis DA, Christakis NA. Do clinical students suffer ethical erosion? Sutdents' perceptions of their ethical and personal development. Acad Med 1994;69:670–679.
3. Forsythe GB, Snook S, Lewis P, Bartone PT. Making sense of officership: Developing a professional identity for 21st century Army officers. In: Snider DM, Watkins GL. The Future of the Army Profession. Boston: McGraw-Hill, 2002:357–378.
4. Colby A, Damon W. Some Do Care: Contemporary Lives of Moral Commitment. New York: Free Press, 1992.

Advice to Others

With respect to reporting impaired or incompetent colleagues, which most dentists are loath to do, Janet says, "Reporting is difficult. My advice to people is that you don't report for small things—for example, overtreatment—but you do report for things where there is real harm. Then you just have to do something." Also, she says, "you can't report anonymously—at least not in my state. The accused always knows who the accuser is. The accused has the advantage, and that is how it should be. If someone is really guilty, the evidence should bear that out."

In considering whether to report a colleague, Dr Johnson says, "You need to be self-assured." Initially, her anger is aroused by acts that harm the helpless and weak. She states that she has always been a patient advocate, and she especially can't stand someone who would take advantage of the weak or elderly. We notice, however, that for Janet, this self-assurance is not a stubborn sense of knowing what is right, but rather a sense of self-assurance that comes not only from convictions about one's point of view, but also from careful investigation and reflection on evidence. We notice, in Janet's account of the story, that she spent hours poring over records so as not to be blinded by righteous indignation. In the end, it was the evidence that kept her from succumbing to the various attempts to discredit her.

Reflecting upon events that followed her various attempts to address the wrongdoing and her final act of reporting Dr Cross to the board, she thinks that once she had gathered the evidence and turned it over to the board, she became too involved in defending her judgments and probably let the board manipulate her into doing more of the work in preparing the case than she should have. She indicated that she spent many evenings preparing evidence, in part because she got caught up in defending herself against the various attacks to her credibility—many of which she thinks were launched to deflect attention from the wrongdoing and reframe the issues as matters of professional judgment. As a consequence of her continued involvement, she thinks that for Dr Cross the case "became a contest—winning, rather than looking at what you did."

Reflecting upon her personal conduct during the years that the case dragged on, she offers two other pieces of advice. She says that were she to do it over again, she wouldn't have listened to the comments of others. For example, things that the assistants told her were represented as hearsay. While her concerns over the criticism she received for using the "hearsay" comments of the dental assistants were ultimately countered by evidence from the records, nonetheless, she says she learned the importance of not relying on hearsay. She also says that she wouldn't have talked with anyone about the case. When a case goes on for a long period of time, it is natural to make a seemingly innocuous remark to those you trust. But, she says, "if your husband makes a comment about the case at his job, it comes back to undermine you."

There is one more piece of advice that Janet Johnson wants to share. It is advice from her grandmother that helps to explain her preference for anonymity. Janet said that during a recent illness, she read the Bible for the first time. As she read Matthew, chapter 6, she was reminded of her grandmother's teachings and better understood why she didn't want attention drawn to herself. This is her grandmother's legacy: "If something is a good thing to do, you should do it. But honor is taken from you if you get credit for doing an honorable thing. The credit must be in the knowledge that you've done the right thing."

References

1. Spreitzer GM, Sonenshein S. Toward the construct definition of positive deviance. Am Behav Sci 2004;47:828–847.

5. American Dental Association Council on Bylaws and Judicial Affairs. Principles of Ethics and Code of Professional Conduct with Official Advisory Opinions Revised to January 2004. Chicago: American Dental Association, 2004.
6. Miceli MP, Near JP. What makes whistle-blowers effective? Three field studies. Hum Relations 2002;55:455–479.
7. Parker LS, Holloway J. Professional responsibilities toward incompetent or chemically dependent colleagues. In: Weinstein BD (ed). Dental Ethics. Philadephia: Lea & Febiger, 1993:101–116.

8. Gundlach MJ, Douglas SC, Martinko MJ. The decision to blow the whistle: A social information processing framework. Acad Manage Rev 2003;28:107–123.
9. Near JP, Miceli MP. Effective whistle blowing. Acad Manage Rev 1995;20:679–708.
10. Morreim EH. Am I my brother's warden? Responding to the unethical or incompetent colleague. Hastings Cent Rep 1993;23:19–27.

Questions for Discussion

1. The real Dr Johnson decided to remain anonymous. Discuss the relationships between her rationale for anonymity and her professionalism.

2. This book is concerned about the development of a professional identity and the development of the moral self. What are the organizing principles that define Dr Johnson? Do the organizing principles that define you include the moral or ethical values of your profession?

3. Dr Johnson certainly took seriously the responsibility for monitoring her profession. As you reflect upon the virtues of professional practice that pertain to the monitoring of a profession, what stands out? How do you assess your own virtues in this regard?

4. What do you think about the fact that many of Dr Johnson's peers did not report what clearly amounted to incompetent use of sedation? How did your professional school prepare you for the affirmative duty for self-regulation and monitoring? What activities do you think everyone in the profession should be involved with?

5. How do you engage in periodic self-assessment to assure that the processes and procedures you employ in your practice meet current standards?

6. What would you like to have happen if someone discovered that something you did resulted in an adverse outcome?

7. Discuss instances that would fit each of Morreim's levels of adverse outcomes as presented in the commentary. Consider ways of approach. Practice the professional stance as the conveyor of wrongdoing and as the wrongdoer.

8. Contrast the strategies used by Drs Echternacht and Owens with the strategy used by Dr Johnson.

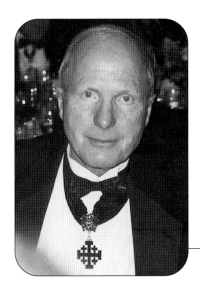

7

Jeremiah J. Lowney

Serving the Poorest of the Poor

Since 1966, Dr Jerry Lowney has practiced orthodontics in Norwich, Connecticut, where he has been active in both community and professional organizations, including the University of Connecticut Board of Trustees and the Board of Governors for Higher Education. Since his first volunteer trip to Haiti in the mid-1980s, during which he provided dental services for the poor, he has returned to that country at least three times each year. Over time the nature of his activities has changed. Through grant writing, personal influence, liaison with a religious order, a huge investment of time, successful fundraising, the seizing of every opportunity, and the expenditure of large amounts of his own money, he has created a multimillion-dollar general health facility in one of the poorest areas in Haiti. Besides dental treatment, the scope of his activities has ranged from creating centers for high-risk pregnancy and malnutrition to the hiring of physicians, the training of local nurse practitioners, and an Save a Family program run by his wife, Virginia. His actions have been influenced by Virginia's caring attitudes and by his conviction that much is expected from those who have received life's bounties.

In August 1981 Dr Jeremiah Lowney had been practicing orthodontics for 15 years when he received a phone call that changed his life. Most Reverend Daniel Patrick Reilly, the Roman Catholic bishop of Norwich, Connecticut, where Dr Lowney had his practice, asked if he would like to join him for a week in Haiti. Pope John Paul II had urged the Roman Catholic bishops from the world's affluent nations to encourage the people of their parishes to help those less fortunate in third world countries. Bishop Reilly responded by organizing an eclectic group of about a dozen people, among whom Dr Lowney would be the only dentist. Jerry told me [JTR] that there was no particular health care orientation to the group. It was merely a broad-based ex-

ploratory trip to assess the problems and perhaps to plan some sort of action to help the poor. Jerry went mainly because of his friendship with the bishop. "We're good friends. I had gotten to know him and like him and respect him. So anyway I said, 'It sounds interesting.' If he had said, 'I'm going to Appalachia,' I'd probably have a health program in Appalachia today. Haiti was chosen just because he was going there."

Jerry said, "I had no idea of what I could do there. I didn't want to go down and be a voyeur for a week—just walk around and observe." To be of some practical use, he thought that if he took some exodontia instruments, there might be an opportunity to do some extractions, the fact that he hadn't extracted a tooth in 19 years notwithstanding. So he asked the help of an oral surgeon friend in reviewing basics, such as the administration of a mandibular block injection and the techniques of dental extraction. He borrowed some equipment and subsequently "spent that whole week taking teeth out by the hundreds." His son, Mark, a pre-med student, went with him and served as a dental assistant.

Dr Lowney's introduction to Haiti was one of the most memorable experiences of his life. In Port au Prince, the group stayed in a home with no water and no bathroom. There was a latrine out back. By the end of the week, the rank odors were pervasive. Jerry said that they were unprepared for what they saw. "We got into these slums. We saw sights we had never ever seen before. I was in an orphanage, and I picked up a little baby, and the baby died in my arms. Just died!" He visited a home for the dying that was attended by the Missionaries of Charity, an order of nuns founded by Mother Teresa.* The sisters brought in the patients "either out of the streets or from the general hospital in Port au Prince. The hospital would put the patients, who were so sick they looked like they weren't going to make it, into a shed behind the facility. The sisters would visit this shed, transport patients to their own building, clean them up, and feed them. Most of them didn't survive. But the whole theme of their outreach was to allow people to die with dignity! [In addition] they all had bad teeth. They were periodontally involved or they were infected. So the day I showed up with the bishop and [our] group, I had my little kit. And I said to one of the sisters, 'If you have anybody here that needs any teeth extracted, I would like to help.' And she said, 'No one ever comes here. God must have sent you.' . . . That was a heavy trip. That comment was a life-changing experience."

Jerry decided to remain at the home for the dying and consequently spent most of the week extracting teeth. Toward the end of his stay, he asked the sisters if he were to come back in a few months, would they be able to find any other places like this. They told him they had a clinic in the slums that was very needy. In fact they had many makeshift clinics in several slum areas. All he had to do was to call a week or two before he came and they would set an agenda.

*The order of the Missionaries of Charity was created in 1950 in Calcutta by Nobel Peace Prize–winner Mother Teresa (1910–1997). Its purpose was to serve the poor, usually the poorest of the poor. The order was inspired by her experience with a woman, half-dead and partly eaten by rats, whom she found lying in the streets. A nearby hospital was reluctant to treat her, but because of Mother Teresa's insistence, they finally treated the woman. From then on, it became her mission to create places where the poor could die in peace and dignity. The functions of the sisters in Port au Prince recapitulated Mother Teresa's original experience.

1981 to 1985: Working in Port au Prince

Six months later Dr Lowney returned to Haiti and has continued to do so every 3 or 4 months. On his second trip he was joined by the pastor of his church (St Andrews in Colchester, Connecticut), Monsignor Ted Malanowski, and Jerry's oldest daughter, Gail, who served as a dental assistant. "We worked in different places," Jerry said, "And I mean we worked. We were doing two or three hundred extractions a day. It was difficult in that you didn't know anything about the health history of these people. Nothing! We protected ourselves with universal precaution. [We used] cold sterilization. We scrubbed the instruments and soaked them in germicide. They would sit down and we'd ask them which tooth hurt, and they'd say 'Tout'—all of them. Then you'd have to do a survey of the mouth, a general physical assessment of the patient, and make a decision. The entire mouth qualified for extraction, but the patient could not be left medically compromised and there was little opportunity for follow-up."

On later trips he usually brought four or five people with him including, as regulars, Monsignor Malanowski and Sister Carla Hopkins, a nun who ran a Catholic Charities program in Connecticut. She spoke French and was therefore able to help communicate with the patients—a major advantage. She also scrubbed instruments. Dr Lowney paid all of her expenses out of his pocket. The sisters in Port au Prince would tell him where to set up a clinic, and he would do it. "We'd arrive at the airport, rent a car, and drive wherever we were needed. The sisters set the agenda, and we'd arrive at 7:30 in the morning. We'd bring a little lunch from the hotel, and we'd bring water and all my instruments and we'd begin seeing patients. The sisters monitored who would be treated." Jerry said that some patients were rejected, even though they looked awful. Once, when he asked why a woman had been rejected, Jerry said the sister replied, "She's not poor enough." He laughed and said, "She looked pretty poor to me. But they knew most people's situations and needs. I don't know how they knew, but they would select them. They would bring in six or seven patients at a time. The others would wait out in the street. They'd sit down in straight chairs, and I'd anesthetize them all at once." On a piece of paper that he gave to the patients, he indicated the tooth, more often teeth, to be removed. One by one they would get care. One volunteer would fill the syringes, and another would scrub the instruments. He used double gloves as a precaution. Although AIDS was not much of a problem then, he was concerned about hepatitis. When I asked if he used a mask, he said, "Most of the time. But by the middle of the day, it would be so damn hot, I'd take the mask off and work with just a baseball cap and a set of scrubs."

1985: Long Distance with Mother Teresa

At the end of each trip to Port au Prince, the sisters, having provided him with Mother Teresa's phone number in Calcutta, would ask him to call her to convey messages—usually requests for more supplies. Phone calls between Calcutta and Haiti were usually impossible for the sisters to arrange, so Dr Lowney would pass the messages on to Mother Teresa, and before each return visit, he would call her again and ask if she had messages for the sisters there.

During a 1985 phone conversation, Mother Teresa told him, "'I'm making arrangements to send four sisters to a very remote area called Jeremie.'[†] Interesting. [That's] my name in French." Mother Teresa said that there were no health facilities there, but sick people were plentiful. Her plan was to open a small orphanage for sick babies and children. Jerry said she had asked him, "Do you think you could go there and help them? They need more help there than in Port au Prince?" He joked that there was no way he could turn down the requests of a living saint for fear of divine retribution. "Anyway," he recalled, "I went to Jeremie. The whole country is mountainous. The first time we went there was an adventure. There was no way of getting there except to rent [an all-terrain] vehicle. It took 12 hours to go 140 miles. The roads were just awful, and we didn't speak the language. When we came to a river, we'd have to ford it—no bridges and no idea of the depth." When they arrived, they found the sisters already at work, building a small temporary facility. Dr Lowney and his helpers set about their usual routine of taking out teeth.

Not long after Dr Lowney returned from his first visit to Jeremie, his wife, Virginia, in an exceptionally

fortuitous encounter, met a Haitian anesthesiologist, Dr Julian Joseph, at the local hospital in Norwich. They met in a dental office in Norwich where both were patients. Jeremie, as it turned out, was Dr Joseph's hometown, and he became excited upon hearing what Dr Lowney was doing. As a result, Dr Joseph, who for political reasons could not return to his homeland, offered Dr Lowney a 10-acre piece of land in Jeremie to use to deliver health services. At that time, Americans were prohibited from owning land. On his next trip Dr Lowney visited the bishop of the diocese of Jeremie and arranged for the bishop to accept the land and in turn provide Jerry with a 99-year lease. To formally receive the leased land, he created a new organization, the Haitian Dental Foundation, having no idea that he would ever have broader health interests. By that time Dr Lowney had already concluded that the idea of becoming permanently located in Jeremie was appealing. He felt that a concentrated effort there would enable them at some point to see the fruits of their labors because the scale was small enough to be manageable. Despite the fact that travel to Jeremie was difficult, Jerry said that the tremendous need for health care made the decision easy. To put his plans into action, he asked Sister Carla if she wanted to remain in Jeremie and build a small dental clinic to provide permanency. She received permission from her superiors and began to work. Dr Lowney made arrangements for an apartment in town for Sister Carla, and she made arrangements to clear the land and build the clinic. The source of the funding for these activities was Dr Lowney's own money.

Beyond 1985: Expanded Scope and Structure

The scale of Dr Lowney's activities in Jeremie underwent a significant expansion, primarily because he had the good sense to listen to Sister Carla. Whenever he visited Jeremie, Sister Carla would talk to him about their desperate need for comprehensive health care. Their dental problems were just one aspect of their overwhelming needs. Jerry told me, "So I said, 'Well, we'll build a little bigger clinic here.'" He decided to add on to the building and create space for some medical examining rooms. However, the construction of the clinic had been done without a written architectural plan. Therefore, when the

---

[†]With a population of 50,000, Jeremie is one of the largest cities in the Grand Anse, which has a population of 600,000. It is located 140 miles southwest of Port au Prince, close to the end of the narrow Haitian peninsula, not far south of Cuba.

time came for a second story, they needed to get a structural engineer from Port au Prince to make sure that proper structural loads could be supported. The engineer's fees also came out of Jerry's pocket. When asked about the support that he and Virginia had given to the project, he said that by that time, "She and I put about $300,000 into this adventure, maybe more, I don't know. I stopped counting at 300."

Because the project was growing rapidly, Jerry realized that he needed more than his own funds to assure its completion. His fundraising efforts launched happily after a serendipitous introduction to a Connecticut businessman. The result was a check for $200,000, and 2 months later, another for $50,000. It was an auspicious start to a successful and continuing program of raising money. Every dollar they received was important. Jerry said that he had been way off on his budget projections. The total cost to build the structure was $1.2 million. At every step of the way there were costly problems: embargoes, changing governments, new requests for permission to build, escalating costs, the greasing of palms, and more. The clinic was completed in 1989, after 4 years of construction. It stands three and a half stories high, one of largest buildings in town. The third floor, with 13 rooms including a living room and kitchen, is essentially for the volunteer residents, Sister Carla among them.

Dr Lowney's program began to assume its present dimensions as a result of another unexpected opportunity. Word of his efforts had gotten around Connecticut, and he was beginning to be known as the state expert on Haiti. Shortly after the new building had been completed, he received a call from a neighbor who was also the district congressman. Jerry was asked to go to Haiti as a guide for a congressional visit. Having now been inserted into a different social group, at an ambassador's reception Jerry talked with a man who happened to be the physician in charge of the medical operations of the United States Agency for International Development (USAID). After describing what he was doing in Jeremie, Dr Lowney learned that USAID might be looking for someone like him to put together a grant on child survival for that area.

With that conversation, Jerry took the first transforming step from clinician to grant writer. Immediately upon returning home, he approached the University of Connecticut for help in putting together a proposal. His request received instant attention, quite possibly because he was a member of the Connecticut Board of Governors for Higher Education. The collaborative result was a 3-year child survival grant for $850,000. Its primary focus was to establish outreach medical programs for the villages around Jeremie that would provide such aspects of the standard USAID program as immunizations and the teaching of oral rehydration.

> When Jerry made his first trip to Haiti, he was looking for something that went beyond his own self-interest.

Jerry made sure, however, that his operations at the new clinic also received some benefits, such as a couple of vehicles, a physician, and a few nurses. Because of the new comprehensive medical orientation, Jerry decided that it was time to restructure his foundation. In doing so, the Haitian Dental Foundation became the Haitian Health Foundation (HHF). At first serving 20 villages, Dr Lowney's program has expanded to cover 98, each village with its own health agent. The foundation provides health care to 200,000 people in the rural villages at $3 per person per year. The idea is to find intelligent villagers, train them as health agents, and send them back to their communities. Jerry said they are excellent liaisons. They understand the essentials of medicine, and they are known and trusted by the villagers. Through their combined efforts, they have immunized 60,000 young children. This is 88% of the child population, which Jerry said is a higher proportion of immunizations up to the age of 5 than in Connecticut.

Meanwhile more and more volunteers arrived, most of them staying for brief periods: construction workers, plumbers, electricians, and others. Of great importance were three new requests from Franciscan sisters who wanted to join them permanently. They are members of the Hospital Sisters of the Third Order of St Francis from Springfield, Illinois. One was just returning from India. Another was a pharmacist working in Illinois. The third was an intensive care nurse who had worked in Taiwan. Their collective experience was phenomenal. Within a few months the clinic was functioning as an integrated medical unit. The sisters remain there today, still running the clinic. Their timely arrival coincided with the expansion of the program and with the fact that Sister Carla was starting to get tired. Sister Maryann Berard, the nun who had recently returned from India, became the administrator.

Soon Jerry began to embark on additional projects with funding from other sources. One of the first was the building of a piggery. On an earlier trip, Jerry had heard from the sisters that an epidemic of swine fever had wiped out every pig in Haiti. The poor asked for his help. He came to understand that the villagers were indeed suffering, "because the pigs were their bank account." USAID had tried previously to replenish the breeding stock, but their efforts failed: The people merely ate the pigs instead of encouraging them to reproduce. Furthermore, USAID denied Dr Lowney's request to start his own pig project, so he began checking around. "Why the hell did they eat the pigs? They told me [that USAID] didn't give them any food for the pigs, and the pigs were grain-fed sows that would eat only corn and soy. The pigs were going to starve to death, so the people figured they might as well eat them." Jerry found a local expert on agronomy to run his project and wrote a funded grant for $40,000 from a Buffalo, New York, foundation to build the piggery. The keys to success, he thought, were the conditions under which the villagers would be given the pig and providing the means for feeding it. His course of action was to bring in an animal nutritionist from the University of Connecticut to develop silage.‡ He also sent a Protestant missionary from Jeremie with an agronomy background to the University of Connecticut to learn how to do artificial insemination. The latter was necessary because the litters of the locally available pigs were too small and the project needed better bloodlines. Semen was brought from the United States to improve the breed and was administered by the newly trained agronomist from Jeremie. Jerry's role was to raise the money and provide leadership. He decided to ask Rotary International for assistance in buying the pigs, which cost $180 each. Some Rotary clubs bought one pig; others purchased as many as 10. They almost all participated enthusiastically. The project was a huge success. Meanwhile, the villagers took courses from the agronomist on the principles of silage and the essentials of caring for pigs, including everything from how to pen them and manage their medical problems to the proper use of pig manure. Everything they were taught was based on what was available locally, and the feed was free. In return, the villagers agreed to give back one female pig from the first litter. Project staff recorded everything on a computer. Usually the sows were pregnant when the villagers received them, and the staffers knew to the day when the litter was expected. Jerry said the villagers were usually compliant about returning a piglet. HHF

---

‡Silage is the conversion of fodder (corn, grass, clover, etc) into feed for livestock by an acid fermentation process that retards spoilage. The process usually takes place in silos.

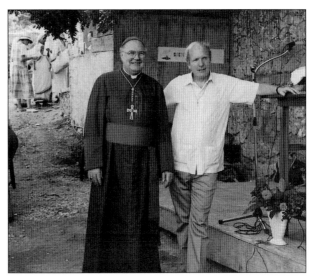

Dr Lowney *(right)* with Bishop Daniel P. Reilly *(left)* at the dedication of the Haitian Health Foundation Clinic in 1988.

would choose a baby sow, then raise it and breed it. "That's how we ended up with 9,000 pigs." Eventually the program became self-supporting, so it was terminated. Jerry said, "The pigs have been returned to the area of the Grand Anse."

Jerry's grant writing continued. Although he had received external help from the University of Connecticut for his first grant, he was now fully immersed in managing the process himself, with occasional skillful help from his youngest daughter, Marilyn, who also was a frequent companion on his trips to Haiti. By this time, money was coming in from various sources. Meanwhile, thinking that it might broaden his perspective for his work in Haiti, he began to pursue a master's degree in public health (MPH) at the University of Connecticut with his daughter Jennifer. Like her father, she had become a dentist, completed her orthodontic training, and joined his practice. They both became part-time graduate students and attended classes together.

Jerry said that his MPH not only changed his perspective, it altered the way that others looked at him as well. "More than anything, when I went to the USAID, it took me out of the mouth. I would write grants or go to see somebody about the public health work I was doing in Haiti, and I think many of these people, especially with some of these agencies, would say, 'This man's a dentist, he's an orthodontist. What does he know about public health?' The MPH degree gave me additional credentials that said, this man has a degree in public health; he must have some expertise in health care." Jerry said the MPH helped in other ways too: the epidemiology, the statistics, the nutrition. "All of that adds to your reservoir of knowledge."

A public health project of which he is proud was the building of latrines in the villages, which was initiated as a strategy to prevent worms and other coliform disease. "There was a tremendous number of kids with worms," Jerry said. "In our clinic we'd clean them up, deworm them, and 2 weeks later they'd be full of worms again. They'd go back home and walk through their own feces." A different approach was necessary. Their idea, made possible with Rotary money and matching Rotary grants, was that if villagers would dig a 25-foot hole, the project would give them the materials to build a latrine and a plan to do it. All went well until a serious and unexpected problem arose. After giving the latrines a try, the villagers gradually stopped using them. They complained that they could not move their bowels. The problem existed even though the village health agents had promoted the use of the toilets and the dumping of ashes from their charcoal fires into the toilet pits to cover the effluent. The team investigated the problem. It turned out that the standard toilet seat, which was set at a 90-degree angle, was excessively high for Haitians, who were used to squatting in the bushes. The seats were lowered, and the use of the latrines resumed.

One of his other successful programs stemmed from a grant Dr Lowney had received from Georgetown University to do a breast-feeding program. To instruct the villagers, they paid trained women, monitrices, who, as Jerry said, "have breast-fed their nice fat babies themselves." The project generated phenomenal data, all stored on solar-powered computers. It has attracted visits by groups from other universities to look at this data and other health data that has accumulated. In addition, dissertations for four or five master's degrees and several PhDs have been written based on this and other data from various projects. Of special interest was the finding that participants in the program showed a longer period between pregnancies than did those in other programs, even those specifically designed to lower the birth rate. The reason was that aggressive and exclusive breast-feeding results in lactational amenorrhea, which suppresses ovulation.

Another hugely successful program is called Happy Houses. On a visit to the villages, the monsignor, once

> Jerry Lowney's most admirable quality is perhaps his ability to inspire others and move them to moral action.

again with Jerry, was shocked by a wretched house made of sticks and a cardboard roof that was occupied by nine people. After learning from a health agent that it would cost approximately $300 to build something respectable, the monsignor gave them the $300. When Jerry returned to the same village 6 months later, the house had already been built. He said that it was a nice house, made of cement, on a slab, with a tin roof, doors, and windows. He took a photograph for the monsignor. As it happened, a couple of Rotarians were with him. Jerry said that one of them remarked, "Look how happy these people are." Another said, "Let's start a program called Happy Houses," and Happy Houses they became. Jerry said, "We got about 125 of them going out of that one house. It just caught on. You know, for $500 you can build a house for a family here. These Rotary clubs were all donating $500. Non-Rotarians as well. Others heard about it in the [HHF] newsletter. One woman sent us $1,500–for three houses." On each house they place a plaque with the name of the donor and a little smile on each side. They take a picture and send it with a thank-you note back to the donor. The donors tell others, and the contributions escalate. Jerry said, "It's a lot of work, but it puts a family into something that can be called a home, not a hovel."

Not all of his projects worked as well. His attempts to raise poultry, for example, fizzled because he could not control the death of chickens that succumbed to the heat. Turning a failure into an opportunity, he transformed the poultry coop, located on the same land as the clinic, into an eye clinic with money from a foundation grant. Previously there had been no place between Jeremie and Port au Prince to get an eye examination or have an infection treated. A Lions Club from Alexandria, Virginia, donated equipment worth $20,000, including an automatic refractor, so that one of the sisters can perform eye examinations without waiting for a visiting optometrist. Jerry has also established a source of thousands of eyeglasses through the cooperation of an opticians' training program and the support of the Lions Club. Although they are not able to treat cataracts at the clinic, Jerry is trying to arrange care with some volunteer ophthalmologists from Connecticut. Patients are charged a fee for any care they receive. Jerry said, "We started off not charging, but found it to be a mistake because, if you don't charge, there is no value to what you are doing. Patients don't value the services. And

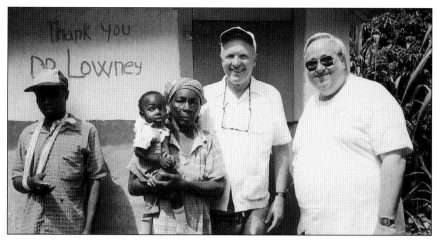

Dr Lowney *(center)* with a volunteer *(right)* at a Happy House that Jerry built for this Haitian family.

there's also a certain dignity with paying a little bit. If they don't have anything, of course, we don't deny them." It is the same with the extraction of teeth or any other service.

New initiatives continue to appear. Based on an analysis of the unmet health needs of the Jeremie population, the HHF has started to address malnutrition and high-risk pregnancies. Previously women identified as having high-risk pregnancies and requiring careful medical supervision as they approached term had nowhere to stay. They, or their unborn children, often died. Now Jeremie has a 15-bed lying-in center for women with high-risk pregnancies. In addition, a malnutrition center has been built for the rehabilitation of children in stages of second- and third-degree malnutrition, primarily with kwashiorkor syndrome.§ Previously there had been no place for them to receive 24-hour feeding services. The center also has 15 beds and a place where mothers can be involved in the child's rehabilitation. Another nutrition program feeds about 1,400 children and perinatal women twice each week. Much of the food comes from Catholic Relief Services, and tuna and Spam are often donated by individuals in the United States. The clinic also provides immunizations, administers vitamin A, and hosts lectures by a Haitian nurse on breast-feeding, oral rehydration, bathing, and general hygiene.

Dr Lowney's programs are all oriented toward caring for large numbers of people, one person at a time.

However, now and then the plight of a particular unfortunate Haitian youngster attracts the attention of the HHF staff. Such is the case with a little boy named Michel. He was 6 years old when he was severely burned after a kerosene lamp fell from a shelf and landed on him as he slept. The fire also resulted in the total loss of the family's possessions. When Michel arrived at the clinic 6 months after the fire, his chin was fused to his chest, his right hand was missing, and he was suffering from third-degree malnutrition. Through the efforts of an HHF board member, his story appeared in the *Boston Globe* newspaper. Because of that article and other coverage that unfolded from it, the HHF raised about $30,000 for the child. In addition, Michel received extensive care during multiple hospitalizations at Shriners Hospital in Boston for the management of his burns. Virtually every aspect of the care was free. With donations from the public, the HHF bought the family a house in Jeremie for $10,000 and established a $20,000 trust fund, which Virginia Lowney manages. Every time Michel flies to Connecticut, he is followed by television newspeople. One even accompanied him as he returned to Haiti. Jerry welcomes the media coverage, which helps the foundation, but said that the real satisfaction came from saving Michel's life and probably his future. Whenever Jerry returns to Jeremie, Michel visits him, often coming to the clinic for breakfast with his friend.

In many important ways Virginia Lowney has made the HHF her life as much as her husband has. Of special importance, Jerry said, "We have the Save a Family project that Virginia runs. It's a phenomenally successful project. I think she just enrolled 1,100 kids in school

§Kwashiorkor syndrome is severe malnutrition in infants and children marked by failure to thrive, apathy, and other serious findings, including fatty degeneration of the liver and severe edema. It is caused by a diet that is excessively high in carbohydrate and extremely low in protein.

in that project. This is the 11th year that over 1,000 children have been enrolled. It probably started in 1988–89, before the clinic was opened. People would come to the gate of the clinic–Sister Carla was there at that time–and they'd have problems, needed money–tuition for a child to go to school, or somebody died, or was sick and had to find medicine." Sister Carla had a limited budget and couldn't really help too many people. So on one of Jerry's trips, she told him, "'With so many of these poor families, it would be nice if somebody could help them.' I said, 'Why don't we start a little family sponsorship program. I'll take a few photographs [of kids and their families], I'll bring them back, and I'll ask people if they want to sponsor them.' I don't know how many I took, maybe a dozen or 20." As a result, Jerry organized a program to which donors could contribute $25 a month to the poorest families in Jeremie. The money is distributed according to the needs of the family, but most often the families use it for food, shelter, tuition, funerals, and seed money for self-supporting businesses. Jerry said, "We put some brochures together, and the whole thing was the $25 for a family. Nobody in the middle–no overhead. People liked that and supported it."

The donors loved the program and often sent clothes, food, and other things in addition to their monthly $25 donations. Jerry said that in every container that they ship to Haiti, they now have perhaps 50, 100, or even 200 boxes that people have brought to his house to send along. In fact, during my visit to their home,

Virginia took me on a tour of their three-level barn, which was filled with everything from the aforementioned boxes to scores of bicycles awaiting transport south. In any event, it is clear that the donors relate strongly to their adopted families. Initially, the program was run by a volunteer in Jerry's office, but it was more than she could handle. As a result, Virginia stepped in and then, Jerry said, "It really took off. I think she has about 1,100 families now. That's US $330,000 going into those slums in Jeremie. A phenomenal amount of money."

In addition to these special projects, the daily work of the people of the HHF continues. This includes the dental care that is now being regularly provided. Although the removal of infected teeth remains the primary service, they are now gearing up to provide restorative care, especially for children. A young dentist from Boston will be volunteering her services. Outreach programs that provide fluoride therapy and emphasize caries prevention through education have already been started. Medically, the work is done by two physicians, two nurse practitioners, several locally trained nurse practitioners, and a Franciscan sister who sees patients. Most of the patients are children, but many adults are seen as well, especially those with prenatal and emergency needs. Altogether the clinic employs more than 60 Haitian professionals with an annual budget of approximately $500,000. In 1992, Alvin Adams, US ambassador to Haiti, called it "a principal agent for change–and for hope."

Commentary

Dr Lowney's story extends the concept of service to society beyond the community in which he practices. In fact, he argued that the service he gave to his immediate community was not "real service." When he assessed his work in professional organizations, in politics, and in his community, he said, "I never really looked at that as a major contribution to anything. Some of that you could look at and say, 'well, if you were on the cancer board, you certainly got some notoriety out of it, and it helped your practice.'" When Jerry made his first trip to Haiti, he was looking for something that went beyond his own self-interest. "Real service," in his view, is the kind of giving for which the only return is the personal satisfaction derived from helping someone who is truly in need. In providing service to the destitute, Jerry willingly immersed himself in what many would find to be unbearably squalid conditions. Whereas today he is not directly involved in the provision of dental care, he is totally immersed in an extensive humanitarian effort to improve the health and welfare of a large segment of the Haitian population.

As with other exemplars, Lowney's concept of service unfolds as he moves through the various stages of life. As a youngster, he was the recipient of the generosity of a Roman Catholic priest who provided tuition to fund his early education. During the practice-building phase of his life, he engaged in local service to his community and profession. It was not until midlife, however, when he had satisfied basic needs, that he saw himself as having a choice: to continue to accumulate personal wealth or to share. At this point, his concept of service underwent an early transformation: "to share my good fortune somewhere else."

Dr Lowney's choice was not, as some have done, the provision of a bit of service in some exotic place. Neither was it a place of poverty in his own country, where his presence could make an impact. In fact he attributed his decision to provide "real" versus "self-interested" service in Haiti to pure happen-

Sowing the Seeds

In 1981, when Dr Lowney received the Haiti invitation from Bishop Reilly, his range of activities already extended well beyond the walls of his practice. By that time he had been active in the Connecticut Dental Association, had held offices in the Connecticut and Northeast Societies of Orthodontics, and had been chief of dental service at Backus Hospital in Norwich. Additionally, he had been thoroughly invested in his community, whether it was the city government, the town board of finance, or the Cancer Society Board. Another focus for his energy was Democratic state politics. In the mid-1970s he had held fund-raising parties on the lawn of his home for then–gubernatorial candidate Ella Grasso, who arrived dramatically by helicopter right behind his house. When he later found that he was being considered for a state position, he told Governor Grasso that the job he would prize most was that of commissioner on the state dental board. Finding that request impossible to meet, the governor instead appointed him in 1976 to the University of Connecticut Board of Trustees. Subsequently, in 1983 he was appointed to the state's newly created Board of Governors for Higher Education, a position that he still holds, and would serve as its chair for 4 years. Jerry said his failure to become a dental commissioner was the best thing that could have happened to him. His entire tenure at the University of Connecticut "was very, very positive for the Haiti experience because it gave me credibility. Resources were there that I could tap into for information. If I didn't have that connection, I don't know whether [the resources] would have been that accessible to me." For example, it was a board of governors member who helped him become aware of the need for a tax-exempt foundation and then helped him organize it. In addition, he became chair of the Health Affairs Committee, which oversaw the University of Connecticut Health Center, a position whose contacts at the dental and medical schools proved to be very helpful in planning and executing programs in Haiti.

Despite his rich array of activities, Jerry indicated that he was looking for something else. He said, "At that time, I think I was looking for something to do that would be of interest and would maybe–I hate to use the words 'pay back' because it's sort of a cliché–share some of my good fortune somewhere else. So many wonderful things had happened to me–at that time I was in my mid-40s–maybe it was time to give back." As to his work in professional organizations, politics, and his community, he said, "I never really looked at that as a major contribution to anything. Some of that you could look at and say, well, if you were on the cancer board, you certainly got some notoriety out of it, and it helped your practice." He was looking for something that went beyond his own self-interest.

stance. He went to Haiti not because of his awareness of its overwhelming needs, but only because a respected friend had asked him to go. Indeed, he noted that if the bishop had been going to Appalachia, he would undoubtedly have developed a program there.

In engaging himself with the poorest of the poor, Dr Lowney dispels a popular stereotype associated with his discipline. Orthodontists typically serve the esthetic needs of families with discretionary income. Critics suggest that for dentists aspiring to a life of ease and high income, orthodontics is the specialty of choice. Lowney's view is different. He sees his specialty practice as a means to an end, the means being financial security, the end being to serve the needs of the people of Jeremie. The practice of his profession, initially a major source of satisfaction, is no longer his primary source of contentment. Even when his daughter joined him in his practice, besides the pride of having her follow in his footsteps, he viewed it as a means to his primary goal. Her presence allows him to spend more time sustaining the work of the HHF.

Let's examine Dr Lowney's activities in light of the selection criteria for moral exemplars.[1] His work in Haiti *"shows a sustained commitment to moral ideals and principles that includes a generalized respect for humanity"* (criterion 1). In approximately 20 years of service there he has functioned on many levels. Initially he worked as a dentist, primarily removing teeth. A short while later he became a facilitator for the work of the Missionaries of Charity serving in Haiti by making calls to Mother Teresa in Calcutta. Next, responding to Mother Teresa's request to establish a health facility in Jeremie, he funded the design of a health clinic and raised funds to build it. During its construction, he began to enlist the help of physicians, thus completing the clinic's shift in emphasis from dental care to evermore inclusive medical care. Experiencing success in the achievement of these objectives, he temporarily shifted his focus to include the economic issues in the community. Responding to the epidemic of swine fever, he brought in experts to reintroduce pigs to the region, an accomplishment of vital economic significance. Again addressing health issues, he implemented public health programs in sanitation,

In October of 1981, 4 months before the first scheduled trip to Haiti, an event occurred that perhaps sharpened Jerry's desires to be of use to others. "I was running a lot at that time," he said. "In fact, I ran the Boston Marathon in '79. I was starting to get hematuria. I went to a urologist and he found a tumor in my bladder." It turned out to be a very rare, but very aggressive carcinoma of the bladder called urachal carcinoma with a bad prognosis. A big man, over 6 feet tall, he had lost more than 30 pounds after surgery and radiation treatments. Nevertheless, going to Haiti in February became a goal to strive for, despite Virginia's concern and the negative opinions of his physicians. As a compromise, his son, Mark, went with him. "He was sent along to sort of watch me. In case I fell, he'd pick me up."

Jerry is uncertain exactly how his experience with cancer shaped what he ultimately accomplished in Haiti. On one hand, he said, "I had a crisis in my life, but I don't think that that had a lot to do with it. The foundation was there before that, because I was involved with other things locally." He said that if he had not developed cancer, he might have gone to Haiti, looked around, and returned home to do nothing, but he doesn't think so. On the other hand, it was clear to him that the cancer "definitely made a positive influence in my life, because I didn't think I was going to live. I was told I wasn't going to live. And I kept thinking, 'Gee, I really haven't done enough.' I kept thinking that, because [the cancer] hovered over me like a sword."

Thus a variety of circumstances converged to set the stage for Jerry Lowney's receptivity to the possibility of doing more—much more—to help others. But why did he feel that way in the first place? A look at his background and the people in his life will provide additional understanding.

Jerry said that he came from a poor Irish family in Fall River, Massachusetts. It was a large family: Jerry is the oldest with eight brothers and two sisters. "At that time my father was a church sexton, which is a fancy name for a janitor in a church." He grew up with more or less constant exposure to religion, mainly because of his mother, who was a daily communicant at mass. His father, on the other hand, was mainly preoccupied with taking care of his family. Jerry said he "didn't go to church except to sweep it," although he nonetheless got the children out of bed every Sunday morning to go to church with their mother. Challenging the family's emphasis on religion was the neighborhood they lived in, where there was a lot of trouble for children to get into. Jerry was a ready participant. He said, "I certainly wouldn't be classified as a real good kid." He had even been arrested once or twice "for doing crazy things like kids do." Both parents, however, preached with great success to their children about the value of a good education, neither having had much themselves. Therefore, it was as clear to Jerry as it was to his brothers and sisters that he was expected to go to college. Working in one of the Fall River textile mills was not a happy alternative. The result was that virtually every one of his siblings achieved a university education, and five became physicians.

Why did he want to be a dentist? Jerry said, "I just thought that it would be a pretty good profession. I liked [my dentist]. He was a very decent fellow. He was nice to me. I was sort of intrigued with his office, with

childhood immunizations, infant survival, and nutrition. A key factor in the success of these programs was the training of Haitian villagers to act as medical personnel.

Turning back to basic survival needs, he facilitated the building of houses in the villages and found individual donors to fund the construction of each house. His wife, Virginia, augmented this effort with her Save a Family program, which provides a helping hand to families with short-term needs. At each phase, Dr Lowney immersed himself in the problems of the community. As goals were realized, new goals were set. Each challenge gave new life to his commitment. Through sustained commitment that included fund-raising and grant writing, he established a stable base of funding for the HHF—at least as long as the Franciscan order continues to supply management of the facilities. Currently, his efforts are directed toward establishing an endowment to sustain and ensure the future of the program.

Coupled with his sustained commitment is a generalized respect for humanity. His respect for the Haitian people is exhibited in his oft-stated concerns for treating people with dignity, regardless of their circumstances, as well as a generalized commitment neither to criticize cultural practices nor to proselytize. This same respect must be extended to those whom he asks for money. He is very conscious of his need to be viewed as authentic, not as a hustler. (We will return to this theme later.)

We also see persistence in his efforts to respond to the human condition in the region he works and a *"consistency between actions and intentions and between the means and ends"* (criterion 2).[1] He seems to turn each of his talents, political connections, and financial assets to achieving his ends. This is not to say that every effort to improve conditions resulted in success, but he demonstrates an uncommon persistence to resolve problems. For example, when the initial USAID effort to replenish the pigs was not successful, Dr Lowney recruited an

the things in his office and the mechanical part of it. He looked like he was doing pretty well and was happy in his life." In addition he said, "My father thought it was a great idea to become a dentist, because it was a wonderful way to make a living. He didn't say to become a dentist so you could go out and help people. He was just a poor guy with a big family. He'd go out on Saturday night to the Corky Row Club, have a few pops with the boys. That's what life was like in those days."

Thus Jerry applied to Tufts just as his dentist had done. He was admitted, worked 40 hours a week in a supermarket in Medford, Massachusetts, and earned grades that were acceptable for dental school. He met Virginia early in his dental school career while she was in nurses' training at a small hospital. They married as soon as he graduated. Together they went to the Pensacola Naval Air Station while he served in the Navy for 3 years as a dentist aboard a carrier. After his discharge he enrolled at the State University of New York, Buffalo, where he acquired his training in orthodontics along with an MS degree. Jerry reflected on the way his life has developed since then. "We have passages in life. The first part of your life is spent with accumulation. You accumulate an education. You accumulate ways of making a living, either with a business or a profession. You accumulate a family, accumulate a house. I think most people experience this at one level or another. Then the next phase of your life is a sort of floating with these things you've accumulated and maybe just tucking them together and making them a little more secure. And then you have a choice. You can continue along that way, or you can say, maybe I should share some of it. I think maybe I took the road of sharing."

Husband and Wife

"It is interesting to consider what influences you to do certain things. I think what influences me the most is my wife." Jerry said the day he married Virginia and his experience with cancer were the turning points in his life. The experience with cancer was abrupt and dramatic; his marriage with Virginia was gradual but more enveloping. He thinks that his accomplishments in Haiti would have been considerably different, perhaps nonexistent, had it not been for Virginia.

Jerry said, "She is a very spiritual person. Just her influence in a very gentle way convinced me that there is a joy in sharing and that the things we have are really things that we are stewards of. Our possessions are a stewardship. They are not given to us to keep. Even our children are given to us to share with others and to share with the world or to share with people who are needy. Interestingly enough, she said, 'I would rather give with a warm hand than with a cold hand from the grave.' Most people deal with the cold hand from the grave after being attacked by the various taxing agencies and probate court. You don't get to experience the joy of sharing. And there is truly a great joy in sharing."

Jerry said that when he returned from his first visit to Haiti, so enthusiastic about what he wanted to do and wanting to commit some of their personal resources to it, "there was never a moment's hesitation from her about it. She's more generous toward it than I am. She is very compassionate, works extremely well with old people. She volunteers in the summertime in a hospice

agronomist (using his university connections and his personal resources) who was willing to go to Haiti to work on the silage problem. When the effort to introduce chickens into the economy failed, he turned the chicken coop into a much-needed eye clinic. When he needed credibility to promote his programs, he obtained a master's degree in public health. When he saw the need for housing, he implemented a fund-raising strategy to buy the houses. When an ally had trouble shipping goods to Haiti, he involved his political contacts to help her resolve her problems.

Sustained by his own good fortune, his supportive family, and his personal faith, he seems more than *"willing to risk his creature comforts, his personal well-being, and personal assets to experience the joy of sharing"* (criterion 3).[1] Dr Lowney sees his bout with cancer as an event that changed his outlook on the risks associated with humanitarian efforts, though it didn't particularly influence his decision to engage in them. He sees himself as less fearful of the ever-present illness or adversity that

accompanies work in a third world country. He also willingly recruits family and friends to join in his efforts to bring hope and help to others.

Perhaps the most admirable quality of Jerry Lowney is his ability to *"inspire others and thereby move them to moral action"* (criterion 4).[1] The story is filled with examples of individuals who were moved by his example and became involved in the work of the HHF. Consider Sister Carla, who was the initial contact, or the three Franciscan nuns, who were inspired to run the clinic, or the hundreds of health care workers who volunteered their services, or the thousands of people who sent money to Save a Family or to build a house, or those who continue to contribute more extensive financial support. Consider also those who were moved to use their vacations to provide physical labor to accomplish the various projects. Finally, consider Dr Lowney's daughters, who are so inspired by their father that one joined his practice and the other became his successor.

given to mothers in the houses as she goes along. That is her pleasure. She writes to a lot of the people and their families. Really, it is now the tail wagging the dog."

Sometimes Virginia's influence has been less gentle and very direct. Jerry said, "When I first went into practice, my wife gave me a report card one day, and it said: Provider–100; Parent–0. I said, 'How did I flunk?' She said, 'You're in the office too much.'" He listened, and their life changed. "I was a workaholic. She made me aware that there were other things in life. I knew that there were other things, but I wasn't practicing the game the way I should have been."

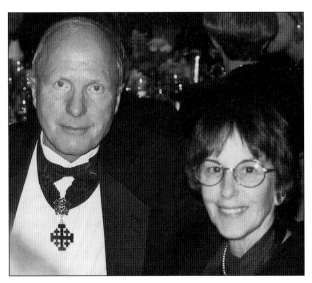

Jerry and Virginia at a dinner for the Order of Holy Sepulchre in New York.

in Massachusetts. She's more of a humanitarian than I am. I just ride on her coattails. When you start talking about Haiti, she'll get so intense she'll take you out to the barn to show you [all three levels packed full of supplies that are ready to be shipped to Haiti]. She calls Haiti her fifth child. She's very committed. In Haiti, she goes down to the slums, the homes, and talks to the women, gives them a few gourdes, and listens to them. And she goes up in the hills and takes blood pressures, takes things and money to the people. She probably spends five or six hundred dollars in five-dollar bills

Acknowledgment and Appreciation

For the sharing of his talents and energy, Dr Lowney has received much recognition, both from his peers and his community. He has even been knighted twice by the Pope. The federal government has awarded him its Congressional Certificate of Merit, and Connecticut has presented him its Jefferson Award for humanitarian efforts. He has received Honorary Doctorate of Humane Letters degrees from the University of Bridgeport and Quinnipiac University and an award for humanitarianism from his classmates at Coyle High School, class of 1954. He has received distinguished citizen awards from the Connecticut Chamber of Commerce and the

Finally, in keeping with criterion 5—"a realistic humility about one's own importance relative to the world at large, implying a relative lack of concern for own ego"[1]—let's consider the personal qualities of this exemplar. Humble? Compassionate? He says he is not. Modest? No. Generous? He says, "not particularly." Aggressive? Impatient? Dominating? Persistent? Unyielding in his conviction? All of the above. Yet these seeming detractors are the entrepreneurial qualities essential for accomplishing his ends. Whereas Dr Lowney, like the exemplars interviewed by Colby and Damon,[1] does not see his moral choices as self-sacrifice, most would judge his contributions as extraordinary generosity of time, talents, and resources. In addition, he is unyielding in his conviction that respect for persons, no matter how destitute the person may be, is a primary value. Furthermore, whether cultivating a donor or treating a destitute patient, no one has a right to tell others how to live or to impose their cultural or religious values on them. Add to this someone who really listens, without reservation or judgment,

to anyone who has something to say. When Virginia gave him a "0" for child rearing, he listened and modified his work life. When Virginia exemplified caring for others in all aspects of her life, he was open to her influence and adopted her as his own moral exemplar. When the bishop said he needed help in Haiti, he listened and responded. When a child died in his arms, he was moved to help. When Sister Carla told him where he was needed, he went. When she needed a place to stay so she could continue to work, he provided it. When a Missionaries of Charity sister said someone wasn't poor enough to receive his services, he respected her judgment. When Mother Teresa said she needed him in the remote village of Jeremie, he made a commitment. When the pigs were eaten rather than used to replenish the supply, he was moved to learn why and then to solve the problem. When Haitians said they couldn't use the latrines because of the seats, he made modifications.

We see in his actions an open-mindedness about new facts and their implications. We see an ability to endure circum-

University of Connecticut Alumni Association and a merit award from his fellow members of the Board of Trustees. Rotary International has twice cited him for meritorious service, and he has received a variety of other awards from local and state organizations.

His profession has also recognized Dr Lowney for his work in Jeremie. This has included the American Dental Association Certificate of Merit and election into both the American College of Dentists and the International College of Dentists. In addition, recognition has come from both dental societies and auxiliary educational institutions within the state.

A different kind of recognition has also provided Jerry with a great deal of satisfaction, even though there is no plaque to show for it: USAID has modeled some of its programs after the successes of the HHF.

Reflection, Resonance, Reasoning

Dr Lowney appreciates all the recognition that has come his way for his work in Haiti. However, he said, "I don't think there is any question that the fact that I have a loving and caring and compassionate family is my greatest achievement. I have been fortunate to have a good wife and good family, and those family values have been a high priority with me." Speaking about his accomplishments from a professional standpoint, he said that what ranks highest is his choice of practicing orthodontics rather than anything else. The context of

this observation appears to be related to the dominant passion of his professional life: his work in Jeremie. He said that he felt very fortunate that when he was introduced to Haiti, he was young enough to respond vigorously and was sufficiently secure economically to be able to take time off and to put financial resources into his work in Haiti. Also from that standpoint he said that he is both proud and privileged that his daughter Jennifer has followed him into the profession and has been able to assume some of the obligations of the practice. He said that often people have to delay the fulfillment of a special interest until their retirement, sometimes not being able to do it then. "I was fortunate that I was able to do it at the young age of 45." For this early start, he thanks orthodontics.

For sustenance in difficult moments, he thanks his Irish sense of humor. "[It] has really supported me. Even with the experiences in Haiti, you know, I can find humor. Sometimes, it's gallows humor. I can find humor to take some of the sadness out of my life, or the sadness I encounter in my life. I'm emotional, no question about that. I can get emotional. I've been reduced to tears many times in the third world. I have to look at things sometimes through the funny side of something that is happening. You have to just have a sense of humor, or it will get to you. I wouldn't be me without my sense of humor. It's a way of coping and it's a stress reliever. And it's my personality. It's me; I am not a serious guy with people."

From a moral standpoint, he said he takes seriously the moral values exemplified in the Gospel of Matthew,

stances that would be dispiriting to others. We see a capacity for finding hope and joy even when faced with dreary truths. It is not that his orientation was so different from the moral concerns of others, including the many volunteers who contributed time and effort to the projects. It is the range of his concern, the vastness of his engagement, and the single-mindedness of his commitment that sets him apart from the many good people who give of themselves for the benefit of others.

Jon Hassler,[2] in a recent book entitled *Good People*, distinguishes dispositional goodness from goodness of activity. Hassler draws on his personal encounters of a lifetime, including characters developed for his novels, to describe persons who were habitually kind, caring, and cheerful in their interactions with others. He distinguishes them from individuals who were engaged in many activities that benefited others, but possessed less admirable personal qualities. Like Colby and Damon, Hassler seems to admire dispositional goodness—it is nice to be around people who exhibit this habitually—but he sees the

altruistic nature, which distinguishes goodness of activity, as the quality he admires most.

It strikes us that Jerry Lowney is an exemplar because he is altruistic. An act is considered altruistic when it benefits another and is performed voluntarily for its own end at some cost to the self, without expectation of personal gain. However, once someone is labeled as an exemplar, there is a tendency to inflate expectations about all aspects of a person's behavior. We not only expect exemplars to be paragons of virtue, displaying dispositional goodness, but we tend to devalue their achievements if they have not personally suffered to achieve them. As Colby and Damon[1] point out, "We confuse altruism with self-denial." We expect our exemplars to lead grim lives of suffering to achieve their moral ends, and "we take personal suffering as the truest sign of moral commitment."[1p300] Yet none of our exemplars or those studied by Colby and Damon saw "their moral choices as an exercise in self-sacrifice." This mindset is only possible when there is a synchrony between moral goals and personal goals.

chapter 23, in which "we are charged with reaching out and helping others, helping neighbors. Those are values important to me. We are not alone in this world, and we do have an absolute responsibility to look to what we can do to make someone who is not as fortunate as others, either health-wise or economically. It is our responsibility to reach out and help them. I think we have a responsibility to show by example to others. Sometimes our actions are the only Bible [lesson] other people need." Even with those strong beliefs, Jerry said, "I couldn't say that my [essential] characteristic is that I am generous or overly compassionate or anything of that nature. There is a little bit of that there, but it isn't overwhelming." Also, he said, laughing, "Humility is not there–modesty and humility."

More to the point, Jerry commented, "I am aggressive in getting things done that I want done. I am a hard charger. I'll work to accomplish something, for sure. I suffer people who are wrapped up in bureaucratic red tape with very little patience. I don't think this project in Haiti would ever have gotten to the point that it's at without somebody being aggressive. You can't be a shrinking violet and let people push you around, because you wouldn't get anything done. I think I am respected by the people that I work with in Haiti and here because they know that I don't take anything out of this. They know that all my wife and I get out of it is satisfaction. We put a lot of our own time and money into it, so people respect that. They say the guy's not a phony. I really never have asked anybody for anything

for myself, but I am not shy about calling and asking someone for something that somebody else needs."

In fact, when confronted with a problem, he appears willing to extend himself as far as is necessary. He told me about an incident that was particularly annoying to him. During one period when the US government was placing an embargo on exports to Haiti, he received a call from a woman in a Baptist mission who was finding it impossible to ship containers of supplies to Haiti. Dr Lowney had encountered no such difficulties, primarily because of assistance he had received from Senator Christopher Dodd of Connecticut. In earlier days, Jerry and Chris frequently had lunch together when Chris was an attorney in Norwich, and Jerry was on Dodd's first campaign committee. Jerry's caller had no such assistance; her organization had been in Haiti so long that they had lost their contacts in the states. Jerry offered to help her work through the Treasury Department to obtain the license that was necessary to ship the container. He submitted the application, but nothing happened. He called but got nowhere. He said, "The people at the Treasury Department seemed always to have an excuse. I was documenting this whole thing–the day and time I called, and what was said. So one day I said I really want to talk to the person in charge of this. This arrogant guy gets on the line, and I said it has been two and a half months trying to get this license. He said to me it takes quite a while to get these things done, and I'm quite busy you know. He was telling me all the problems involved on his end, giving me the usual government litany, the

While Jerry Lowney has not led a grim life of suffering and self-sacrifice himself, he is intimately involved in the circumstances of the impossibly grim lives of others. How does he sustain himself in situations most of us would find deflating? He said, "It is very important that you don't look at the big picture in Haiti or in Jeremie. You have to concentrate on the fact that you are dealing with one person at a time. One person who will not be in pain because you removed their infected tooth. One person for whom you built or repaired a house. It is not saving the whole country, not even saving the whole village." The magnitude of the problem is such that Jerry has come to see his sense of humor as his greatest asset. "I've been reduced to tears many times in the third world. [You] have to look at things through the funny side, or it will get to you. I wouldn't be me without my sense of humor. It's a way of coping and it's a stress reliever. And it's my personality."

Despite his extraordinary commitment, he is not a perfect person, perhaps too aggressive for some tastes. Yet there is a modesty in his denial of his generosity and compassion and in the recognition of his less admirable traits. There is generosity of spirit in the way he acknowledges the contributions of others, particularly his wife, to his personal development. His self-disclosure reveals insights about his motivations and convictions. What stands out for Dr Lowney and other exemplars, and what sets him apart from ordinary good people, is a unity of the self with moral concerns. It is a unification that is directed by his faith and his conviction that his responsibility in life is to mobilize his multifaceted talents and energies in the service of others.

References
1. Colby A, Damon W. Some Do Care: Contemporary Lives of Moral Commitment. New York: Free Press, 1992.
2. Hassler J. Good People. Chicago: Loyola Press, 2001.

usual line that 'I'm doing the job six people used to do before the cutback.' So I said, 'You know, the time you used in explaining this to me, you could have typed that license out and sent it to me.' He said, 'I suppose I could have, but I'm not going to!' And he hung up on me. So, I called Dodd. I always keep him in reserve. [Senator Dodd] said, 'So, what's the phone number down there? Stay on the line and I'll put a conference call in.'" The result was predictable. Senator Dodd introduced the Treasury Department official to Dr Lowney, one of his dearest, closest friends, and with great assurances that the license would be sent by fax that afternoon, the business was completed successfully.

Dr Lowney enjoys the influence that he is able to wield that is usually associated with affluence and social status. However, he said that his experiences in Haiti have considerably altered his and Virginia's point of view about material things. "We don't spend a lot of things on ourselves. We have a nice car and a house. But when you go into the third world and see how little people have, I can't get excited whether the stock market goes up or down, even though I have some stock. I'm still better off. I'm better off than so many other people." He said that his experiences with cancer also heightened that perspective. Parenthetically, Jerry said, "It also changed my outlook, in that I am not frightened of anything anymore. Nothing bothers me. Worrying about AIDS never bothered me after that. I don't feel like I'm invincible, but nothing worries me anymore. I can't get nervous about issues like that."

Jerry said that the Haitian experience "has been phenomenal for my family and my kids. They have all been inoculated with the importance of serving others. They all go down at least once a year. And so many other friends and acquaintances have brought their children along with them to Haiti." He said that it has been a positive thing for everyone who goes there.

There is no problem in finding people who want to volunteer. In fact, Jerry said that he has a waiting list of all types of people who want to volunteer their time in Haiti. "There are so many people out there that I've met who want to do something. They're dying to do something positive for others. A man that was here this morning—he just retired as a policeman—is going down there for a month. He used to go down for a week." That man, like all the others, wants to make a contribution. Jerry

> "Virginia's influence in a very gentle way convinced me that there is a joy in sharing and that the things we have are really things that we are stewards of."
>
> *Dr Lowney*

said, "My experience is that there are tremendous numbers of good people who want to get involved with something. And it's too bad that there are not more avenues for them to wander down, because everybody doesn't have to go to Haiti or should go to the third world. When you are involved with something like this, you find some great friends, because these are people who have the same values that you have and feel the same as you do. So you form relationships with nice, solid people."

Jerry is particularly struck by the number of dentists who want to volunteer their services in any number of places. He said, "I think that people in the dental profession don't have the opportunity to interact with people's lives to the point where they can say they've made a major difference. I'm talking about the life-changing differences that maybe people in medicine or in law can make. Dentists are confined to a narrow area of interest and expertise, and I think that might be why many dentists are interested in volunteering. It gives them an opportunity beyond dentistry." Jerry added, "If you have that nature of wanting to do things and you are not able to do them, you reach outside the profession and do them somewhere else, even in politics." In his experience dentists tend to be involved in many more community-oriented activities than physicians. He noted that ten times more dentists than physicians have volunteered to go to Haiti through his organization.

When Jerry talks to his volunteers, he tells them, "It is very important that you don't look at the big picture in Haiti or in Jeremie. You have to really concentrate on the fact that you're dealing with one person at a time. One person who will be not be in pain because you removed their infected tooth. One person for whom you built or repaired a house. It is not saving the whole country, not even saving the whole village. But it's important to that one individual you're dealing with. It's a lot of work, and it builds. There is a vast ripple effect."

The other admonition he gives to volunteers about working in Haiti has to do with respecting the people who are being served. Jerry said, "In the third world this is very important. You can't invade another person's culture with yours. If you have money, and you're giving them things, they're going to agree with you. And they're going to take what you've got." It is the same with other cultural issues. When Jerry goes into the vil-

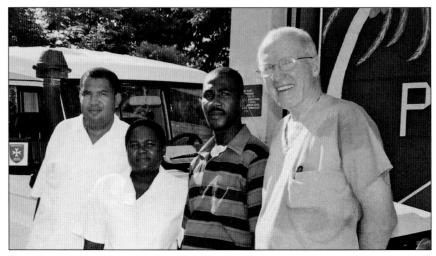

Dr Lowney *(far right)* with an ambulance crew at the HHF clinic in Jeremie.

lages, people often asked him what he is doing about population control. Although he privately agrees with their concerns, he tells them he is not doing anything about it. "You don't walk into somebody's village and say to them, 'You've got too many kids. You're going to have to stop having children.' No one counted my children. . . . It's the same when you're going in and proselytizing with religion. From day one, that was something I said I would never, ever do." The HHF board is a mix of people and is definitely nonsectarian.

Preparing for the Future

Jerry said, "In the beginning I was a clinician. I don't do much of that anymore. Most of the time I am in administration. The personal relationship with the poor has changed from my being a dentist for them to being more of a program coordinator. There is a different type of satisfaction."

There are also major challenges, and they all involve the future of the HHF. Mostly they involve finding money. There is, of course, always the risk that he might lose USAID funds altogether. However, Jerry said, "Our program is one of two premier programs, so we would be the last to shut down because they use us as a model. You know, when a congressman or senator comes through Haiti and USAID wants to show off something, they take him up to Jeremie to see HHF."

Over time, however, USAID has increased the number of people that the HHF takes care of from 50,000 to 200,000 without increasing their budget very much. He said, "I'm fighting with them all the time. They haven't given me a new vehicle for 5 years. We've been buying our own vehicles or getting people to donate vehicles. One of our main problems for the future is sustainability." He worries about how to keep all of his programs going and fears that some will have to be cut back. Some agencies, such as CARE and UNICEF, upon which he had depended for funding, no longer provide financial support. Therefore Jerry has no choice but to search for new money.

"They say Jeremiah is a prophet, and a prophet is someone who makes the comfortable uncomfortable, and the uncomfortable comfortable. So I go out there and tell them what they are missing and tell them I have the answer for them." Jeremiah J. Lowney said he has become a fundraiser, and he spends much of his summers raising money. "I do raise quite a bit, maybe $50,000 in the summer [speaking at] churches." He arranges to be an invited speaker on Mission Cooperative Sundays. On that day, each church in every diocese invites a speaker from the mission field: a priest in Africa, a nun from the Philippines, or perhaps Dr Lowney from Haiti. At the end of the talk, the congregation takes a collection; the amount "depend[s] on how convincing you are, how well your sermon goes, and the financial ability of those attending." He covers the diocese in Norwich, the archdiocese in Hartford, and the dioceses in Bridgeport and Fall River, Massachusetts. "My weekends are pretty much taken up in the summertime. I go to four or five masses on a weekend and give the same talk at every mass. So I'm just loaded with sanctifying grace."

Occasionally he gets invited to a different part of the country. Once when he was in Springfield, Illinois, where the sisters in Jeremie are from, he was asked to speak to the hospital staff. Jerry said that among those attending was a man seated way in the back, who "had been interested in how we concentrate our efforts on child survival and maternal care. HHF could not be everything to everybody. The future of Haiti was the children. As a group in 1989, the HHF directors decided on this policy." Jerry discovered later that, based on his presentation, this man made a trip to Haiti, fell in love with the program, and gave $1,000,000 to the Franciscan Sisters for their use in Jeremie. Jerry said, "That's how things happen. Strange isn't it? Maybe I might have blown it if I had known this gentleman was so wealthy. I might have tried to polish him up a bit, and he might have mistaken me as [a hustler]."

Often, as with the man who donated the million dollars, the use of the money is designated by the donor. Otherwise, Jerry said, "I'm building an endowment now with any funds I can get my hands on that isn't designated for something specific. I've been building it over the last 8 or 9 years, and I've been investing it in the stock market on my own, so HHF has a fair amount in the investment account." His goal is to accumulate an endowment of $5 to $8 million. The purpose of the endowment is to sustain the HHF after Dr Lowney is no longer in the picture. It is intended to be a reservoir of money to keep the programs going in case the environment for funding deteriorates. In 2001, as of this writing, Jerry, now in his mid-60s, has cut his practice back to 3 days a week, but still spends many hours each week on HHF business.

Three years ago, at the time of this interview, his concerns about the sustainability of the program were even deeper than they are now. He was preoccupied with finding a successor. Jerry knew that it would be impossible to find someone like himself who would elevate the Haiti experience to the self-sacrificing position that it occupies in his life, presuming of course that he or she could afford to do it in the first place. In the future, the person who runs the program would have to be paid, that realization being part of the need for the endowment. Jerry said, "The problem is, beyond the pay you have to have someone who really wants to commit to do it. If someone is doing it just for a paycheck, it isn't going

to work. We need someone who is committed to wanting to do this type of work." His hope at that time was that his youngest daughter, Marilyn, would do it. She knew the program, having previously been active in grant writing. Furthermore, he said, "She's been going to Haiti since she was fourteen. I can groom her to do it. I'm waiting for her to say she wants to do it. I hate to say to her that this is what I want you to do. I have a strong influence with [all the children], and she probably would do it to please me. But I wouldn't want that. I'd like it to come from her–something she wants to do."

The problem of Dr Lowney's successor is now resolved. Marilyn Lowney is already at work as an employee of the Haitian Health Foundation, serving as its executive director. This does not mean that the HHF personnel problems are resolved. At the time of the interview, Jerry spoke about his struggle to maintain on-site personnel, which continues to this day. This problem gives him sleepless nights. The Franciscan order, which administers the program in Haiti, is having "the same problems every religious order is having: they don't have many new vocations. They don't have many sisters that they can say can take over this project. They don't know how long they will be able to continue sending sisters to Jeremie." To alleviate part of the problem of finding staff to work in Jeremie, Jerry has been encouraging more full-time volunteers who would like to spend a year or two there. As an inducement, the HHF has built a separate house for them to live in. The effort continues.

Continuing Efforts

The HHF occupies most, but not quite all, of the Lowneys' attention. They share their good fortune in other ways as well. One of the great debts that Jerry owes is to his mother–for many reasons, but in particular for her persistence in finding a way for him to go to parochial school. He has always felt that the quality of the educational experience, if not the discipline, made the rest of his life possible. "There is no question that my mother did me a great favor. She didn't have any money, though it wasn't very expensive. . . . We could walk to Catholic grammar school, but high school was 15 miles away. She had the money for the bus, but not for tuition. She went to the pastor of our parish church, and he gave her the money for tuition. A few years ago they asked me to give the commencement speech at this high school, and there was a whole list of awards named for different people. And when I perused the list I noticed memorial awards, but there was nothing for the priest who had given the money for all of us to go to this high school. Virginia and I set up a scholarship in his name. It was a way of giving something back and honoring somebody important. I wouldn't have gone to this school without him. There wasn't just one tuition either. At any given point in time there were three or four of us in high school."

One gets the impression that even in the few moments when Jeremiah Lowney is not directly involved with the concerns of Jeremie and the HHF, he cannot seem to avoid looking for problems that need resolution, particularly those where he can make a difference. And when he finds one, he steps in to fill the void.

Questions for Discussion

1. Dr Lowney describes the people who were important role models in his life. Who were his role models and what important lessons did they impart? Think about your own life. Are there individuals who influenced you to act in particular ways?

2. Many professionals conceptualize "service to society" as serving those who pay for your services. Dr Lowney's definition is far more expansive. Describe it.

3. The commentary includes a definition of altruism. How does Dr Lowney's concept of service fit that definition? Is this a concept that should be incorporated into the practices of all American dental professionals? Into your practice?

4. Dr Lowney has a coping mechanism for sustaining himself in situations most of us would find repugnant if not unbearable. How does he manage it? How would you manage it?

4. What are some of the ways in which Dr Lowney demonstrates "a generalized respect for humanity"?

5. Dr Lowney observed that in Haiti, if you do not charge at least a small amount for your services, patients do not value the service. In addition, he feels that there is also a certain dignity that comes with paying even a little bit. Discuss these observations in relation to the philosophy of the US Medicaid system.

6. What virtues of professional practice does this story illustrate? Assess yourself and the professionals closest to you in terms of these qualities.

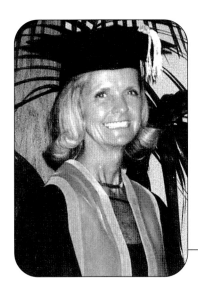

8

Donna J. Rumberger

Organized Dentistry
As an Agent for Helping Others

Dr Donna Rumberger graduated from the New York University College of Dentistry in 1980 and has practiced dentistry in Manhattan ever since. Even before her graduation, she was active in organized dentistry, always viewing it as a conduit for helping other people. Working with the American Association of Women Dentists, she was cofounder of the Smiles for Success Foundation, a program started in New York City that helps women advance from welfare into the workforce with restored, healthy smiles. That program now has expanded to 14 other cities. Working with organized dentistry in New York City, she has been instrumental in initiating and running the Skate Safe program, which provides mouth guards and oral home care education for inner city children in Harlem. In addition, she has worked with the dentistry merit badge program for the Boy Scouts of America Jamborees, helped coalesce women's dental organizations in New York City, and led her dental society to collaborate with Columbia University in a program to improve access to dental care. As further evidence of her ability to get things done, she also has served as president of the American Association of Women Dentists, the Midtown Dental Society, and the New York County Dental Society—one of the largest dental societies in the country.

On September 11, 2001, Dr Donna Rumberger was president of the New York County Dental Society (NYCDS), an organization of some 3,000 dentists located in Manhattan, a borough of New York City. When the news broke about the World Trade Center, her immediate thoughts were of the thousands of people working in the towers—and their families. Walking home from her dental office that terrible afternoon, she passed by the firehouse on her block and was shocked to see no fire trucks and the usually immaculate building in complete disarray. She said that she never thought the firehouse on her block would have responded to the alarm because it was so far north of the World Trade Center. Desperate for news that the firefighters were safe, she entered the firehouse and, apprehensive about how to ask the question, inquired if the trucks were out on a call. Donna said, "This is when I learned that 'our' trucks had indeed responded, and of the 12 men who went to the [World Trade Center], only 3 returned. I lost 9 very special people that day, including a firefighter patient." Dr Rumberger had many patients who lived or worked near Ground Zero. When they came to her office, she says, "They relived their experiences with me, and we cried together."

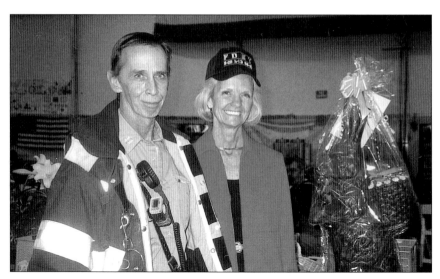

Captain Timothy McKinney of Ladder 13 and Dr Rumberger with one of the 30-pound chocolate rabbits.

As the impact of the tragedy continued, Donna wanted to do something special for the firemen who returned to let them know they were not forgotten. With the Easter holiday approaching, she arranged to have thirteen 30-pound chocolate rabbits delivered to the firehouses that had lost the most men, and another to Ground Zero, where the work continued. On the evening before Easter, four firemen volunteered to help Donna deliver the gifts using a NYFD van. Donna stayed in the background but said that "seeing the smiles on the faces of our hero firemen who had very little to smile about was, to me, the true meaning of Easter. It was my best Easter ever."

Dentists all over New York City were affected. For scores of them, the impact was devastatingly personal. Many relatives, friends, and patients were lost. Thousands of patients left practices because their jobs were relocated. Numerous offices closed because of fear, emotional trauma, feelings of devastation, and an inability to function on the part of both dentist and staff. Some offices were crushed by collapsing buildings. Others closed because access was impossible. Smoke continued to emanate from the attack site, and streets were closed. Many offices were covered with dust, with much of the equipment and records therein irretrievably damaged. One dentist on vacation was watching television during a leisurely breakfast and saw the second plane hit the tower just above where he practiced and lived. The personal and economic consequences to all practitioners in New York City were enormous.

After 9/11, Dr Rumberger's priorities at NYCDS changed. The goals she had set for her yearlong presidency now seemed less important. Immediately she began to work with her dental society to arrange for a $20,000 donation and with the New York State Dental Association to establish a disaster assistance fund. The goal was to help members who had lost their practices and who had been most affected. Money came in from individual practitioners and from other dental societies in the state, and a large contribution was made by the New York State Dental Association, all of which totaled about $250,000. Contact also was initiated with the American Dental Association to enlist their support. As a result, the fund eventually increased by an additional $350,000. In addition, contributions came from dental manufacturers, laboratories, and organized dentistry (including the California and Ohio State Dental Associations, to name just two), and from individuals all over the country. Donna said, "I will never forget that generosity—we were frightened and our sense of security damaged, and any act of kindness from fellow colleagues was hugely welcomed." In January 2002, when her term as president of the NYCDS ended, her successor publicly acknowledged Dr Rumberger for having personally raised about $600,000.

This was not the first time that Donna Rumberger had worked hard for the benefit of others. Dr Margaret Scarlett, then president of the American Association of Women Dentists (AAWD) and her nominator as a moral exemplar in dentistry, said, "From the minute she graduated from dental school, she believed in contributing back to society in the only way she knew how: using her skills, her dedication, and hard work to volunteer to help as many people as possible."

Bringing People Together

Donna's introduction to organized dentistry was an unexpected consequence of winning the New York University College of Dentistry student table clinic competition. Donna, along with the winners from each of the other dental schools, traveled to Dallas for the selection of the best student table clinics in the country. Although she did not win the competition, she caught the eye of Dr Dushanka Kleinman, then president of AAWD and now chief dental officer of the US Public Health Service and deputy director of the National Institute of Dental and Craniofacial Research. Dr Kleinman invited Donna to attend one of the AAWD board of directors meetings and afterward asked for her help on a pressing problem. Three women's organizations in New York City were competing for the favor of the women dentists. They included the 57th Street Study Club, the AAWD of New York District 2, and a New York Women Dentists Organization. A woman dentist in New York might choose to belong to one of these organizations, but certainly not to all three. As a result, none of them was doing well. Dr Kleinman asked her to bring all three groups together.

Even though Donna had spent several years as a nurse and was mature in work experience, in dentistry she was a novice. Nevertheless, she agreed to take on the challenge, thinking that she could promote the move toward unity with a major lecture sponsored by all three groups. Obtaining their agreement turned out to be remarkably easy, and the lecture was a big success. The only problem Donna encountered came from the male-dominated Greater New York Dental Meeting, which urged them to limit the presentations to women's issues. However, in 1982 there weren't any defined women's issues in dentistry. Donna said, "What were we going to talk about? Fingernail polish in the dental office? Menopause?" She preferred mainstream issues. In the end, her committee decided to circumvent the problem by asking an expert to speak about prenatal fluorides, which was arguably both a women's and a mainstream issue. She figured that once the subject of fluorides was on the floor, any aspect of prevention was fair game for

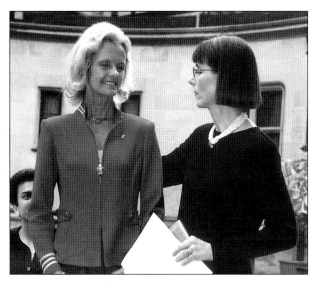

Dr Dushanka Kleinman *(right)* installs Dr Rumberger as president of AAWD.

discussion. In addition, with the presence of a woman psychiatrist, a psychologist, and a speaker on occupational hazards, it turned out to be a pre–women's health conference–before such events became popular. Everyone worked hard to have a big turnout. They were rewarded with an audience of approximately 350 people. The effect was lasting. The organizations united, and they have had successful lectures ever since. The membership of the AAWD began to consider Donna as a rising star and, some years later, elected her as its president. To complete the circle, at her inauguration, Dushanka Kleinman conducted the installation.

National Jamboree

Another opportunity for volunteering came in 1981, just after Dr Rumberger graduated from dental school. A colleague had asked her if she would help with the dentistry merit badge program at the quadrennial National Jamboree of the Boy Scouts of America. Sixty thousand scouts from all over the world, mostly the United States, were scheduled to descend upon Fort A.P. Hill, an army base in Bowling Green, Virginia, in late July. They would all be scrambling to have some fun and to pick up some new merit badges. Agreeing to help was an easy decision. It sounded exciting, and Donna liked what scouting represented. She said they were "good kids, drug-free kids, but they did not come from wealthy

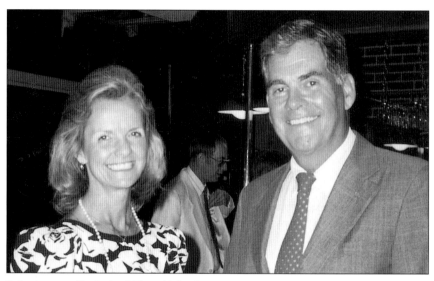

Dr Rumberger and her husband, Clinton M. Hamilton.

families." To cut costs, scout troops often would travel long distances by bus, even across the country, to reach the Jamboree site.

Boy Scouts who wanted to complete the dentistry merit badge had to fulfill some 30 requirements. Among other tasks, they kept a 3-day diet history; took alginate impressions on each other; identified dental instruments; discussed dental anatomy; and demonstrated the basics of reading radiographs. They also were expected to show up with a dental prevention or health poster that would compete for American Dental Association (ADA)–sponsored prize awards.

Besides helping with the merit badges, Donna volunteered to arrange for all the supplies that were needed, which were considerable. In addition, thinking that boys traveling and camping may not know or care where their toothbrushes might be, she convinced dental suppliers to donate toothbrushes, toothpaste, and floss. This was her first taste of organizational leadership, and it wasn't a bad one, despite the hot weather.

Fort A.P. Hill in Virginia in July was miserable—first heavy rains and leaky tents, then heat and dust. Regardless of the discomforts, Donna loved working with the scouts. She also met Clinton Hamilton, who was president of the Boy Scouts of America's Southeast District. Along with various army personnel, Clinton would stroll by to check out the young woman who was helping with the dentistry merit badges. In his uniform, he finally approached Donna and requested a toothbrush. She refused the request, telling him that the supplies were

for the kids. "Aren't you big for a Boy Scout?" she asked him. Unrebuffed, Clinton persisted. Four years later, they returned to the next Jamboree as a married couple.

Since 1981, Donna's experiences in volunteering, virtually all of which have been connected with organized dentistry, have been extremely important to her. "Doing good for others is doing good for me," she says. "My volunteerism is my life."

Smiles for Success

The AAWD, like the ADA, is organized into districts. Long before Dr Rumberger became president of the AAWD, she served as the chairperson of District 2. At that time, the organization wanted to undertake a worthwhile project that would have an impact in the community. They considered establishing programs for prisoners, for the homeless, or for victims of abuse, but none of those ideas met their criteria. Finally, they were referred to a broadly based program in New York City called Suited for Success (now renamed "SuitAbility"), with which AAWD might be able to collaborate. Suited for Success is a New York City–based nonprofit program that was created to help low-income women find employment by providing them with clothing, accessories, and shoes to wear on job interviews. Because of Donna's reputation for getting things done, AAWD asked her to help set up a program in New York City that linked dental care to the larger goal of helping women emerge from public assistance and achieve independence. In 1996, Donna met with another AAWD member, Judith McFadden, who was also the editor of the *Pennsylvania State Dental Journal*, to discuss a possible pilot program. Together they laid out a plan, named the project "Smiles for Success," and submitted it to AAWD, where it was approved. They wanted Smiles for Success to be more than just another welfare program. Donna and Judy McFadden were concerned that unless the program was carefully designed, the free dental care that would be offered might not actually be a factor in helping the participants move away from public assistance—it might just be an extension of the welfare program. Participants also needed other skills and attitude changes in order to have productive lives. Therefore, besides formalizing their relationship with Suited for Success, they decided to work with a job training and placement organization that would help the participants qualify for more sophisticated jobs than housekeepers or babysitters.

The two women wrote a brochure, set up a foundation, created a constitution with bylaws, achieved nonprofit tax status, submitted successful grants for start-up money, and made "Smiles for Success" a trademarked name. Much of the work was done together, but Donna was the prime mover.

Dr Rumberger treated the first patient and then found other dentists to volunteer for the program—with the caveat that they had to be members of AAWD. She said that it was easier to find volunteers than she thought. All she had to do was ask them. A few men joined AAWD just to participate and give back to the community.

Except for not having to pay fees, the participants were treated as private patients. The basic idea was simple: restore attractive smiles and dental health. However, Donna discovered that legal guidelines were required to manage expensive or extensive treatment such as orthodontics, multiple endodontic procedures, and large amounts of fixed prosthodontics. The practitioners took responsibility for all costs of treatment except laboratory fees, which were covered by the Smiles for Success Foundation.

Before dental services could be provided, a program applicant first spent 2 weeks at the job training and placement service, where she was given instruction in writing resumes, handling interviews, some basic work with computers, and tips on how to be viewed as a responsible person. Donna said the job-training people were "fairly hard-nosed. For 2 weeks the applicant had to show up at 8 AM—a half hour late twice, and she was out."

The applicant then was interviewed by Suited for Success. If she was accepted, she joined other applicants for a year-long program that met once a month for 3-hour seminars and workshops designed to orient the women to what were essentially middle-class concepts. Sessions addressed everything from money management and mental health counseling to tattoo removal, and from dental home care and finding legal aid to instruction on "how to wear a scarf 30 different ways." Attendance was mandatory.

The participants became eligible for dentistry after 3 of the 12 months they spent with Suited for Success. Initially, the plan was to provide dental care and new clothes simultaneously. This, however, did not work. The participants tended to disappear after receiving the clothes—the same with dentistry. As a result, additional safeguards of demonstrated responsibility were introduced.

Donna went to every one of the workshops. She did so because even if her program was wonderful—which she was sure it was—it would be meaningless if there were no participants to take advantage of it. She felt that since fear of dentistry is so widespread, especially among the disadvantaged, her presence and her contributions might help them accept dental care.

At one of the early workshops, Donna initiated a discussion with one of the participants, a woman named Carmen Encarnacion, who eventually became Smiles for Success's first patient. During their entire conversation, Carmen covered her mouth with her hand in embarrassment over some badly fractured anterior teeth. Donna offered her the opportunity to come to her office, but Carmen was reluctant. She agreed to come only if Donna promised not to do any dental work! From that tenuous beginning, Donna says they are now at the point where Carmen calls her for the smallest chip on a tooth. With her anterior teeth restored and an attractive suit for her interview, Carmen secured a good office job with the Girl Scouts of America.

To let others know about the program's success, Carmen accompanied Donna to a meeting of the

> "From the minute she graduated from dental school, she believed in contributing back to society in the only way she knew how—using her skills, her dedication, and hard work to help as many people as possible."
>
> *Dr Margaret Scarlett*
> *Dr Rumberger's nominator*

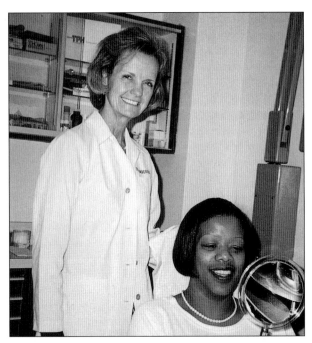

Dr Rumberger *(left)* and Smiles for Success participant Carmen Encarnacion.

AAWD in Orlando, and Donna arranged for Carmen to tell her story (afterwards, Carmen was her guest at Disney World for 2 days). Donna described Carmen's presentation. "She spoke at a breakfast meeting, and she had them all crying. To see someone who picked herself up and went forward and made something of her life is very touching. She didn't mean for them to be overwhelmed, but they were." Carmen has told her story in an appearance with Donna on a New York City television program. The Smiles for Success program has also been featured in the *ADA News*,[1] the *New York State Dental Association Journal*,[2] and the *Pennsylvania Dental Journal*[3] and written about several times in the AAWD *Chronicle*,[4-6] along with receiving honors at the ADA meeting in Kansas City in 2001.

Even though Carmen's story represents a paradigm for the Smiles for Success program, it does not mean the participants are without problems. Destructive life patterns are difficult to overcome, and even some of the most successful women occasionally failed to keep dental appointments, lost their jobs, or reverted to drug habits. Dr Rumberger's relationship with Carmen goes far beyond the dental office, and from the standpoint of support, she is Carmen's mentor, as formally designated in the program. Only one mentorship for each volunteer

dentist is suggested. Mentoring is taken seriously, and if one were a mentor to more than one participant, it could at times be challenging. Donna said that although "Carmen has done very, very well, she's fallen by the wayside at times. I've had to pick her up." It occasionally has been necessary to have rather pointed conversations with Carmen about her responsibilities. In fact, the participants sign a contract that outlines their responsibilities.

Mentoring is manifest in other ways as well. Once when Donna was on her way to a dental society meeting after work, a call came in from a frightened Carmen. Her sister was seriously ill and hospitalized, and she asked Donna to be with her at her sister's bedside. At the hospital, Donna functioned not only as a provider of emotional support, but also as an interpreter of the physician's medical terminology—none of which was good news. When Carmen's sister subsequently died, Donna attended the funeral.

Six months later, Carmen called again saying that her mother was in the hospital. Donna went and stayed with Carmen for 6 hours to help her sort through the problems created by her mother's illness. Donna explained, "I am her mentor. I am there to help her." In the context of the program, helping means encouraging responsibility. For example, with respect to the guidelines for dental fees, the participants get free care only in the first year. Afterwards they pay increasing proportions of the fees, until year 5, when they pay it all. Donna said that the Smiles for Success aspiration is that the women will stay with their dentists (or some dentist) for the rest of their lives.

The program faces other problems besides those of the individual participants. One of the biggest is raising money. Although the program's interdisciplinary structure contributes mightily to helping women in difficult circumstances make significant changes in their lives, by its very nature, it can benefit only scores of participants rather than hundreds or thousands. One-on-one caring takes a lot of time. Granting agencies prefer to invest their money in larger projects even though Smiles for Success is demonstrably fiscally efficient.

Even with their funding difficulties, AAWD has also set up programs in 14 other cities. Donna's vision is to set up programs in major cities all over the country. However, to do so would mean becoming deeply immersed in the particular circumstances of each site. Suited for Success is not a national organization and neither is the job-training agency with which they work. Therefore, other organizations with differing goals and practices would have to be utilized, with differing outcomes as a result, some of them problematic.

"So there are humps," Donna says. "But it is a good program, and there's nothing like it in the world." In an interview with the *ADA News*, Donna commented, "Working with the Smiles for Success participants is one of the most gratifying experiences of my life. It is a wonderful way to give back some of the many benefits that dentistry has given me. Dentistry opened up a world of professional opportunities for me, and I feel that I am doing the same for other women."[7]

Skate Safe

Dr Rumberger's interest in helping people is not limited to women only. By chance, at a meeting of the Suited for Success Board of Directors (of which she is a member) she met the education director for an organization called Ice Hockey in Harlem (IHIH). IHIH was created in 1987 by two men, one of them a New York Rangers ice hockey player. Their aim was to use ice hockey as an incentive for children in low-income neighborhoods to participate in educational opportunities. If children attended after-school tutoring sessions once a week, they would be allowed to take advantage of weekly ice hockey clinics. The genius of their approach was that they taught math with ice hockey statistics, and taught reading and geography with information about the home cities of hockey teams. IHIH started with 40 children and has expanded to the point where it now provides annual help for 275, approximately 30 percent of whom are girls. In addition, about 50 children are provided the opportunity to attend a summer hockey camp. IHIH also helps students obtain high school and college scholarships, provides counseling, and assists in coordinating with other community service agencies. On the ice, they provide almost everything that the children need, from ice skates and hockey sticks to uniforms and pads. The education director told Dr Rumberger that the only thing they needed was mouth guards. Donna had previously read about IHIH and had toyed with the idea of being involved. So, with this new information from the education director, Donna exclaimed, "Mouth guards! My gosh! Why can't we make mouth guards for these kids! What if I propose that the dental society make the mouth guards?"

Dr Rumberger immediately established a budget to cover an anticipated 250 children and got approval from the dental society. She called the program "Skate Safe." Getting it started was at least as complicated as it had been with Smiles for Success. Dr Rumberger negotiated a formal agreement between NYCDS and IHIH, insured the purchase of liability insurance, and made arrangements to acquire formal parental/guardian consent. Because of the large number of students involved, it became clear that everything would have to be done on school property rather than in dental offices. Considering the constraints of working in the field, she had to decide what kind of mouth guards to use, whether to fabricate them from impressions, and what to do about the ever-changing mixed dentitions. And on top of everything else, she needed to buy the supplies—white lab coats, gloves, masks, hot water, and mouth guard materials—and arrange for them to be delivered to some suitable place. It was also necessary to plan how to handle 250 children scattered around Harlem in nine different schools and how to do it all in 2-week teaching sessions. In the first week, the dentists taught home care and nutrition with the help of videotapes, while giving the students toothpaste, brushes, and multiflavored floss. "We wanted it to be fun," Donna said. "And it was fun." In the second week, they performed limited dental examinations and fitted the mouth guards.

Donna was also concerned about another issue. "I did not want the parents or the schools to see us as white men, white women—white dentists—from Manhattan coming up to Harlem to 'do good.'" So Donna worked hard to achieve diversity by enlisting the help of women and different ethnic groups with the collaboration of the NYCDS. The result was that 67 dentists agreed to be Skate Safe volunteers, and Donna scheduled them for each time slot and at each school. Besides asking them to work in the schools, she also asked them to provide free care for the children, and many did. Some children were supported by Medicaid funds, but most of the care was donated.

Two television stations were at the first class, along with one of the hockey players on the New York Rangers team. The program was written up in the *ADA News*, the *New York State Dental Journal*, and the NYCDS newsletter. The organization received calls from other dental societies about how to set up similar programs. Skate Safe has been in existence since 1996, except for a disruption in 2001 from the aftermath of September 11.

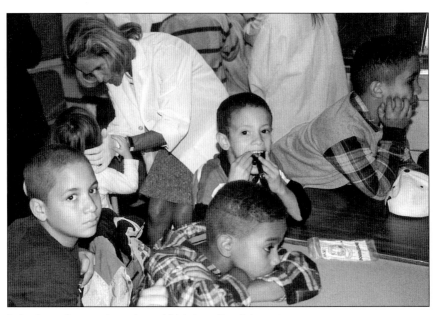

Dr Rumberger fits a mouth guard on a child during a Skate Safe event.

Dr Rumberger loves this program. She says, "I needed to do more than just practice dentistry. If you have free time, do something good!" It is the perfect example of organized dentistry's potential for doing good for others. She hopes that other dental societies are doing similar projects. Outreach programs such as Skate Safe can counter public perception that dentists organize simply to promote their own interests.

Early Years

How did Dr Rumberger's interest in helping others through organized dentistry develop, and what makes it so important to her? The experiences of her early life provide partial answers. They show that she finds new and difficult challenges almost irresistible. What is less clear is why her most satisfying challenges are those that benefit others.

Donna grew up in a large family on a dairy farm in Warriors Mark, not far from State College in central Pennsylvania. Of the nine children in the family, she was the second youngest. Her parents were 39 when she was born, and at that age, being a parent was even harder than when they were younger. Donna thinks that after those long years of child rearing, her parents were

simply tired. In order to invite her parents' attention, she felt that she had to be extraordinary. Doing well in school, which she did, wasn't enough, so she tried to excel in everything. She said, "I had to outperform everybody."

A story about Donna in ninth grade illustrates the point. She attended a small community high school. There were 28 students in her class. Just about all the boys joined the Future Farmers of America (FFA), and the girls–Donna included–joined the Future Home-makers of America (FHA). The FFA boys decided to have a tractor-driving contest at the school. In order to have enough participants to make it interesting, they asked the girls to enter the contest. After the boys (untruthfully) said that several other girls had signed up, Donna agreed to join them. "I volunteered, and I had to be the best." However, to be the best required mastering several maneuvers that were unfamiliar to her, even though she had often driven the family's tractors. It was necessary, for example, to attach a manure spreader to the tractor and back it carefully into a roped-in slot, with only three inches leeway on either side. Furthermore, in connecting the tractor's hitch to the spreader's hitch, one had to back up the tractor perfectly on the first attempt, so that the tractor's pin would drop into the spreader's hitch–no maneuvering was allowed. Everything had to be carefully aligned. Then one had to take the manure spreader through an S-shaped obstacle course with very little margin for error and once again back it in to the slot and unhook it. And that was just one part of the exercise. Donna said, "I practiced and practiced and practiced at my home. I was going to be good." On the day of the event, she discovered that there were 25 participants, and, as the only girl, she was the last to compete. Donna said, "I did the thing perfectly, except that when I backed the manure spreader in, I hit the back rope, so that took off 3 points." But she won anyway. "I beat all the boys."

Donna felt that she always was in competition, especially with boys. "I was a tomboy," she said. She was better than the boys in baseball, and in softball, where she threw a no-hitter. "I had to be—to be understood and appreciated by my parents."

In some respects, Donna's life on a farm made her competitiveness more effective, since she knew what hard work was all about. Every morning at 5:30, she milked their 28 Holstein cows. After school she did the same thing all over again. The work was relentless, and Donna viewed it as "harsh." She had few girlfriends and not much of a social life even though she had been elected president of her class and president of 4H, another organization to which she belonged. Time was scarce, but in the evenings, she could do what she wanted, so she read. Her goal was to read every book in the school library. Given the size of the school, it was almost an attainable aspiration, and she made fairly good progress. She also wanted to read her family's set of encyclopedias from cover to cover. "I started, and I got pretty far. Reading was important for me, perhaps taking me to worlds I dreamed about."

Asked how she equated her competitiveness and desire to excel with her compassion and concern for others, Donna said, "I think that comes through animals—pets. We had lots of pets." Donna spent a lot of time with her animals. She took care of them, nurtured them, and became attached to them. She said, "I identified a lot with animals, because I had no close friends." In addition, Donna's sisters, with whom she was very close, were older and interested in dating, and she was increasingly left on her own. Although Donna feels that her concern for animals taught her valuable lessons about caring that were later transferred to humans, she said, "I'd never, ever live on a working farm again."

The dominant figure on the farm and in her family was her father. Besides running their farm, her father

> "Doing good
> for others is
> doing good for me.
> My volunteerism
> is my life."
>
> *Dr Rumberger*

was an inventor and also found time to be an officer in the local bank. Donna remembers a big shop on their property where he turned his inventions into reality. Because of all of his accomplishments, he was widely known and well respected. His dairy farm was a model for the latest available technology. Donna said that her father was driven to excel in whatever he did, including making sure that his milk had a higher butterfat content than did anyone else's. Yet despite his creativity and competitiveness, his income was rather modest.

In many ways Donna admired him greatly, and she is like him in certain respects. She said, "He was very, very bright, and he taught me a great deal." She remembers having discussions with him in his den about "how to speak well and conduct myself." He excelled in math, as did Donna, and she remembers her joy when she once worked out a very complex problem faster than he did. Her delight, she said, was based more in the hope that it would please her father than in the satisfactions of competition. She didn't compete with older people, only with boys. Older people were to be respected.

As with many men of that era, Donna said that her father had trouble showing his feelings, and it seemed hard for him to give praise. She found herself wishing for these sentiments. She says that while she benefited enormously from him intellectually, she craved expressions of his love and support. Because she missed these things, she considers him a mentor, but never a role model. Donna said that from her father she learned the lessons of understanding and forgiving—but by deduction, rather than by example.

Donna said that her parents enjoyed a harmonious relationship, but she thought it was because her mother accepted a subservient role. She never knew her mother to be an autonomously functioning person until her father died, which was several years before her thoughts turned toward dentistry. "And then, she became a person! A beautiful human being who could function on her own!" But even before her transformation, Donna's mother had an enormous influence on her life. "My mother was a wonderful person with a heart larger than the chest it was made to fit inside." She was a nurturing mother who was always there when her children needed her. In addition, she opened their house to everyone, especially children. Three or four children lived with them every summer. These were the offspring of family friends who were busy doing other things, and she took no compensation for her generosity. "I will never understand how she raised her family along with other families' children without going insane—and she never once complained of being tired. [Her generous actions] were perhaps the building blocks that explain why I enjoy reaching out and helping others."

Mainly, however, Donna feels that she had no paradigm role models available to her while she was growing up. As a child, she distinctly remembers looking for role models, but not finding any. She now thinks she was the role model for herself. Her archetype developed gradually during dental school and in her working years under the influence of diverse circumstances and several influential people. The next section will help us further understand these influences.

Life As a Nurse

Donna Rumberger didn't even think about dentistry as a career until her late 20s. In high school, more than anything else, she wanted to be a plastic surgeon. She also wanted to be a seventh grade math teacher and a lawyer—all three of them, in fact. As a teenager, she thought she could do it all. "Not a problem," she said. "I just had to work it out when." Nonetheless, plastic surgery was what she had her heart set on. Unfortunately, it proved to be an impossible goal. Donna's father wanted her to be a nurse and would not finance a medical education. To back up his position, he took her to a local surgeon who told her that medicine was not for women. At school, she went to her guidance counselor, who was of no help in finding scholarships, even though Donna was a standout. As a result, Donna had very little help and no support in finding her way into medicine.

As a career alternative, she said, "I became a nurse, because that's what my father said I had to be." Nursing was the only education that he would finance. He went so far as to complete Donna's application for the nursing program at nearby Phillipsburg State General Hospital and arrange for the interview.

Mr Rumberger was proud of everything Donna did in nursing. Anything having to do with nursing was the exception to her father's failure to praise. He was delighted when she became president of the student body. Any time the school of nursing had a function, he was there. One night he took the whole school caroling in one of his trucks. "He was so proud! I could have whatever I wanted in nursing." When Donna graduated from nursing school, she worked for a few months in a nearby hospital and then was selected to go to Costa Rica as part of the International Foreign Youth Exchange Program. She was one of three young people from Pennsylvania who were chosen. It clearly was an honor. There was a problem, however. The program had nothing to do with nursing, and her father seriously objected. Undeterred, Donna spent the next 9 months in Costa Rica.

Commentary

The concept of selfhood has an honored place in psychology because it represents a widespread perception that the self is a master control system that guides how we live and affects how we feel about what we do.[1] As such, it explains why two individuals—both aspiring to be skillful dentists, respected by patients and peers, earning good livings, contributing to their community, and functioning as good friends, parents, and spouses—may have vastly different responses to their relative successes or failures, even if their accomplishments were similar. Depending on how their achievements measure up to their concept of self, one of them might proclaim success, the other failure.

Augusto Blasi,[2] a theorist who studies identity formation, states that the self is not simply a collection of characteristics, dispositions, or traits. Instead it is a process by which self-related information is organized according to certain key values: those that help the individual maintain consistency. The core self of any given individual, for example, may identify with self-actualization, achievement, power, and wealth, or with compassion and fairness—or with some combination of these or other values. Among groups of individuals, however, values that are important enough and consistent enough to serve as organizing principles for personal identity vary widely.

These organizing principles define the core self. Without them, one's view of oneself would be radically different. When Dr Rumberger states, "my volunteerism is my life," she makes a powerful statement about an identity that is at the core of her being. Notice that this is not the only identity that occupies her consciousness, nor the only identity that contributes to her concept of self. Asked to reflect on her life's work, its origins and significance, she reveals multiple identities. She has been a daughter, a nurse, a writer, a dentist, a companion, a fashion consultant, a wife, an organizer, a leader, an athlete, and a volunteer. Each of these contributed to her development as a moral exemplar.

Viewed from a developmental perspective, we see two values contributed by two individuals that make significant contribu-

Her experience in Costa Rica was culturally shocking but extremely rewarding. She stayed with the people of the country, an experience that was difficult and not always fun, but one that "I'll always remember with love." They lived on dirt floors, read by the light of oil lamps, drank rainwater, and took 5-mile trips with donkeys. Her new friends were "proud, hard-working, good, honest people," and she felt honored to be among them. When she returned to Pennsylvania, as required she talked about her experiences at elementary schools, high schools, Lions Clubs, Rotary Clubs, and other community organizations all around the state–61 lectures altogether. By her own choice, she wrote a column for the local newspaper, which appeared every 2 weeks for 9 months.

After her Costa Rican experience, Donna decided that working full time as a practicing nurse was not for her. Perhaps teaching would be more satisfying. So, at age 20, based on the friendship of a classmate from nursing school who lived in New York City, she moved there and enrolled at Columbia University. Her goals were to earn a BS degree from Columbia's Teacher's College and then to teach nursing.

Donna was a successful teacher. In her first year, the students gave her the outstanding teacher award and a dozen red roses. Pleased as she was with her success as a teacher, she knew that she didn't want to teach nursing the rest of her life. It wasn't long before she started taking courses at New York University. What she would do with them, she was still uncertain–perhaps teach

math courses for seventh graders like she had dreamed about as a child.

After 2 years of teaching, Donna switched to retailing, which she enjoyed for another 2 years. She had always been interested in clothes, and it was fun and glamorous. Even so, she was looking for a more permanent career choice.

Dentistry emerged as an extension of her interest in the cosmetic aspects of plastic surgery. She said that dentistry would enable her to "make someone else pretty, and help another person be dentally healthier." She had considered plastic surgery once again, but concluded that the 12 years it would require would make her older than she wanted to be by the time she established a practice. With dentistry, she could enter in only 4 years. Her stockpile of credits at NYU now had perhaps a different purpose. To fund her dental education, she started to do some private duty nursing at Mt Sinai Hospital in New York City.

Working at Mt Sinai proved to be an unexpected piece of good fortune for Donna, mainly because it resurrected some earlier aspirations about writing she had had while doing her newspaper columns on Costa Rica. Those efforts were very rewarding, and she thought that the challenging cases she was seeing at Mt Sinai would provide an even more dramatic opportunity for testing her skills as the writer of a book. One case, for example, provided the following dramatic elements: a patient who was placed on a respirator after an unsuccessful

tions to her emerging self: achievement (her father), and selfless service (her mother). Challenged by her ninth grade peers, her identity as a competent competitor emerges in the story of the tractor competition. What attracts our interest in this story is first her intuitive understanding of what it takes to win, and then her focused ability to get the job done. She recognizes that winning isn't just a matter of luck, but of skill and concentration. To master the skill, she devotes hours to practice. Consider how many 13 year olds you know who are able to maintain the focus to practice a skill to perfection. This story of a child's achievement, modeled after her father, is a paradigm for her later actions. At this point, her success is designed to benefit herself alone. Turning her skills to the service of others—her mother's contribution to Donna's self-identity—will appear later and often and are the foundation for the development of the moral self and for her nomination as a moral exemplar.

The value of selfless service obviously has greater intrinsic moral implications than does that of achievement, though Dr Rumberger's story is a clear demonstration of how they can inter-

act. Blasi notes that for some individuals, moral concepts seem to penetrate to the very essence of who and what they are. For others, such ideals appear to be only glancing acquaintances.[2]

In describing ways to "forge a moral identity," Cerine et al[3] incorporate Blasi's view that the development of a person's moral identity is more than an accretion of disciplined habits that automatically and reliably become right action. It is also more than the nurturing of compassion that results in the bestowing of care and generosity, and it goes further than a deliberative stance toward decision making that promotes the weighing of the implications of everyday choices. Beyond good habits, compassion, and reflection, moral identity "is partially captured by words like will, resolve, and aspiration. It is as much searching and striving as coping and adapting; it is a way-of-being-in-the-world rather than just a response-to-the-world."[3]

Moral identity shares features with other identities. Each of us has multiple identities: as a scholar, a professional, a child, a parent, an athlete, a student, and so on. We tend to be preoccupied by our major identities, in that we monitor their adequacy

attempt at suicide; a brother who tried to hasten her demise by reprogramming the respirator; and a successful intervention by Donna.

Even though Donna has begun work on that book, her involvement with organized dentistry has placed her writing efforts on hold. She says, however, that the writing will get done. In fact, she plans to write three more books. One will be based upon her experiences at Bellevue Hospital while taking a residency in general dentistry, which she dictated every night into her tape recorder. And as Donna said, "You see all aspects of humanity at Bellevue!" Another book will be for children. Despite Donna's clinical preference for treating adults, she nonetheless finds the intellectual appeal of writing a book for children to be challenging and fascinating. Initially, the final book was to have been an account of the indecorous experiences of the student nurse–the beds made, urinals emptied, dentures cleaned, and faces washed. Now, however, the intended book will probably be an account of her life. "It's been an interesting life," she said. The book would be true, but written as fiction.

Fledgling Dentist

Donna's first definitive step in becoming a dentist also was linked to an experience she had as a private duty nurse at Mt Sinai Hospital–albeit an exasperating one.

She had been assigned to a floor where there were a number of celebrity patients. One morning, while her patient was sleeping after her breakfast, Donna noticed a commotion in a patient's room across the hall. When Donna went to investigate, the nurse there frantically told her that the patient had stopped breathing. The nurse had placed the bed and patient in a seated position, a forbidden posture for a nonbreathing person. Furthermore, while the bed was moving to its upright position, the electrical cord to the patient call bell had been pulled from the wall, thereby severing communications with the front desk. Donna told the nurse to recline the bed and get help. Then she jumped onto the bed and performed CPR. After a short time, the patient started to breathe on her own, and at that point an intern arrived. Trembling from the experience, Donna returned to her own patient's room. Her patient was still asleep, and Donna said nothing about the incident to anyone. Later that day she saw the grateful family hugging the attending doctor, who shamelessly was lapping it up. Right then Donna decided that it might as well be her, rather than someone else, who received the credit for her honorable work. Whether it would be as a physician or a dentist was something to be dealt with later.

Although it may have been her competitive spirit that brought her into dental school, Donna said that while she was there, her need to rise to the top underwent a modification. She had no interest in running for office. Dental school was interesting and challenging, and that was all that concerned her. In addition, paying for her

and resist challenges to them. The point is particularly well made by Cerine et al[3] with the example of the athlete. "[S]omeone with a genuine athletic identity, as compared to someone who merely enjoys exercise or engages in sports for the adulation or profit it brings, is on the lookout for opportunities to play his sport. He expresses his athleticism off as well as on the field by staying in shape and avoiding temptations. He monitors his skill level and seeks to improve. Faced with a setback, such as an injury, he goes through rehabilitation eagerly and earnestly." Similarly, someone with a strong, as compared to a weak, moral identity "is alert to opportunities for expressing moral statements and actions, sees the moral implications in seemingly neutral situations, questions the adequacy of his responses, and courageously resists invitations to be amoral or immoral, despite the cost to his self-interest (as perceived by most)." The analogy seems particularly appropriate given that Donna was a distance runner. She has devoted the same sustained commitment to her volunteering that she dedicated to developing her ability to complete a marathon in 3 hours and 20 minutes.

In recounting important events of Donna Rumberger's life, we see the shifts in identity formation that are characteristic of a "developmental trajectory" that ends with the mature moral identity described by Blasi[2] and Robert Kegan[4] as the goal of development. In the early phases of identity formation, characteristic of childhood and early adolescents, individuals are "self" rather than "other" centered. The development of the self-oriented self is critically important work and is well demonstrated in Donna's story about the tractor-driving contest. It isn't that adolescents don't understand that others have perspectives and agendas different from their own, but the focus is on achieving personal goals, and the need for approval is high. Only after achieving self-confidence and competence can an individual make the transition to the phase that enables them to view experiences from multiple perspectives simultaneously, and to be able to adopt values and make decisions in the absence of positive social feedback.

The transition from a self- toward an other-centered identity begins when Donna enters nursing, though the initial

education with evening and weekend nursing duties cut significantly into her study time. Consequently, her grades were not as high as she had hoped. However, her performance was good enough to get into a general practice residency program. In any case, Donna said that excellence in treating patients was her goal, not the accumulation of high grades from written tests. Nevertheless, she loved the didactic part of dental school, and everything about it, from the science courses and the laboratory work to taking care of patients. She simply loved being a student. Had she been able to afford it, Donna thinks she could have been a perpetual student. She also realized that it was important to be as good a dental student as she was a nurse for patients. And as a result of her dedication and caring, she received the award for outstanding clinician for the class of 1980.

> "If you have free time, do something good!"
>
> *Dr Rumberger*

The "Granduncle"

After her graduation from New York University College of Dentistry and the completion of her general practice residency program at Bellevue Hospital, Dr Rumberger opened an office in New York City for the practice of dentistry. This event provided the base for almost all of the work for which she was selected as a moral exem-

plar in dentistry. Perhaps just as important, it gave her the opportunity to meet Henry Quade, her adopted "granduncle."

Mr Quade came to Dr Rumberger as a patient at the suggestion of his wife, Henrietta, who had been under Dr Rumberger's care for several years. A handsome gentleman in his early 80s who had a huge, frightening presence and weighed in at 300 pounds, Mr. Quade was a self-made man who, as a high school dropout, became an attorney by taking a correspondence course and had risen to prominence as an executive for General Motors. He was impatient with everyone, including Donna. According to him, women should not be college educated, and they certainly should not become dentists. Their relationship was strictly formal, despite their growing friendship with each succeeding visit. He was Mr Quade, and she was Dr Rumberger.

Their relationship deepened after some years when Mrs Quade was hospitalized for what was thought would be a short stay. By that time Mr Quade's health had also deteriorated to the point where it was difficult to take care of himself. Thus, he, too, entered the hospital as a "guest," but also to receive some general medical care. The Quades had asked Donna if she would help them when Henrietta went to the hospital, so she did. For example, each morning before she went to her office, she visited them, taking them each copies of the

decision is motivated, at least in part, by an unwillingness to defy her father's wishes. She continues to achieve, and her leadership skills are recognized—an early indicator of the emergence of an orientation toward helping others to achieve. Upon graduation, she asserts her independence and goes to Costa Rica, where she has a developmentally broadening experience that enables her to see the needs of others from multiple perspectives. More importantly, she takes time to reflect, write, and talk about her experiences, thereby incorporating these perspectives into her emerging identity. Her next step toward the value-generating self is to consider what she wants to do. Not surprisingly, she settles on another helping profession, teaching. Kegan[4] identifies this sort of independence as critical to the growth of autonomous professionals capable of exercising judgment in the face of the ambiguous and uncertain situations that characterize professional practice. This level of functioning is rarely achieved before midlife and is attained by less than half of all highly educated adults.[4]

We notice another atypical transition in motivational forces as she enters dental school. We observe the emergence of a value-generating self that enables her to set personal goals for achievement. No longer bound by the approval of others, she is not only able to see the perspective of others, but can consistently give priority to the interests of others. This capacity is perceived by her instructors, and she is recognized as an outstanding clinician. As she enters dentistry, we see the emergence of the fully formed moral identity. It is exhibited in the sustained caring for Mr Quade and her consistent volunteering to help others through dentistry, coupled with her emergences as a leader who mobilizes others to assist with helping.

In reflecting on her life story, Donna expressed some concern that the early "tractor story" casts her as overly concerned with competition and bettering others. We see this somewhat differently. We see it as the essential development of competence and self-confidence—without which one cannot move on to effectively help others (through nursing and dentistry). Many people offer help to others. What distinguishes Donna is the degree to

New York Post and the *New York Times*. In the evening, after office hours, Donna visited them again. During her hospitalization, Mrs Quade's condition became dramatically worse, and before her death, she asked Donna, who had become one of her favorites, to promise to take care of her husband.

Mr Quade became Donna's "granduncle" as a countermeasure to the restriction that only relatives could see patients outside regular visiting hours. Being a "grandniece" had another benefit as well. Mr Quade's medical condition had worsened, and there was discussion in the hospital that in the absence of a "relative"—and he had none—there was a risk that the state might step in to help manage the affairs of a seriously ill gentleman in his 80s. Once Dr Rumberger began to refer to herself as the "grandniece," no one ever questioned anything.

Donna remembers their time together with great fondness. Even before Mrs Quade died, Donna would go to the Quades' massive but deteriorating Manhattan apartment frequently, sometimes in the evenings and once a week for a few hours during the day so that Mrs Quade could spend some personal time away from their apartment. After Mrs Quade's death, Donna visited Mr Quade for about an hour and a half every day, except perhaps on Sundays. Occasionally she would be called with an invitation for dinner. Especially important were her evening visits. He would ask her to write a few checks and take care of any other rudimentary financial business that was on his mind. Then he would enjoy his nightly cigar and cocktail while they visited. They would talk about wide-ranging topics, and often he would quote poetry from well-known authors. Even into his 90s, he received her visits seated at his huge desk, dressed in a white shirt and a smoking jacket—both gifts from Donna. During his illnesses, he had lost about half of his body weight and badly needed a whole new wardrobe, which Donna bought at Brooks Brothers after measuring him. Donna said dressing well was "important for his self-esteem, his pride."

Besides the social aspects of their relationship, Donna helped with other important practical necessities. For example, when the plaster started to sag and collapse—the Quades' home had been without renovation for 35 years—Donna arranged to have the apartment plastered and painted.

"It was a wonderful experience," Donna said, "and it was so important for me to make him happy." For a time, she arranged for a pianist from Juilliard to give a concert every Wednesday. To make the concerts more festive, the housekeeper served cookies, and Donna encouraged others to attend. Usually the concertgoers were older people, and some of them were patients from her dental office. Donna's sisters joined them when they were in town. In addition, Donna organized open house parties at least twice a year. One was at Christmastime. A home care aide helped with the wheelchair, and they all went out to select a 12-foot-high tree.

At Donna's suggestion, Mr Quade agreed to withhold money from his housekeeper's salary so that she later could use it to pay her college tuition. The housekeeper was delighted, and the plan worked. Mr Quade attended

---

which the help is effectual. The drive to perfect one's competence is particularly essential for a leader who hopes to mobilize and sustain the collaborative efforts required to accomplish large-scale projects. The first job in identity formation is the development of the self. With respect to the development of the moral self, the incorporation of moral values into identity is an obvious requirement. However, without competence, one may be a kind and nice person, but one is unlikely to be effectual. Mobilizing a large group of independent practitioners to achieve a common purpose when the purpose is purely service to others requires enormous competence and a whole range of skills that are developed only by a strong drive to succeed. Without competence, the moral self achieves only what Hassler[5] refers to as dispositional goodness, but not the goodness of activity that is characteristic of the moral exemplars we have studied. (See the commentary on the story of Jeremiah Lowney in chapter 7 for further discussion of this distinction.)

Reflecting further on this exemplar, we see an individual who is clearly and consistently centered on the interests and needs of others. In the early stages of leadership in her profession, rather than being critical of the contributions of one's predecessors—which so often defines beginning leaders—she appreciates their contributions and sees that they are honored for them. Perhaps more remarkable is her clear vision of the profession's collective responsibility to put the oral health interests of others before the interests of the profession. Too often the public sees organized dentistry actively involved in promoting their own interests (eg, assuring adequate reimbursement for their services), rather than in activities that benefit the community—especially the disadvantaged community. Professionals are socialized to see the responsibility to put the oral health interests of their patients before self-interest, but relatively few articulate, act upon, or contribute to the profession's collective responsibility. Notice that each of the activities to which Donna devotes energy is inexorably linked to dentistry. There seems to be an implicit recognition that anyone can volunteer their services to benefit the less advantaged, but only dentists can fix teeth, make mouth guards, and contribute to self-esteem by improving smiles.

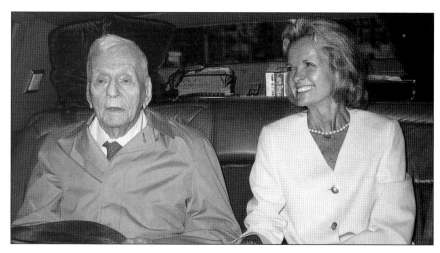

Mr Henry Quade and Dr Rumberger on one of their many outtings.

the commencement ceremony—the first time he had been in a car in 25 years. After that initiation, other outings were possible. They especially liked to go to the Bronx Zoo and the botanical gardens. "We did things to make him happy, to get him out." Whenever Mr Quade needed to see a physician, Donna was the one who took him, along with his home care aide.

Donna said, "He was one of the most marvelous people I ever met in my life." Although she had undertaken the responsibility of his care with trepidation, "It worked out well. He taught me a lot. He was a big influence in my life."

Some years after his wife died, Mr Quade established the Henry and Henrietta Quade Foundation, which was to be used for worthwhile charitable purposes. Donna was the president. In 1997, the foundation granted $250,000 to the New York University College of Dentistry to be used as financial aid for worthy dental students enrolled in the school. In receiving the grant, Dean Edward G. Kaufman said that, "Donna Rumberger embodies the finest qualities of the humanistic health professional. . . . She has set a marvelous example for other alumni."[8]

We can hardly leave this story without looking at the roadblocks (ie, gender bias) that women like Donna have had to overcome. Recently, a highly regarded female dental leader was granted an outstanding achievement award by the American Dental Association. When asked to what she attributed her success in such a male-dominated field, she quipped—in good humor—that it was her ability to "work like a horse, think like a man, and act like a lady." The spontaneous laughter and thunderous applause reinforced the underlying truth: Gender bias makes achievement more difficult for women.

Let's think about succeeding under the adverse conditions Donna has experienced. She seems to feel like she hasn't done enough—perhaps based on a "late start" occasioned by her father's opposition to her career aspirations and the failure of school counselors to come to her aid by providing either information or support for her aspirations. So, first she has to demonstrate superior competence, all the while hiding any resentment she may feel for the lack of equal opportunity and fair treatment. She says that in those early years she felt like

she had to be like a boy to be understood and appreciated. We see at an early age a tremendous drive to compete and to succeed and a need for approval, especially from the father figure, since males seemed to be valued. We notice that each significant male in her life was an accomplished person—her father, the physician who advised against a career in medicine, and Mr Quade. Yet each disapproved of her career choice. Though they may not be role models in the strictest sense, they are her models for what she feels she ought to be: competent, competitive, and accomplished. Despite the prejudice she experienced, she doesn't display resentment—as many who have experienced discrimination do—and she doesn't take a separatist view. Even in working with organized women's groups, she works for gender equity that is inclusive of her male colleagues.

Whereas males appear to be her model for competence and achievement, her mother emerges as the role model for generosity and caring that her consistent volunteerism requires. Donna remarks that her mother cared for others without complaint, playing a subservient role in order to maintain harmony.

Perspectives on Dentistry

It was not long after her graduation that Donna became active in her component dental society, having been primed with her first organizational experience with the AAWD as a student. She had attended a lecture and meeting of the Midtown Dental Society, one of two subdivisions of the NYCDS. During the meeting, she discovered that the Midtown newsletter was without an editor. No one appeared to be interested in the job, so Donna volunteered. The publication was floundering, and she agreed to see if she could turn it around. Based on her ability to persuade her colleagues to submit articles to the newsletter, it became a publication with some substance. Donna said, "So they noticed me. And before I knew it, I was going up the chairs in the Midtown Dental Society, and ultimately became the president."

During that period, Dr Rumberger began to be recognized as someone who not only had good ideas, but also worked hard to implement them. For example, she came to appreciate that among the three branch societies of the First District Dental Society, now the NYCDS, there had been many illustrious leaders who had contributed greatly to the profession over the years. Believing that they should be remembered, she identified all the past presidents back to 1900 and designed plaques to honor them. The idea was approved by the parent society.

Not all of her ideas went as far as she would have liked. Based on questions she was hearing from her patients about what she put in their mouths, she realized that there was no disclosure of ingredients on the labels of dental materials. As a result, she worked to get her society behind a movement that would require such a listing. Although the Midtown Dental Society, NYCDS, and the New York State Dental Association endorsed the idea, it was turned down at the national level.

Dr Rumberger has put her talents to work in other activities as well. She has written a dozen or so articles for publications of the organizations in which she has been active, primarily in the AAWD's *Chronicle*. She also has been a delegate to the annual meeting of the ADA, a member of the Dental Commission for the 1994 World Cup Soccer Tournament, and a member of the Advisory Board for the New York University College of Dentistry. In addition, she has served for more than 15 years on the Committee on Dental Health of the US Olympic Committee, giving pro-bono dental care to many Olympians.

Donna's ability to make things happen has been a source of some—albeit restrained—satisfaction for her. To begin with, when asked how she feels about her ascendancy to leadership of organizations, Donna said, "Being president of an organization is an opportunity to make a difference. If you have something that needs to be done, and you can't do it alone, you do it as a group." Dr Rumberger's nominator believes that the way she gets groups to work together is by inspiring them. Dr Rumberger says that she doesn't see that quality in herself, and views such things as a team effort. "It's not just me. If I do it, other people will follow, and we work as a unit." She is pleased,

Yet, when the occasion arose, she adapted and became a fully functioning autonomous person. Like her mother, Donna doesn't see unremunerated service as self-sacrifice, but rather as a core activity that sustains her. As she says, "Doing good for others is doing good for me."

One gets the feeling in reading her story that she sees achievement as what is most valued. She sets for herself ever-more challenging goals (writing books). There is a kind of optimism about what is possible and what can be accomplished. As a child she said she was going to become a doctor, lawyer, and a math teacher—all three of them, in fact. This kind of optimism is what makes possible the development and sustaining of programs like Smiles for Success. Most who have worked with individuals who grew up in circumstances of extreme poverty recognize the low probability of success and the challenge of working out contingencies that make some level of success possible. Perhaps it is her optimistic outlook that sustains her in situations most of us would find impossible.

When we look at just one of her accomplishments, like the Smiles for Success program, we recognize the enormous amount of competence, drive, persistence, and attention to detail required to accomplish, sustain, and then expand such a program. Many of us aspire to, but few of us achieve, what this remarkable woman has done.

References

1. Goodman JF, Lesnick H (eds). The Moral Stake in Education: Contested Premises and Practices. New York: Longman, 2001.
2. Blasi A. Moral identity: Its role in moral functioning. In: Krutines W, Gerwitz J (eds). Morality, Moral Behavior, and Moral Development. New York: Wiley, 1984.
3. Cerine A, Comfort C, Knox H, Laszlo M. Forging a moral identity. In: Goodman JF, Lesnick H (eds). The Moral Stake in Education: Contested Premises and Practices. New York: Longman, 2001.
4. Kegan R. The Evolving Self: Problem and Process in Human Development. Cambridge, MA: Harvard University Press, 1982.
5. Hassler J. Good People. Chicago: Loyola Press, 2001.

however, to reflect that her major accomplishment at NYCDS has been to advance the practice of volunteerism. Skate Safe is a good example of what people working together can do in this area. She is also happy about her role in the dental society's collaboration with Columbia University in a program to provide care for the underserved.

Her satisfaction is mitigated by her attitude that once a project is completed, "It's done. To be learned from and move on to the next project." Besides that, her view is what she does is nothing special. She only does what everyone ought to do. Furthermore, she feels that she should have accomplished much much more. She considers herself to be a late developer who "should have done all this a long time ago."

Whatever hard line she adopts with respect to her self-assessment, Dr Rumberger views organized dentistry as a vehicle for activism on behalf of other people. And when she makes her choices of things that call for action, it is characteristic that they primarily advance the interests of the people whom dentistry serves. The interests of the organizations she represents come second. She says, "A lot of people are in dentistry because it's a good way to make a living, and you're respected." As important as these factors are, she feels that they are not enough. Dentists need to embrace their special skills and responsibilities to serve the public. "Dentistry is a hands-on profession where you help improve a person's self-esteem by enhancing his or her smile and by restoring and maintaining oral health. To me, that's what dentistry is about."

At the core of Dr Rumberger's beliefs about professions is the view that they are different from other occupations. Donna said, "A profession is something that you really want to do. I don't look at what I do as a job or as an occupation. The distinction between jobs or occupations and professions is that a profession is something a little more important, or a little more to the heart. I'm not looking at it from the [dictionary] point of view. I'm looking at it as something very special."

Currently

In late January 2002, at the time of this interview, Dr Rumberger, like all New Yorkers, was still deeply affected by the events of September 11. Though she was reluctant to make the trip, early one quiet Sunday morning, before the tourists came, she went to Ground Zero. She found herself mesmerized by a single fluttering piece of paper that was still attached to a street sign weeks after the attack. "I just couldn't take my eyes off of it. I didn't want to go, but once I got there, I didn't want to leave." As president of the NYCDS, she had not had much time for that kind of reflection. Raising money for disaster assistance for the dentists of New York City became an immediate and time-consuming priority. Now, at the time of the interview, her presidency had been over for 3 days. She was happy for the privilege of having served as the leader of the NYCDS.

The work of the dental society continues, however. Donna was one of eight people who organized the 2002 Greater New York Dental Meeting. With 38,000 registrants, it is the largest dental meeting in the United States. In particular, she was in charge of workshops and table demonstrations. There were scores of speakers to contact, competing dental and dental hygiene students to organize, and trunks of supplies to be managed. It kept her busy, to say the least, and it would be the same for the 2003 meeting.

Apart from her work in the dental society, Donna is uncertain about what she will do next. She will have more discretionary time than she did in earlier years, and not all of it is welcome. Some of her freer schedule is because of the death of her husband several years ago. His last illness was the aftermath of a cerebrovascular accident that had occurred years before his death. Donna remembers it vividly. She and Clinton loved to sail and were anchored on their boat off the shores of the Florida Keys. When the attack came, and with it his cessation of breathing, it was obvious to Donna what was happening. She called on the radio for help from the Coast Guard and started mouth-to-mouth resuscitation. Clinton's breathing resumed before the Coast Guard arrived, and he recovered enough to go back to work for several more years.

Some of Donna's increased available time comes from less disturbing changes in her life. Previously, she had spent much of her time training for and running New York City marathons. Altogether she completed five of them, clocking her best time at 3 hours and 20 minutes. Those days are over, however, and she now contents herself by working out regularly. One thing she says she would like to do is to make Smiles for Success a more recognizable national program. Or perhaps she will find a totally new service project in which to invest herself. On the other hand, maybe she will use her time to write one of the books that are waiting for her. She says, "I would love to publish. That is probably my next challenge."

We'll see. Don't forget, she has also said, "My volunteerism is my life."

References

1. Dentist volunteers help other women. ADA News. February 5, 1996:34.
2. Clark LB. Smile. You're on the road to success. N Y State Dent J 1997;63:28–30.
3. McFadden J. Reconsidering the reasons why we volunteer. Pa Dent J, 1997;64(5).
4. Rumberger D. Smiles for Success–Suited for Success. AAWD Chronicle, May-June 1995.
5. McFadden J, Rumberger D. Smiles for Success. AAWD Chronicle, March-April 1996.
6. AAWD. AAWD's Smiles for Success wins Pierre Fauchard Grant. AAWD Chronicle, Jan-Feb 1997.
7. Luz C. Smiles for Success pushes ahead. ADA News. January 7, 2002:18.
8. NYU College of Dentistry receives $250,000 grant for scholarships from the Henry and Henrietta Quade Foundation [press release]. New York University Public Affairs; July 10, 1997.

Questions for Discussion

1. The commentary for this story speaks of the development of the self. The core self may identify with any one of a number of organizing principles: self-actualization, achievement, power and wealth, compassion and fairness, or some combination of these or other values. What core organizing principles define you? What really brings you satisfaction and happiness?

2. Consider each of the multiple identities you have assumed. What does each contribute to your understanding of the organizing principles that define you?

3. This book is concerned about the development of a professional identity and the development of the moral self. What do you think are the organizing principles that define Dr Rumberger? Do the organizing principles that define you include the moral or ethical values of your profession?

4. Dr Rumberger's story illustrates ways to exercise the collective responsibility of the profession to put the oral health interests of society above the interest of the profession. Think of some examples from your own community in which you and your colleagues are similarly engaged. What else might you do to promote the public image of dentistry as a caring profession?

5. Think of some actions by your profession that undermine its public image. What countermeasures could be taken?

4. If Smiles for Success were your project, how would you react to the high rate of participants quitting after receiving free clothing or dental care or falling back into old habits like drug abuse? Are there changes you would make in the program? If so, would you make them on the basis of efficiency or justice?

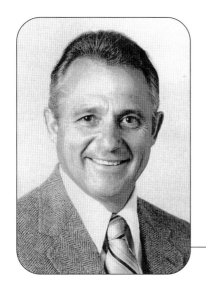

9

Camille B. Capdeboscq, Jr

The Good Teacher

Dr Camille B. Capdeboscq, Jr taught operative dentistry at Louisiana State University School of Dentistry from 1972 until his retirement in 1996. Before that, he had practiced for 9 years, partly in Louisiana's bayou country. With a reputation for clinical excellence, he became a legendary figure at LSU for his humility, his generosity of spirit, and his humanitarian dedication to students. Despite his demand for the highest of standards and his toughness in grading, his students nonetheless loved and revered him for his ability to inspire confidence, stimulate learning, and instill a sense of dignity at each encounter. Dr Capdeboscq also inspired his colleagues to look at their own character and values.

Dr Capdeboscq's nomination came in the form of an open letter from Dr Allan Rappold to the dentists of Louisiana entitled "The Person I Would Most Like to Emulate." A former LSU colleague of Dr Capdeboscq's and then–acting chair of the Department of Operative Dentistry and Biomaterials, Dr Rappold had published the letter in Louisiana's state dental journal. It painted the picture of a man who is immeasurably more concerned about generosity, kindness, dependability, and honesty than he is about money and appearance. Dr Rappold said, "The beauty of the complex nature of Dr Cap lies in his simplicity. He wants and desires mainly the simple and good things in life, the things that have the greatest real value. These are the very things he already possesses in abundance."

Before meeting Dr Capdeboscq at his home in Tickfaw, Louisiana, I (JTR) visited the LSU dental school on a Friday afternoon to talk with some of his former students and colleagues. Both groups had enthusiastic stories to tell about "Dr Cap." Some of the stories were legend-promoting. For example, it appears to be true–or close enough–that Cap never missed a day of work in his 24 years at LSU. In addition, according to Dean Eric Hovland, the story is told that Cap even made it to work during the great New Orleans flood of 1989, despite the fact that no one else showed up. For Dr Cap getting to work meant driving the 64 miles from Tickfaw to New Orleans, something he accomplished by 6 o'clock each morning. From then until his departure at half past 5, his job was to help students. Cap figured that if students needed extra help, they could do a lot of remediation in the 2 hours before classes started at 8 o'clock.

A favorite subject that afternoon at LSU was Dr Cap's generosity with his time. A typical example was given by a student who had problems with his first casting late one afternoon. Dr Cap had just finished grading some lab work, but stayed to see if the student had any problems. The student said, "He stayed close to an hour. That's his time, you know. He could have gone home, and he had a long drive. I guess he knew I was a little nervous about what I was doing. That's just the type of guy he is. If you were having problems, you could come catch him anytime out of class. He was always available." Apparently, it has always been the same. A former classmate of Cap's remembers that Cap "had the best hands in our class and was always willing to help anyone who needed assistance." A current student said that his own dentist, who graduated 20 years ago, remembers Dr Cap in the same way.

Cap was as generous with his knowledge as he was with his time. It was obvious to everyone that it gave him great pleasure to see students flourish under his instruction. Cap himself often expressed the idea that "Teaching is sharing." Whatever knowledge Cap had, it was yours if you asked for it. Allan Rappold said, "He is the most giving individual I've ever met. If you ask Cap to do anything for you, it's done." In addition, Dr Rappold said that Cap's expertise "that was yours-for-the-asking" extended beyond dentistry to electrical work, plumbing, carpentry, hunting, fishing, cooking, airplanes, automobiles, gardening, and farming. "I've never seen anybody that could do as much." Cap was also generous in more traditional ways. He gave meaningful gifts that were connected with the things he valued in his life. A friend said, "In my backyard I have trees that he gave me–persimmon trees and fig trees. And every year when they bloom, they remind me of him."

Not only was Cap available to his students, he was also concerned about what they learned and how well they learned it. A student said, "Rather than just sitting down and doing something for you, or just telling you the quick way to do things, he really was concerned that you learned what you were doing–I mean, [both] how to treat your patient and how to do the procedure." Furthermore, "He's not intimidating at all. If you did something wrong, he could tell you about it in such a way that you weren't afraid he was going to degrade you." Another student said, "Dr Cap knew students

pretty well. When he worked with you, he always knew what you were weak in, and he concentrated on that with you." And he did it in a nice way. The student said, "Dentistry can be frustrating for a student. Dental school is hard, and he's one of those instructors that, [when] you've had a bad morning and you're scared about the procedure you're going to do, if Dr Cap is your instructor, you know you always walk away with a positive attitude about dentistry." In fact, one student had a good friend and classmate who changed his mind about quitting dental school because of the encouragement he received from Dr Cap. From his account it seemed that, more than anything else, it was Dr Cap's subtle availability that made the difference. At 5 o'clock when patients were discharged and other instructors had left, "Dr Cap would always stick around in case you wanted to ask him something while your patient wasn't there. Or in case you wanted to talk about something, or if you had a rough time, and you just wanted to say, 'What did I do wrong?'" This student had been feeling very frustrated, but a month with Dr Cap turned things around for him.

Dr Capdeboscq treated patients with the same sensitivity that he did students. Patients were delighted to have him work with them and were known to request him as an instructor. One student said that it was not that Dr Cap spent a lot of time with the patients–none of the instructors were able to do that, "He just had a demeanor about him." With a smile and a few words of greeting, he was able to convey an atmosphere of reassurance that relaxed everyone. As the student said, "Some of the patients probably can sense that you're nervous, and they're nervous too. But when you had Dr Cap, when he sat down, it just put everybody at ease."

Allan Rappold said that students who found that they were assigned to Dr Cap for the sophomore laboratory course were overjoyed. This was remarkable from my perspective, because many faculty members who are popular with students are widely known to be pushovers when it comes to grading. Dr Capdeboscq, on the other hand, was of a different breed. The departmental secretary, Cathy Daigle, who logs in the faculty's grading statistics, said that Dr Cap was the toughest grader in the department. When students got the top score from him (which was rare), they knew that they had truly earned it. When she asked students why Dr Cap was such a favorite, given his tough approach to grading, they again affirmed that he never belittled them or made them feel inadequate. At the same time, he successfully demanded excellence.

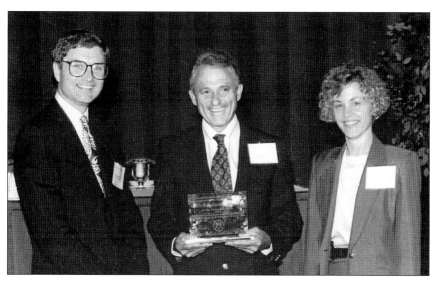

Dr Capdeboscq *(center)* receives a Dr Ernst Lederle Award for Excellence in 1993.

Any discussion with students or faculty invariably comes around to Dr Capdeboscq's unassuming nature. His modesty is a trademark, and despite his talents and accomplishments, he does not like to talk about himself and is never self-promoting. Some faculty speculated about whether he would be willing to spend hours talking about himself. Dean Hovland had told me in a letter that I "would really have to spend some time with Cap to understand how special he is and how quietly, yet strongly, he inspires you to do the right things."

Without a doubt, Dean Hovland expressed the feelings of everyone in the following paragraph: "Cap might be a simple man in his lifestyle, but he is a giant in character. He demonstrated incredible moral strength. He was a superb clinician, one of the best I have ever encountered, and yet he never bragged about or ever mentioned his extraordinary skills. He was demanding of students, yet always fair, understanding, and patient. He never wavered in his moral approach to patient care and his humble honesty. He quietly went about his business of sharing his skills with students and demonstrating moral character through example. Over time his actions inspired both students and colleagues to look at their own character and values as their respect for Dr Cap developed."

A close colleague said, "I think everyone around here learned a lot from him. Not only clinically and professionally, but just from being around him. It was a lesson in honesty and kindness, and humility." One of the things she liked best was that he showed respect for everyone equally, regardless of station in life, gender, or race. At his retirement party, besides his colleagues and dignitaries, the janitorial staff attended and were specially greeted by Cap. Dr Rappold said, "The world is a better place because of the existence of Camille Capdeboscq, and although I don't have the power to be exactly like Dr Cap, I am a better person and teacher because of his influence."

Toward the end of the afternoon, a former student and now part-time faculty member, Dr Rick Henry, made a suggestion for the interview with Dr Cap. He had planned a hunting trip on the banks of Lake Mary, a former oxbow of the Mississippi River, located a couple of hours away, across the border into Mississippi. He had invited Cap to go with him and stay at his cabin, as he often did. (I later learned that Dr Henry paid $1,500 per year for each hunter who used the facilities. He considered this a small payback for what Cap meant to him.) Cap, however, had turned down the invitation because of my meeting with him that weekend. So Rick invited me to conduct part of the interview at the cabin. It was there that Cap began to talk about himself and share how he came to be the person he is.

Hard Work

Camille Bernard Capdeboscq, Jr, was born on January 16, 1933, in the city of New Orleans, but he grew up working on his father's mostly rented farms located slightly south and west of the city—first in Marrero, then in Plaquemine's Parish, back to Marrero, and finally in Waggaman. Except for one stretch as a vegetable farmer, his father was always in the dairy business. The moves were precipitated by the encroachment of civilization. Cap said, "Too many people were moving into the area, and you couldn't dairy there. You had to get away. The property was too valuable to be used as a dairy farm."

As the oldest of four brothers and a sister, the natural course of things was that Camille was expected to work harder than all the others. With nearly 100 cows to milk every day, dairy farming was a 24-hour enterprise. Beginning at age 14, "we used to get up at 2 o'clock in the morning and milk the cows. We'd finish probably by 5 o'clock or 6 o'clock, time enough to go in and bathe—you get all dirty fooling with cows. I'd eat, and it would be time to catch the bus at 7 o'clock. And when I got out of school, I went back home, and I worked again until we were finished." Even when he was 9 or 10, he had helped out in the mornings cleaning up the barns after the cows had been milked. Cap said there was "no time for foolishness or running the streets." In fact, he hardly participated in any after-school activities. He would have enjoyed baseball, but it was out of the question. Camille never protested his workload; it was just the way things were. Wondering about the impact of all that work on his studies, I asked if he did well in high school. Cap said, "No, not at all. I just passed. I was worn out by the time I got there."

Life was not particularly easy, but it was not devoid of fun either. He enjoyed going to an occasional dance, and Cap recalls the one high school stage production in which he participated as an actor. He initiated his reputation as a prankster by surreptitiously pinning a crepe paper tail on a fellow actor just before he went on stage. "Prankster" might have been too benign a word for some critics. During high school a principal had punished him and two other boys with a whipping. The other two boys had been whipped for fighting. Camille had been whipped for being the instigator. Cap said that he received similar punishments from his father. "If I didn't behave when I was growing up, he whipped me." It wasn't that his father would "brutalize anybody." His father's attitude was simply, "'How do you raise five kids and keep them all in line if you don't spank them occasionally?' And he did. He'd give you a couple of whacks, and you knew he meant business." Cap felt that his father's approach to discipline was nothing more than what most people did in those days and under those circumstances.

He remembers with pride that his father's greater legacies were an abiding respect for honesty and the hard work necessary to responsibly look after a family. Cap remembered one of his brothers saying, "I've never seen anybody more honest than Dad, and have as little as he had, and work as hard." Cap agreed. "He would work as much as two or three people. He wasn't the fastest, but he just never stopped. And the type of a business that he was in, that's all you did was work." Cap said he was once shocked to hear his father say he loved to hunt. "I didn't think he liked anything like that. . . . They didn't have time to do anything."

Camille would help his father deliver milk in the early mornings. Other milk processors were on the road as well. Some of his father's competitors would steal the empty glass milk bottles that his customers had placed outside their doors to be picked up. The thefts made the elder Camille furious, but he never stole milk bottles in retaliation. Instead, he would face the likely perpetrators and inquire about the bottles. He would not go out of his way to be confrontational, but "he would stand his ground, and they would leave him alone. They wouldn't fool with him." Cap said that at 5 feet 6 inches, an inch shorter than himself, "[My father] wasn't big, but it was just his manner, I suppose. He could look fierce."

The family household was not fierce, however. Cap said that his parents, Camille and Rosalie, "had a good relationship." For both parents the central theme of the household was work. They saw life similarly and had similar values, but his father was the dominant figure. "He was quieter than she. She made more noise, but when it came to the showdown, he was the boss. [Yet he was] a very kind-hearted person. I remember people coming over and telling him stories in the barn. They would start crying, and he would cry with them."

> "He is the most giving individual I've ever met. If you ask Cap to do anything for you, it's done."
>
> *Dr Allan Rappold*
> *Dr Capdeboscq's nominator*

His mother made her own special contributions to the family. Cap remembers that the only family vacation he ever had was with his mother and siblings. He was to report to the Air Force in Texas on July 10, 1952–he remembers the date well–at the age of 19. They all rode the train to Biloxi, Mississippi. His father could not leave the farm. It was Cap's first train ride and the first time he had ever left Louisiana. They rented a cabin on the Gulf Coast for a few days and, also for the first time, luxuriated in doing nothing. It is a very special memory.

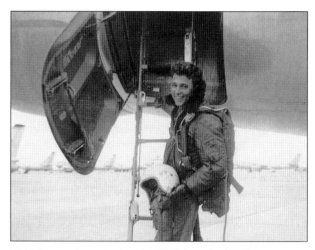

US Air Force engine mechanic and AERO Club member (1955).

Neither of Camille's parents had expectations for his education beyond high school. No one even spoke about it. When he graduated from high school in 1950, he stayed in the dairy business with his father, even though his father had never asked him to stay. As the oldest son, Cap said he just had the feeling that he had no other choice. Furthermore, "I didn't know anything. I knew nothing. All I knew was cows, chickens, hogs, and growing vegetables." It never entered his mind that he might be able to do anything other than farm. However, after a year or so, Camille had had enough and told his father that he wanted to quit. Cap still remembers his father's famous response: "You can't quit, and I won't fire you." The Korean War provided a timely and acceptable solution to the problem. It was either enlist or be drafted, so Camille joined the Air Force.

Awakening

Camille's 4 years in the Air Force were a continual process of transformation. Among the least consequential changes was the nicknaming of "Capdeboscq" to "Cap," something that had never happened to his father. Cap's makeover began when he took the Air Force's aptitude tests, which, because of his background with farm machinery, showed that he was well suited for mechanics and heavy equipment operation. He was sent to Wichita Falls, Texas, for training in the mechanics of reciprocating propeller engines, then to a bomb squadron near his home, followed by assignment to Amarillo, Texas, for training in the increasingly used jet engines. Along the way he took advantage of free flying instruction offered by the Air Force's AERO Club. He became a pilot and maintained his license until his marriage, when his wife thought better of it.

Cap was seeing the country, having altogether new experiences, and enjoying it immensely. The Air Force changed his life. Good grades in mechanics school earned him his first two stripes on his way to staff sergeant, and he saw himself move ahead of others with whom he had arrived. Though he had lacked confidence in his abilities in his early days as an airman, now that he had had widespread dealings with instructors and others who were college educated, he realized, "'Well, gee whiz, I'm as competent as they are.' It made me see that I could do things other than just fool with cows and grow vegetables and plants." Within a year or so, he was convinced that he wanted to get a college education. He was especially certain that he was not going back to dairy farming, or to mechanics for that matter, but he was not exactly sure what he would do. "The only thing I was sure of was that I should go to school." Cap took advantage of the Air Force's offer to get some college credits. His grades were better than in high school: "I was applying myself and I wasn't worn out."

Cap had given veterinary medicine and geology some thought. He already had had a lot of experience with large animals, and geology would position him well to be part of Louisiana's early but ongoing oil boom. Dentistry was nowhere in sight until a fellow pilot and member of the AERO Club who was also a dentist mentioned the idea. The dentist suggested, "Working up in these little access holes in the sides of these engines is like working in a mouth." Furthermore, he pointed out that dentists, just like mechanics, use little mirrors to see into difficult places. With about a year left in the Air Force, the seed was planted.

Entering His Profession

Discharged from the service in 1956, Cap took advantage of the GI Bill, which offered financial support to discharged military personnel, and entered both the pre-veterinary and the predental programs at Southeastern Louisiana College close to home. He also became interested in a new neighbor, the daughter of another dairy farmer who lived across the street from his father's new farm. Her name was Conjetta (Connie) Terrase. She would attend nursing school while he was a dental student, and they would eventually marry in his senior year.

Within 3 years, he had accumulated enough credits to apply to both schools. His application to veterinary school at Texas A&M—Louisiana had no such school—was approved, but only as an alternate. However, his application to Loyola (now Louisiana State University) Dental School was accepted, and he became a freshman in 1959. By this time his parents had become wholly enthusiastic about higher education for their son. They helped out whenever they could, but support from the GI Bill had run out, and Cap essentially financed his own dental education. Sometimes he worked on oil rigs in the Gulf of Mexico, and late in his student career he took a job doing supervised dental treatment at Hope Haven, a home for unruly boys and, more recently, Cuban refugees.

Cap's experience in dental school was like that of many students. He enjoyed learning techniques, he put up with those teachers who taught by fear, and he enjoyed his patients. What set him apart from his peers, however, was his reputation for perhaps having the "best hands" in the class. Classmates frequently came to him for help, and instructors often asked him to help them teach. Cap said that sometimes he thought, "I was like another teacher in my class." In fact, Cap first considered a career in teaching while he was still a student. A classmate told him that he ought to go into teaching right from the beginning, but Cap thought he needed to get some experience first.

Dr Capdeboscq graduated from dental school in 1963 and set up practice in Arnaudville, located west of New Orleans in the bayou country and close to some of the only wild areas left in the country. Cap said, "When I first left school, I figured I was going to do good for humanity. That's why I went there. I was going to cure the world's dental problems." In Arnaudville there were few dentists, loads of patients with untreated disease, and various other problems as well. Most of the residents believed in the fatalistic inevitability of dentures at an early age. Many children spoke only Cajun French. Adjustments to racial integration were still ongoing. Cap said that when he first opened his practice, most places in the region were still segregated, with separate waiting rooms for whites and blacks. "But I didn't. I just had

Commentary

The story of Dr Capdeboscq helps us comprehend the inner life of a highly regarded teacher. In it we see the characteristics of good teaching and the virtues of a good teacher. For US dentists, especially older practitioners, the story resonates because it too often represents the exact opposite of some of their own experiences. Almost every dental school in the country seems to have had its own notoriously legendary "Czar," who was known as much for draconian pedagogy as for technical competence. The irony of this approach to teaching is that, just as the concept of excellence is ground into students' repertoire of professional behavior, so is the model of interpersonal interaction by which the concept was conveyed. Unfortunately this particular model promotes long-lasting and often damaging attitudes and tends to reinforce paternalistic patterns of relationships that endure for caregivers as well as teachers. In addition, the dentist-teacher often seems driven by a need to inflict on students the same wounds that early academic life had inflicted on him or her for deficiencies of habits, knowledge, or abilities.

We do not think that most teachers of dentistry model the tactics of The Czar in Dr Capdeboscq's story. Even so, the qualities and characteristics of Dr Capdeboscq clearly set him apart in the minds of both students and peers. We all want to learn, as did his colleagues, why he was repeatedly nominated as an outstanding teacher. What does the testimony of Dr Capdeboscq's students and peers reveal? What can we learn through Dr Capdeboscq's reflections on his life, the forces that shaped his character, and the way these forces influenced his assumptions about teaching and learning—assumptions that influence the doing that is so highly regarded?

When his colleagues asked him to share with them what made him such a good teacher, he could not respond. He was unable to reduce a way of knowing, being, and doing into a handful of tips or techniques. Some might say he lacks an ability to engage in reflective practice. Others, like Palmer,[1p10] would say that "good teaching cannot be reduced to technique; good teaching comes from the identity and integrity of the teacher." Dr Capdeboscq's resistance to reducing the concept of good teaching to good technique, or to telling others how to do it, speaks volumes about who he is and how he thinks of himself in

one waiting room." People told him that it would not work. "But in a place like that, way out in the sticks, it worked out fine. All these people knew one another. They had the best time in the waiting room that you could want. I was amazed."

Cap liked living in that region of Louisiana, and he liked the good-natured generosity of the Cajun people. "They were very, very nice. They would give you the shirts off their backs." Nonetheless, Cap stayed in Arnaudville for only 2 years. He became discouraged: "They could afford dentistry, but they didn't want dentistry. It wasn't important to them. A 16-year-old would get off the school bus wearing a denture, and you'd wonder if you were in the Stone Age." He grew weary of having to explain why he refused to extract sound teeth and initiating futile attempts to change their perspective on oral health. "I figured that I would spend my life there and die and these people would still be ignorant toward dentistry, so that's the reason I decided that I would get out. I wasn't doing what I was trained to do. I wasn't satisfied."

Cap bought a practice in Hammond and an 11-acre farm in Tickfaw, where he still lives. The practice had a huge number of patients and enabled him to do everything he ever wanted to do in dentistry. He enjoyed the relationships he had with his patients and the friendships he made. Cap also enjoyed performing the work of his profession, "very much so. It was a gratifying experience. Especially to fix things that people thought were unfixable." After several years though, "I got to the point where all I did was work, and when I got home I often had to go out at night." Patients would call with toothaches and other problems, and occasionally even showed up at his door, "and I never refused anybody," he said. Cap felt like he was being used up. Having had five children within 7 years, "I just thought that I could have a little more time for family affairs and relaxation." Therefore, with the idea of teaching always having been in the back of his mind, he decided that for "a little relief, I'd get a part-time job" at the dental school. In 1972 he started working 2 days at the school, and a year later the chair of the operative department asked if he would consider coming on full time. Cap asked Connie for her opinion before he agreed. He said that he considered himself fortunate that she had always been so supportive.

The Good Teacher

Concern and Generosity

In the 1985 student awards assembly, the LSU seniors inaugurated an award for the faculty member who had been most influential in their careers as dental students. Dr Capdeboscq received it then and also for the next 2

relation with others. The gift he has given instead, through assisted autobiography, is a picture of an exemplary teacher's inner life. By openly and honestly sharing who he is, he helps us reflect on our own inner lives as teachers or caregivers: who we are, who we want to become, and how we might further discover our own identity. To assist this reflection, Palmer points out that "[identity and integrity] are subtle dimensions of the complex, demanding, and lifelong process of self-discovery. Identity lies in the intersection of the diverse forces that make up my life, and integrity lies in relating to those forces in ways that bring me wholeness and life rather than fragmentation and death."[1p30]

The wholeness of Dr Capdeboscq's identity and integrity is best revealed by the perspective of his students and peers. Each of the qualities his students valued is admirable in itself, but the constellation of qualities is truly impressive. *Available.* Dr Cap was the first teacher to arrive and was accessible to students from then on. *Generous.* He sees teaching as sharing, and he freely shares what he knows. *Engaged.* He was present for students. He truly knew them, not only by name but also by their needs and weaknesses. As one student put it, "Rather than just sitting down and doing something for you, or just telling you the quick way to do things, he really was concerned that you learned what you were doing—I mean, [both] how to treat your patient and how to do the procedure." *Reassuring and encouraging.* He created an atmosphere in which students developed faith in their ability to learn and a willingness to reveal their insecurity and ask for feedback. *Inspiring.* He demanded excellence, held students to high standards, and believed that they could achieve them. *Respectful.* Even while demanding high standards, he evaluated without being intimidating and judged without being judgmental. He gave useful feedback and left students' dignity intact. On graduation day he treated each student as a respected colleague, no matter their level of competence at that time. *Fair.* He was considered the hardest grader, yet students respected him because he was scrupulously fair. Students felt they had earned their grades. *Understanding.* Despite his own extraordinary skill, he was able to view the students' work from their perspective, asking himself if he would be able to do better in similar circumstances. This enabled him to focus on the positive element of performance and offer constructive comments. Further, he allowed students who were having problems with certain procedures to

years, after which the students discontinued it because the same person received it every year. The award lay dormant until 1996 when it was presented to Dr Rappold, Cap's nominator. Having been designated for the first award, Cap's suspicions kept him away from the assembly the next year, just in case. Dr Rappold accepted the award on his behalf. The same scenario was replayed the following year.

Cap did not like the attention, and to make matters worse, during a faculty retreat he received a request to discuss what he did that made him such a good teacher, perhaps so that his colleagues could become better teachers themselves. Cap felt extremely uncomfortable. "I told them I don't know why I got the award, and they left me alone then. It was a terrible spot to be in. They asked me questions, and I didn't know what to tell them. I said, 'You should ask those who gave it.' I didn't appreciate that at all, you know."

Dr Capdeboscq actually has a lot to say about teaching. One of the characteristics for which he was so revered was his respect for, and concern about, the feelings of others. "I always thought that once you do something to somebody, or say something ugly to them, it's hard to retract, even though you apologize. You can't retract it. Never. So I tried awfully hard not to do that to anybody. I didn't like to beat people down,

> "Cap might be a simple man in his lifestyle, but he is a giant in character. He was a superb clinician, yet he never bragged about or even mentioned his extraordinary skills."
>
> *Dean Eric Hovland*

because I had been beat down occasionally, and I knew how it felt." Therefore, when students came to him for evaluations, he consciously looked for ways to avoid being destructive. He said, "There was always something that I could tell them that was good about what they did, even if their overall projects were failures." In addition, he said, "I always offered them an avenue of retreat with dignity." No matter how severe their difficulties, he would always give them the opportunity to explain what had happened without launching such admonitions as, "Don't tell me. I don't want to hear about it." Dr Capdeboscq intuitively wanted to provide a positive start for what then could become a learning experience.

Cap's positive approach was in direct contrast to many of his own experiences as a dental student. One of his own professors, known as "The Czar," had spread terror in the hearts of students. His standards were of the highest order, but he ensured their fulfillment by humiliation and intimidation. Cap said, "I liked the results he got, but I didn't like the method." According to Cap, there are still some people on the faculty who were taught by The Czar, and they still go a little crazy when his name is mentioned. Cap did better than most with this professor, perhaps because he had had "a drill sergeant who was as tough as he was. . . . Once I knew what he

save face by encouraging them to explain what had happened and even to offer excuses for their performance. Recognizing the lasting damage from negative remarks, he was able to restrain his anger and allow the other person an avenue of retreat with dignity. *Trustworthy*. Because the student needn't worry about what he will say or do, especially in front of a patient, Dr Cap was able to calm the anxieties of both student and patient. *Patient*. He was able to wait for the student to develop and then celebrate the student's achievement.

The qualities his peers valued were similar to those of the students: generosity, kindness, dependability, honesty, and his propensity for sharing whatever he has with others. His peers were especially impressed with Dr Capdeboscq's *technical competence*, which is perhaps the trait most admired in dentistry. Endowed with these great talents, he has done what few teachers have been able to do: He has figured out how to maintain high standards and still be decent. It is his exemplification of this concept of teaching that established Dr Capdeboscq as one recognized by his colleagues as standing apart from all others. In addi-

tion, his colleagues recognize that as much as they wish to be kinder, more humane teachers, it is the rare individual who can do so, as did Dr Capdeboscq, by learning from reverse example. Above all, however, without his trademark *modesty*, Cap would not be so widely admired by his peers. He is neither a braggart nor a self-promoter, he rarely turns the conversation toward himself, and he intuitively recognizes that giving advice on how to teach or how to practice is likely to be not only unwanted but essentially unhelpful. Last, his peers admire him for having lived his life well. They respect the simplicity of his lifestyle and admire him for who he is—an outstanding teacher and an outstanding human being. As his dean stated, "He quietly went about his business of sharing his skills with students and *demonstrating moral character through example*. Over time his actions inspired both students and colleagues to look at their own character and values as their respect for Dr Cap developed." This clearly applies to the colleague who nominated Dr Capdeboscq as a moral exemplar: "Although I don't have the power to be exactly like Dr Cap, I am a better person and teacher because of his influence."

expected of me, I did it. And I got along fine with him." In more recent years he heard that The Czar had even liked him. Nevertheless, Cap emerged from the experience with the conviction that it would be desirable to maintain The Czar's standards, but not his philosophy of teaching.

In contrast there was an instructor named Dr Darrell Jobe; students searched for him if they wanted a more humane approach. Dr Jobe's view was that no matter how hard you strived for perfection, it was the nature of dentistry that you might not always achieve it. Cap said that Dr Jobe had a "lot of compassion for the students. I think I learned a lot from him [because of his compassion]. . . . I was tougher than he was, but I used the same approach."

Part of Cap's toughness as an instructor reflected how he evaluated his own skills. He said that when he looked at what a student had done, "I always asked myself, could I do any better as a practitioner? I would always look at that point, and I used it as a determining factor." He often used this assessment to the student's benefit. Sometimes a student's treatment might not look as skillful as one would have hoped, but Cap looked hard for explanations and mitigating circumstances.

Until 1985 Cap had never thought that students might consider him as anything "other than a regular teacher. I never thought of myself as anything higher or greater than that. I just thought that my job was to teach. I had a responsibility, and I tried to fulfill it in the best way I could." To listen to Cap, one would think that the basic concept was simplicity itself and hardly worth mentioning. Explaining himself, he said, "Well, I was obligated to be there to do the cows. And that was something you did twice a day, and you could not ever miss. We were drilled, 'You cannot miss a milking.' Otherwise, they get mastitis, and sometimes they never recover. You end up sending them to the slaughterhouse. That was that! I guess that's where the sense of obligation first got deep-rooted." After that experience, whether it was keeping an airplane in top shape, taking care of a patient, or nurturing a student, the fulfillment of obligations was something that just came naturally. Furthermore, as far as students were concerned, it was clear to Cap that students would learn better if their experiences were positive. Therefore, he tried his best to express his obligation as a teacher with that conviction in mind. What makes Dr Capdeboscq's achievements so distinctive is how much more successful he has been than most of us in dental education. The culture of American dental education, though improving, has too often been symbolized by "Czar" look-alikes.

Cap's reputation for generosity is something that also relates to his days on the farm. The family had a big garden, he said, mainly because of the superabundance of manure. "We had beans and everything you could think of. And my father, the generous soul that he was, would make me go out there and pick all this stuff, after we had been working in the dairy from 2 o'clock in the morning." Then after picking bushels of vegetables, they gave much of it away. This annoyed young Camille

---

If, as Palmer[1] suggests, one's identity derives from understanding the diverse forces that intersect in one's life, and one's integrity derives from relating to those forces in ways that bring wholeness and life, what can we learn about the forces that shaped Dr Capdeboscq's character and the way those forces influenced his approach to teaching?

For Dr Capdeboscq, the diverse, intersecting forces began with a work ethic instilled early. Dependability and responsibility grew from the grinding daily necessity of tending to a dairy farm. The consequences of failing to meet one's work obligation were serious: Cows would die and the farm would fold. One tended not to spend time arguing with oneself about whether the obligation could be postponed or sidestepped. The habit of meeting one's obligation became firmly ingrained. From this early experience with work, Cap also seems to have learned a critical sense of balance. Too much work left one too worn out to learn. Whereas our first impression might be that Dr Cap's 11- or 12-hour days as a teacher were excessive, it pales in comparison with his 16-hour days as a youth, when the morning milking began at 2 o'clock and the evening milking was finished in time for bed. Whereas his father milked cows 7 days a week, Dr Capdeboscq taught class only 4 days a week. He could have enriched himself through private practice on the 5th day of the workweek but chose instead to spend time with family. Further, when presented with opportunities to be an administrator, he declined because it would upset the balance of responsibilities to self and family. Certainly, he could have achieved more as a scholar—he has a modest CV by today's standards in high-pressure universities—but he preferred to devote himself to teaching and to do it well. Dr Capdeboscq's concentration on teaching and family are examples of temperance and balance in foregoing academic advancement for goals that he considered more important.

Honesty and self-control stand out as well as he tells of his father's reaction to stolen milk bottles. Rather than retaliate, his father would confront. In other circumstances, however, his father demonstrated sensitivity to the needs and hardships of others. It is an unusual man who reveals that he

because many of those receiving the vegetables were better off than they were. Furthermore, they did not have to work for it. Not surprisingly, the older Camille ignored his son's suggestions that people who wanted vegetables should come and pick them themselves. In addition, his grandfather did the same thing. Even though he sold vegetables to make a living, if anyone came to his house, he would fill their trunk with vegetables for no charge. Cap said, "That was just the way we did it, and I do the same thing today. I pick I don't know how many vegetables and give them away. I go out on the street looking like a peddler, and I just give all this stuff away." Cap reasons prudently, "I want to make sure that I'll have a sufficient crop. Sometimes you have failure, so I always plant more than enough. And then if everything works out real well, I can give it away. I won't waste it. I keep what I need and I give the rest away."

Part of the reason for Cap's generosity with his vegetables is an affirmation of his heritage. He said that some of the people in his area grew up on strawberry farms, but now, "They hate their past. I don't hate my past. I still grow vegetables, and I have cows. God knows I had a tough time [milking] cows in my life. It was hard. But I still have them, and I still grow stuff, [whereas] these people won't grow a twig."

> "There was always something that I could tell them that was good about what they did, even if their overall projects were failures."
>
> *Dr Capdeboscq on his students*

A Concern for Balance

Dr Capdeboscq was heavily involved in teaching and had contact with students during every year of their program. He taught in the freshman morphology course, the sophomore operative dentistry course, and all the clinical operative dentistry courses. For many years he offered a gold foil technique course to seniors. His colleagues thought he was a good lecturer; he kept his audience's interest. One colleague said, "He wasn't what you'd call real polished. It was like listening to an interesting folktale." Dr Cap also spent many hours each week teaching in the clinic. In his spare time, which was not much, he managed to put together seven publications, including three that were refereed.

At one point in Cap's tenure at LSU the chair's position was open. The acting chair at that time wrote that everyone, himself included, tried their best "to convince Dr Cap to put his name in the hat for head of operative. It is my opinion that he would have gotten the job had he just put his name in." He went on to say, "Dr Cap knew that [administration] was not his calling, but teaching was, and he did a fantastic job of [it]." Cap's evaluation of that opportunity was somewhat different. He said that the primary reason he chose not to apply for the position was not that

was influenced by a father who could elicit the stories of friends and neighbors and "cry with them." Perhaps this same sensitivity heightened Cap's awareness of the insensitivity and hurtful comments he experienced as a youngster. He learned that a negative remark takes on a life of its own and lives on in memory. As he said: "Once you say something ugly, it's hard to retract—you never can." The destructive legacy of negative remarks was reinforced by his own teachers and became a pivotal factor in the development of concern for the feelings of others.

For many dentists of Dr Capdeboscq's era and some today, insensitive and hurtful comments from teachers served as models for interaction that were assumed to be appropriate. Many of us, unlike Cap, are unable to identify why such hurtful comments are inappropriate, let alone how to consistently frame evaluative information in ways that are positive and constructive. When students are observed in the clinic pointing out the faults of their patients, or offering unyielding directives, we see negative modeling in action—whether learned in dental school or in other aspects of life. When students defend these models, arguing that patients want to be scolded for their negligent behavior, we see the insidious effect. Cap was fortunate. He was able to combine the concept of high standards that he learned from The Czar with the human decency he saw modeled in Dr Jobe. Intuitively, Dr Capdeboscq achieved what Fisher and Ury[2] describe as the art of negotiation: Be hard on the problem, soft on the people. They point out that many softhearted people fail because they care so much about interpersonal relationships that they are soft on the problem. To gain respect, one must maintain high standards, but treat people respectfully. Doing so requires exceptional skills in interpersonal communication, in problem solving, and in creating an atmosphere of respect for persons.

Often when teachers assert high standards and demand student accountability, they are viewed as having a form of moral rectitude. Dr Capdeboscq sees it as something much simpler. He said, "I just thought that my job was to teach. I had a responsibility, and I tried to fulfill it in the best way I could." The Czar had taught him about high standards, and when it

he did not like administration. "No, I could have handled that. But I just didn't want to [work] 5 days." At LSU, as in many institutions, the workweek was 4 days with clinical practice being allowed on the 5th day. If Cap had been chosen to be the new chair, he would have received a higher salary, but it would have meant at least another day required for administration. "I wanted to stay home that [5th] day. I was satisfied with what I was doing." He preferred taking care of his farm and the additional time it allowed him with his family over the extra income that a 1-day practice would provide. His father had never had time to play with his children, and Cap wanted to make sure that he would not be put in the same position. In addition, if he were chair, he would have had to buy a briefcase for the first time in his life. He had never needed one before, and he prided himself on being able to handle any preparation time during regular hours, which were substantial anyway. As it was, driving 128 miles each day cut severely into the rest of his time.

One wonders, if Dr Cap had become an administrator, would he have felt constrained to change other aspects of his life? No longer considered a prankster, he was more often described as mischievous. For example, Cap once tied a 20-foot string between a gift bag of habanero peppers and the purse of a colleague who kept forgetting to take them home. She was out of the office and down the hall before she felt the tug. Would he have felt that this was unseemly behavior for a chair? People claim they never saw Cap on an elevator. If he

were the boss, perhaps he would have to stop racing elevator-taking colleagues to lecture halls. In addition, though not exactly an act of mischief, he might have felt it necessary to discontinue his modest showing off of his ability to attach names to faces, last names especially. Often he could remember them for decades. Colleagues said that when examinations were being given, if a count determined that some students were missing, Cap could look out over the assemblage and in a minute or two identify who was missing. Cap confirmed the story and said that he could also do the same thing with cows. He had given each cow a name, and he knew which ones still needed milking.

Dr Capdeboscq clearly felt highly rewarded by his choice of teaching as his primary professional option. He found great satisfaction in being part of the progress that students made during their 4 years in dental school, including the students who had a rocky start during his freshman morphology class. In Cap's view even though some of them might have barely passed, they completed the course satisfactorily. "No matter how difficult it had been through their years in school, after they would graduate and get their diploma, that was it. My job with them was finished, and I would congratulate them and shake their hands. I did that with all of them. . . . I would show them respect as a dentist, as a fellow colleague."

During our time at the cabin on Lake Mary, I learned what it felt like to be a student of Dr Cap's. One morning, I greeted him as he returned from an unsuc-

came to teaching, it was common sense to teach the students to be as good as they could be. Furthermore, from his personal knowledge, offering them a positive experience was smarter than being punitive. As far as grades were concerned, Cap's only concern was that students receive the grades they earned. Why do otherwise?

Dr Capdeboscq never worried about whether his reputation as a tough grader would negatively affect his relationship with students, and current research suggests that he was right—not that he would have cared. The premise that faculty members will receive negative student evaluations if they are perceived as "hard-nosed" has been refuted. Research on college students' perceptions of fairness suggests that fairness is invariably a primary factor in describing the "best teacher" they ever encountered.[3] Such research has shown that students are concerned with three kinds of fairness: interactional fairness, procedural fairness, and outcome fairness, in that order. Students consider that showing partiality or unrestrained anger (including profanity), embarrassing students with sarcasm and insults,

exhibiting an uncaring attitude, and failing to respond to student questions are the most serious interactional offenses that faculty can commit. They judge procedural fairness as more important than outcome fairness. Students assume, as does the general population, that if the procedures are fair, then the outcome will be fair. Consequently, a "tough" faculty member (one who is very strict and gives low grades, but is scrupulously fair) is viewed as more caring, worthy of respect, likeable, and appealing than a professor who is lax and gives high grades. Further, students are deeply concerned about procedural fairness related to the monitoring and regulation of cheating and plagiarism. Students also expect courses to be challenging, and they want the results to discriminate between various levels of performance.

Palmer[1] asserts that persons choose to teach for reasons of the heart, because they care deeply about their students and about their subjects. People who choose to be caregivers come to feel the same way for their patients and their profession. In this story, Dr Capdeboscq has shown how, in Palmer's[1] terms,

cessful 3-hour wait in a tree, hoping a deer would come by. He was carrying a climbing deer stand, a complicated piece of equipment used by hunters to scale trees, and he proceeded to explain it to me. The essential component for using the stand was first to loop a cleated strap around the base of the tree so that the cleats dug into the tree. Then you put your foot into an opening that was attached to the strap and braced against the tree. The opening for your foot served as a stair step. At that point you loop another cleated strap around the tree at about shoulder height, to stabilize your body while you take another cleated-strap step all over again. On it goes until you get to where you want to be. True to form, Dr Cap downplayed my ignorance as a nonhunter, and with great joy in the process of explanation, taught me the procedure. Clearly Cap just loves to teach.

Currently

Despite his love of teaching, for 10 years Cap had planned to retire at the age of 62, although he finally decided to work for one more year. The daily travel had begun to wear on him. He said "I had enough. . . . There comes a time when you have to move, and I told them it was my time to go." He was sent off with a retirement party that was especially noteworthy because of who came. It was attended not only by the customary group of university dignitaries and faculty, but also by some dental students and a sizeable number of the janitorial staff, with whom he had shared early morning greetings for so long. Having attended countless university retirement dinners, I cannot remember such a broad-based tribute.

When I first met with faculty and students upon arriving in New Orleans, it was striking to hear several of his colleagues say almost the same thing: Dr Cap was the only person they knew who had never been the object of unkind words. Having met him, I now understand the meaning of their tribute. His modesty, his giving nature, and his willingness to accept other people on their own terms promote the warmest of feelings in return. Even so, Camille Capdeboscq has high standards and cares about what other people do. This is quite obvious in the high expectations he has for students, as well as those he has set for himself. Over the course of the interview he spoke about the guidelines and rules that he strives to follow. It is a list that he is serious about: honesty, fairness, compassion, kindness, restraint of anger, the Golden Rule, and high moral standards. Although Cap keeps his judgments largely to himself, he is troubled by many things that he sees around him. A partial list of concerns that emerged during the interview includes incompetent colleagues, politicians who accept graft, political systems that encourage graft, people who ignore you when you say good morning, people who don't work hard, people who are lazy and don't work at all, crime in the city, and faculty who say disparaging things about students.

Cap said he misses being with the students. "I miss being there when a new class comes in. I used to like

"to think together" two apparently paradoxical dimensions of good teaching: high standards and decency. The joining of apparent opposites in Cap's pedagogical approach links the student's intellect with his or her emotion, the head with the heart. Learning to honor that paradox can help teachers become more whole. The paradox can be honored for practitioners as well. Consider the similarities between the healer and the teacher in Pellegrino and Thomasma's[4] account of the good healer. To be healed (or to learn) the patient (student) must subject him/herself to the authority of the healer (or teacher) and hope that the healer (teacher) will use his skills to promote the other's welfare. To ignore, override, repudiate, or ridicule the patient's (or student's) ability or person is to assault the patient's (or student's) dignity. This aggravates the disintegration that already exists as a result of illness (or ignorance). The good healer (or teacher) co-suffers with the patient (or student), and out of this co-suffering comes the ability to use one's competence—the cognitive and technical aspects of heal-ing (or teaching and learning)—to fit the unique predicament of the patient (or student).

Whether as a caregiver or teacher, Dr Capdeboscq was able to integrate caring with healing, dignity with high standards. This is what sets him apart from his peers and inspires our admiration.

References

1. Palmer PJ. The Courage to Teach. San Francisco: Jossey-Bass, 1998.
2. Fisher R, Ury W. Getting to Yes: Negotiating Agreement Without Giving In. New York: Penguin Books, 1981.
3. Rodabaugh RC. Institutional commitment of fairness in college teaching. In: Fisch L (ed). Ethical Dimensions of College and University Teaching: Understanding and Honoring the Special Relationship Between Teachers and Students, no. 66, New Directions for Teaching and Learning. San Francisco: Jossey-Bass, 1996:37–45.
4. Pellegrino ED, Thomasma DC. The Virtues in Medical Practice. New York: Oxford University Press, 1983.

that, getting them to start fiddling with wax, and most of them had a difficult time." The freshman students would ask him how he ever learned to master the art of carving wax teeth, and he would tell them, "The only wax I [worked] with before [dental school] was birthday candles," and he just kept trying. Now that he is retired, he said the only time he uses wax is when he grafts trees and uses it to coat the cut surfaces to keep them from drying out.

Reporting on his current activities, Cap said he had just finished grafting a pear tree. His orchard also includes persimmon, apple, plum, peach, black walnut, cherry, and sweet olive trees. A new key lime tree had just been planted as well. His muscadine southern grapes need drastic trimming, and he had just finished disking the garden, getting it ready to plant broccoli, beans, corn, melons, turnips, and garlic. Indoors he is learning to play the piano, having started lessons as soon as he retired. He is now on his own because his piano teacher moved away. She was from Russia and, although her approach to teaching reminded him of The Czar, he had been comfortable with her. Her general attitude was that she could make concert pianists of all her students. Cap said he felt as humbled by her as he had by The Czar.

Early in 2000 Cap attended the annual banquet by Omicron Kappa Upsilon, the national dental honorary society. Each year the banquet honors the new group of students elected to OKU. Cap has gone to each banquet since he retired simply because he wanted to maintain contact with the students and to honor them. The banquet he attended this year was for students who were freshmen the year he retired, the last group he will have known personally. He said, "This is the last year I will go." It's time to concentrate exclusively on the farm.

Questions for Discussion

1. What virtues of professional practice does Dr Capdeboscq illustrate? Assess yourself and the professionals closest to you in terms of these qualities.

2. What are the paradoxical dimensions of good teaching that characterize Dr Cap? What are the similarities between the healer and the teacher?

3. Dentists often focus more on their role as healers and less on their role as teachers. For patients to accept treatment recommendations it is essential that the practitioner be a good teacher. How could you assess your effectiveness as a clinician-teacher?

4. Who were Dr Cap's role models? Were there negative aspects to the modeling that he experienced? If so, how did he overcome them? What strategies have other exemplars used?

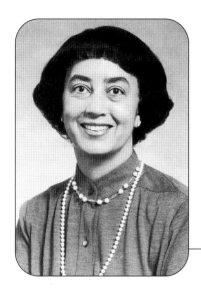

10

Jeanne Craig Sinkford

Moral Leadership in Academic Dentistry

Jeanne Craig Sinkford graduated from Howard University College of Dentistry in 1958 and there began a career in academic dentistry as a clinical instructor. Six years later, armed with specialty training in prosthodontics and a master's degree and PhD in physiology from Northwestern University, Dr Sinkford returned to Howard expecting to develop a research program and continue her clinical teaching. Instead, she was immediately made head of the Department of Prosthodontics and in 11 more years became Howard's dean of dentistry. After 16 years as dean, Dr Sinkford retired and took a position at the American Dental Education Association charged with developing and implementing policy on issues involving gender and minorities in dentistry. In addition to her reputation for her principled approach to getting things done, Dr Sinkford is widely recognized for her dedicated sincerity, her warmth, her concern for others, and her "reasoned reasonableness."

In 1991, after 16 years as dean of Howard University College of Dentistry, Dr Jeanne Sinkford took early retirement and accepted a position as special assistant to the executive director of the American Dental Education Association (ADEA)* in charge of gender and minority issues. Since 1986 recommendations pertaining to these concerns had been lying dormant. Dr Preston A. Littleton, then ADEA executive director, told us that he was "extraordinarily high" on Dr Sinkford's capabilities and her accomplishments. He had expected her to make a good start, but she had been "phenomenally effective" and furthermore had done so "without being obnoxious." Essentially, Dr Sinkford

has become the ADEA's prime mover for minority and gender policies and programs. Dr Littleton described her as "a dedicated, sincere, warm, and gracious person with concern for others, and who is nonetheless highly principled in her approach to issues." He said she possesses the quality of "reasoned reasonableness," which I (JTR) interpreted as a sensible, well-balanced, and persuasive pursuit of her goals.

During her years as dean at Howard, Dr Sinkford had been skeptically aware that the ADEA had not been active in minority and gender issues, even though minority recruitment was a serious problem and about 37% of all dental students were now women. As a result, she had taken the position with some concern about whether the organization was serious about these

*The American Dental Education Association (ADEA) was, until 1999, the American Association of Dental Schools (AADS). It will be referred to throughout as the ADEA.

issues. Not only that, becoming an ADEA employee had meant giving up her temptation to investigate other opportunities, including a university presidency or a deanship in a women's college. (Jeanne Sinkford loved working with young people.)

Therefore, in 1995, when her area of responsibility at the ADEA was formally elevated to the status of a division, she was relieved: she knew they were serious about institutionalizing women's and minority programs. Later, in 1999, another sign of their interest was her promotion to the rank of associate executive director. Her responsibilities were no different, but the recognition was rewarding.

Dr Sinkford said that until she came to the ADEA, she had never been able to work specifically on women's issues. As dean, "I couldn't be partial or do anything special for women that I was not doing for males. When I came to ADEA, that was one of the things that I was charged to do—promote the advancement of women. It was a good fit."

Dr Sinkford's general approach to gender issues was influenced by her own experiences as a dental student. A few of her clinical teachers were women from the Baltic States who freely advised her "not to separate myself out as a female, but to compete as the males would compete, so they would see me as someone with the same skills and the same credentials." More succinctly, one piece of advice was, "Just make sure they don't see you as a 'skirt.'" For the same reason they suggested that she not join the American Association of Women Dentists, and for years she took their advice. However, while she was dean, Dr Sinkford said, "when I saw the large number of female students coming into the school, and saw that they were feeling isolated and that they needed to be able to discuss problems they were having, I felt the need for the student women's association." Even then, she said, "I wanted to be sure that everybody was invited to their activities, so that they didn't isolate themselves in a minority school. I wanted the women to be accepted as colleagues." Through it all, she said, "I've tried not to be a feminist."

Just as important was the prospect of being nationally involved with minority concerns. As an African American and as dean of a minority school, one of the most important problems she faced was minority recruitment. In fact, because of the small pool of minor-

ity students, it was as pressing an issue at Howard as it was for any other school. Nationwide, during most of the 1990s, the number of African American dental students was only about 200, and they were selected from a pool of less than 500. More recently the pool has fallen to below 300, and in 2000 it took a sharp drop to 174. Dr Sinkford said, "We are at a very critical point." Half of the dental schools have seriously underrepresented minority enrollment, with 15 or fewer minority students for the combined 4 years of the program.

During her tenure at the ADEA, Dr Sinkford has left no doubt in its membership that the central office cares about diversity and equity. With respect to minority issues, she has led efforts to help dental schools secure funding for creative recruitment programs, has held national conferences on minority issues, has published a handbook on opportunities for minority dental students, and is currently working to have culturally competent care accepted as a mainstream approach to dental education. Her most important effort is that since 1998 she has been working with the American Dental Association (ADA) in an evolving partnership between practitioners and dental schools that is designed to increase minority access to careers in dentistry.

Dr Sinkford's leadership in gender equity in dental education has included both recruiting women for academic dentistry and then increasing their numbers in leadership programs. In 1998 she organized an International Women's Leadership Conference in France. She established a registry of available dental faculty positions, institutionalized the invitation of female administrators to deans' conferences, and created women's liaison organizations in each dental school. In 1999 the ADEA published the first-ever major study on women's oral health and is now following up with curriculum development. Finally, she helped create the Enid A. Neidle fellowship program (named after a former ADEA president) that offers a 3-month ADEA fellowship on a gender-related academic issue.

The picture that emerges from this brief account of Dr Sinkford's current activities is of a highly capable and principled person who wants to make a difference in important and challenging issues. However, it gives limited insight into the distinctive quality of her career in academic dentistry that has been characterized

> "Jeanne Sinkford is a dedicated, sincere, warm, and gracious person with concern for others, and who is nonetheless highly principled in her approach to issues."
>
> *Dr Preston A. Littleton*

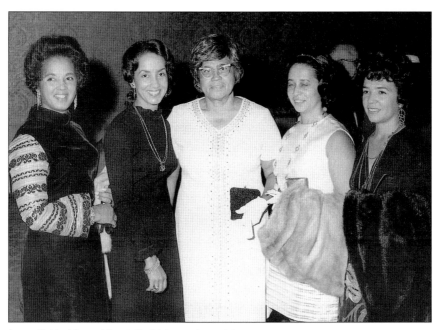

Jeanne Sinkford *(second from left)* with her mother and sisters.

throughout by a concern for ethical leadership. A chronological look at both her career and the influences on her moral development will help our understanding of Jeanne Sinkford as a moral exemplar in dentistry.

Early Years

Much about Jeanne Sinkford's life seems to have been precocious or unprecedented. Born Jeanne Frances Craig, she grew up in an integrated Capitol Hill neighborhood in Washington, DC, where the Craigs were the only African American family on the block. Jeanne's best friends were white. She remembers, "It was a very nice community that we grew up in. We were just like a family. All the parents looked after everybody else's children. They would come to my house and play, or we would go to their house and play and have dinner together. It was really very, very nice."

Jeanne also grew up in a devoutly Methodist family. Her father was a deacon and her maternal grandfather was a minister. For his primary source of income, her grandfather worked a tobacco farm in Sunderland, Maryland. On Sundays, Jeanne said, "He would take off his overalls and perform his function as pastor." Since her mother worked, Jeanne spent summers on her grandparents' farm, reading the Bible, memorizing Bible passages, and on Sundays sitting in the front row of church as insurance against bad behavior. Nevertheless, after attending public school through grade six (skipping fourth grade), she and two of her three sisters attended junior high at a Catholic school, Jeanne skipping eighth grade. The Catholic school was not only closer to home than the public school, Jeanne's mother, Geneva, thought it was better. The academic standards were higher, as were the expectations for discipline. In Jeanne's case this was a good idea. She said, "I think that discipline was absolutely what I needed, because I always wanted to push the envelope. Whatever I was supposed to be doing, I was going to be doing the opposite. I wanted to do what the boys did. I was a tomboy." She loved to go fishing with her father, Richard, and work with her hands around the yard (which she still enjoys).

In Catholic school, Jeanne discovered that a lot was expected from the students. They went to mass every morning and did their catechisms. They never showed up dressed improperly or without having completed their homework. Since the school had no janitor, the students shared the responsibilities for cleaning up. Scrubbing the floors was reserved for those who ignored the rules. Jeanne's discipline improved, but she did a lot of scrubbing, too. The whole experience, Catholicism included, was a good fit with Jeanne's basic orientation to life.

In fact, while still in Catholic school, Jeanne became a Roman Catholic. What she liked about Catholicism was its discipline. "It was an orderly way," she said, "and I guess that was what I needed." She joked that maybe she liked the shorter services, too: "Nine o'clock, out at ten." Despite the humor, it would be a mistake to think that Jeanne did not take religion seriously; for a while, she considered becoming a nun.

At first, her mother was concerned that Jeanne was too young to make such an important decision to become Catholic. On the other hand, Jeanne said her father's views were, "She's always had her own mind, and if that's what's going to get her in church, let her convert." Once her mother was sure that this was what Jeanne really wanted, she acquiesced. Jeanne said that even her Methodist grandparents felt comfortable about her decision.

Jeanne explained why her mother eventually relented and approved her conversion to Catholicism. "My mother was so *evolved*. All of her life she was thinking that there are so many things that would influence your life that you aren't aware of, and there are many gates to heaven. She had friends who were Hindu. She had friends who were Baha'i. She had friends who were every religion. I think that was why I didn't get that much resistance from her. She just wanted to be sure that we had a religious linkage in our lives, so that whatever came up, it was going to be something that would sustain us, no matter what hardships or what challenges were presented."

Jeanne went to Dunbar High School, which was the premier high school for African Americans in Washington, DC, at that time. She loved it. The school accepted only the best students from across the city, and 95% of its graduates went to college. Dunbar was a no-nonsense school that was strictly oriented toward academics. It also had a cadet program, with separate curricula for boys and girls, and Jeanne said, "Of course I was in it." The program developed leadership skills and discipline with a military flair. Once a week, the cadets, dressed in uniforms, arrived at school at 7:30 AM for classes taught by military personnel and based on military-type training manuals. Jeanne felt very much at home. She was designated the captain of her company. The big event of the year was a citywide drill competition that was judged by military officers. Acknowledging that she was "very competitive," Jeanne said her company came in first.

From College Through Graduate School

Jeanne graduated from Dunbar High School at the age of 16 armed with several scholarships, both for Howard and for schools further away. Although she had wanted to go to Syracuse, the family's finances would not allow it, so she chose Howard. Her father worked for the federal government, first as a cook in one of the large hospitals and ultimately as procurer of culinary supplies. Her mother had a short career as a teacher, but soon took a job in the Department of Commerce, which offered a significantly higher salary. It took hard work to put Jeanne and her sisters through college. At one point all four sisters were in college at the same time. After her two older sisters graduated, they pitched in to help Jeanne. "It was kind of like the Marshall plan for the family. They thought I would never graduate."

Jeanne graduated from college in 1953 with a dual major in psychology and chemistry and a husband, Stanley Sinkford, who was a medical student at Howard. When Jeanne was in high school, she had wanted to be a psychiatrist, but by the middle of her junior year in college, it was clear that she intended to be a dentist. Jeanne said that unfortunately "science majors at that time were not directed to careers in dentistry." Nonetheless, her family dentist had encouraged her to study dentistry. It was when her relationship with Stanley matured that she made her final decision to pursue dentistry because "He was already in medical school, and I did not want to have a conflicting profession." Although Jeanne had planned to enter Howard University College of Dentistry in the fall of 1953, the August birth of the

> "Discipline was exactly what I needed, because I always wanted to push the envelope. Whatever I was supposed to be doing, I was going to be doing the opposite."
>
> *Dr Sinkford*

first of her three children resulted in a year's delay. Jeanne entered dental school visualizing a career that included both research and practice. When she graduated in 1958–first in her class and senior class officer–she stayed at Howard for 2 years as an instructor in prosthodontics and also ran a part-time practice. Meanwhile, her husband, now a physician, completed his military obligation and training in pediatrics. Together they spent the next 4 years in Chicago, where Stanley completed a cardiology fellowship at the University of Chicago and Jeanne pursued training in prosthodontics and a PhD in physiology at Northwestern University. She was now fully committed to an academic career in research and teaching.

Unexpected Opportunity

When Jeanne returned to Howard in 1964, she expected to initiate a research program in oral physiology. Instead she found a vacancy in the chairmanship of the Department of Prosthodontics and a request for her to fill it. Looking back, Jeanne attributes this exceedingly early opportunity to the fact that because there were so few minorities in training programs, when someone with a broad background came along, career-altering demands were placed on her. To make the offer attractive, the university appointed her as associate professor; thus she once more skipped a "grade"–this time the rank of assistant professor. Jeanne took the position despite an initial reluctance, stemming from the fact that there would be no time to do research. (Later, as dean, she sublimated her personal research interests by helping faculty and students find money for research, developing research training programs, lobbying the National Institutes of Health for money to support minority research programs, and serving on the advisory council of the National Institute of Dental Research and the Institute of Medicine. Additionally, during her 16-year tenure, she read every advanced education thesis to monitor quality and as a commitment to research.)

Another concern Jeanne had was that the department, which included both fixed and removable prosthodontics, "was the largest [department] in the school, and it was having difficulty merging the two specialty areas." The "fixed" people and the "removable" people were constantly at odds with each other; the patients were affected, and the students were caught in the middle. Jeanne said that for her to survive, she had to be

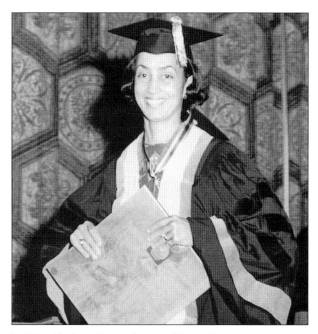

Dr Sinkford is elected into the American College of Dentists.

effective in "getting people to work together, putting the patients' needs ahead of individual likes and dislikes, and retraining the faculty so that people could teach across disciplines."

Jeanne was chair from 1964 to 1968 and apparently survived quite well. During her tenure, the already large department was made even bigger by the merger with the operative dentistry department to create the Department of Restorative Dentistry. In addition, beginning in 1967, she was promoted to professor and took on the added duties of associate dean, which included the responsibility for research, advanced education, and special programs. It was a catchall position that gave her extensive experience in program development, implementation, and oversight. A year later she devoted essentially all of her time to the associate deanship.

An important issue surfaced while Dr Sinkford was chair that lasted through her years as dean: the special challenges of teaching minority students. As she described it, since many Howard graduates would be serving populations that had little access to specialists, the faculty had an obligation to prepare them to handle most of the problems that would present in their practices. It was an obligation that was essential to recognize but almost impossible to fulfill given the time it takes for a dentist's clinical judgment and skills to

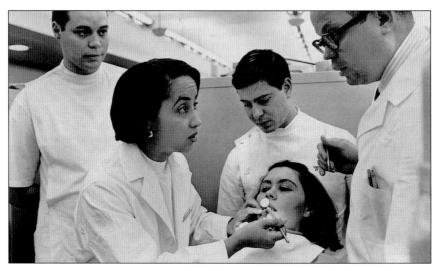

Dr Sinkford in the clinic.

mature. In her 5 years as chair, however, Jeanne recognized that her practical concerns were similar to that of every other chair in the country. She spent much of her time elevating the standards of faculty performance and finding qualified full-time teachers who were committed to dental education.

Deanship

Style and Substance

Dr Sinkford's selection as dean came in 1975–the International Year of the Woman–while she was on sabbatical leave at Children's Hospital in Washington, DC. It was the first time a woman had ever been appointed dean of a US dental school, and it would be nearly a quarter of a century before it would happen again. At the time, she was working on the development of a curriculum for adolescent dentistry. Her intent was to structure the adolescent curriculum as a "subspecialty" of pediatric dentistry such as had been done in medicine. She thought that pediatric dentistry would be the discipline of choice to contain this effort, since it already included groups such as the handicapped, the institutionalized, and other special needs patients that others were not trained to care for. In acquiring this experience, she decided to be certified in pediatric dentistry, mainly because she wanted to be sure that her

colleagues would accept her efforts in curriculum development.

When she left for her sabbatical leave, she had no idea that her dean, Dr Joseph Henry, had plans to retire. Jeanne said, "Being a dean was not on my mind, was not on my radar screen. In fact, I didn't want to be the dean. I had my doctorate in physiology. I wanted to develop the research programs at Howard, which needed someone to be there and just do it. And as the dean I couldn't do that. That was one of the things that I always regret. I don't know whether, if I had not accepted the deanship and had stayed strictly in research, would we have been able to build up the basic sciences/clinical interface that I think all dental schools need, and they need them critically now."

Nonetheless, Dean Henry convinced Dr Sinkford that, given her background, she was the person most prepared to succeed him. As associate dean, her experience was extensive. Dean Henry had been on the road often and had left her in charge. She had the reputation of getting things done. She had had experience handling emergencies, negotiating salaries, articulating the school's programs at the president's level, and had been active in maintaining good alumni relations, although some alumni had asked if she was tough enough.

A deficiency of toughness did not seem to be a problem. Jeanne said, "I was hard-nosed, and I was determined and persistent. I knew where I was coming from. I was very clear." For example, a time arose when due process became important for problems involving both students and staff. Dr Sinkford tried to make sure that the dental school was on its toes. Whenever a case came up, they were always prepared. Documentation was complete. The university's attorneys viewed the dental school as a model from which others could learn. Dr Sinkford said, "I made sure that the department chairs knew what they were supposed to do." Her view was, "Don't come to me telling me that you don't know what the policy is. And don't tell me that you haven't followed it and then expect my support. I think they respected that, because I was like that with everybody. It also raised their level of expectation." Asked if she was more hard-nosed with faculty or with students, after a pause, she said, "Faculty, because I thought they should know better." Jeanne was aware that her firmness might have its price. When I told her about Preston Littleton's judgment that she was effective without being obnoxious, she responded, "I try to be. But that's not what some of my colleagues would say. If you are going to insist on trying to do what's right and insist you've got a goal, then a lot of people are going to stand in the way, drag their feet, and not do what's right. I think I was appreciated, but I am always for excellence and I think sometimes you can't achieve what you want to achieve. But if you set standards low, then achievements will be low."

Despite her firm approach to maintaining the standards of the institution, she wanted to be thought of by students and faculty as approachable when there were problems to solve. She avoided the caustic remarks and overpowering demeanor that some persons of authority exude. That was not her style. Instead, she valued eye contact, patience, and observation of nonverbal communication as entrées to understanding. Jeanne's concern was, "How do I get people to respond in a positive way so that they accept it [as their own] doing rather than something that I am demanding." Her goal was to encourage others to participate in decision making in a way that "doesn't change the standards, and it doesn't change my expectations of what you do. It just changes how you respond and how you assume some responsibility for change or for your actions." From Jeanne's standpoint, there is no dichotomy in being hard-nosed and in maintaining "reasoned reasonableness."

Jeanne said, "My mother was very much the same way. She was loving and caring [just like my father, who was] maybe gentler than my mother." However, her mother was the one who "had to see that things got done . . . She was going to see that you did what you were supposed to do. You did not overspend. You bud-

geted your time. You washed your clothes; you ironed. It meant order. I don't like chaos and disorder. I can do a lot of things at one time, but there's got to be a certain amount of order and priority. That's what I learned very early, and it is not contrary to being gentle and kind." Jeanne's Grandfather Jefferson had left his mark as well. On summer weekdays at the tobacco farm, he got the Craig children and their cousins up before dawn to help with the chores. Jeanne said, "We were city kids according to them, and we were lazy." Despite their perceived deficiencies, the thing Jeanne remembers is "the gentle nature in which he corrected us." She said he was a wonderful role model.

For Jeanne Sinkford, her professional life and values are intertwined with her personal values and her religious beliefs. She thinks that the Golden Rule and the need for honesty—obviously important concepts in religion—are also the bases for professionalism. She says, "It's almost a feeling of being in balance when you have your religious beliefs in sync with your behavior. I just have a good feeling that I'm doing right, that I'm doing what I am supposed to do."

Jeanne thinks that in some way her professional involvements and how she conducted them were influenced by her religious beliefs. "I think so, but I don't think it was a conscious thing. I was always concerned about whether it was the right thing to do, or whether it was just and fair. [However] I don't think I had time to think about whether it was religious. I just had the religious background that gave me the strength to fight opposition or put in long hours or whatever the job required."

The job frequently required long hours, and it was often necessary to find a way to gain perspective. Jeanne says, "I pray every day, and I meditate. I pray all the time. I pray for other people and I pray for myself. I think that communication with God is important. I think so many good things come to us that we don't take time to appreciate them. When I come down here to get in my car, before I start the motor, I say a prayer. When I'm driving up the street, I might be listening to music, and then all of a sudden I realize that I'm praying again. It's kind of a part of me, and it makes me feel good." She also meditates each day for about 15 minutes. "I think that meditation is a very important part of my life. Sometimes you just need to hear what is there, but you are too busy to get it. A sense of what's right and wrong comes to you when you distance yourself from all the things around you, and you're quiet, and you're not being distracted." At times, when Jeanne meditates, passages from the Bible emerge. Now and again, she hears her mother's voice reacting to her current state of mind, sometimes in a memory of a childhood reprimand for a willful act.

The Pleasure of Being a Dean

"The pleasure of being a dean," Dr Sinkford said, "is being able to see the students with fresh young minds, that don't even know what they are going to be, come into your environment. And in 4 years you've got to be sure that they are able to step out there and assume the responsibility for all the patients they're going to treat for the rest of their lives. It was such a challenge to meet those responsibilities of providing the kind of experience they needed. I love students."

It seems that the sentiments were reciprocated. During her years as dean, she received 10 awards from either the student council or one of the classes (an extraordinary acknowledgment from the point of view of one with almost four decades of employment at four dental schools). Jeanne Sinkford explained, "I tried to keep an open-door policy, and I think that's what the students respected. I didn't have a lot of time to spend with students, and I hated the fact that most of the time students [came to] my office was when they got in trouble. So I

> Dr Sinkford's professional values are intertwined with her personal values and religious beliefs. She thinks the Golden Rule and honesty—two important concepts in religion—are also the bases for professionalism.

tried to have an open-door policy during the lunch hour. . . . They always knew they didn't have to make an appointment if they had something that was pressing." Sometimes they did come with pressing problems, such as complaints about faculty whom they felt were not grading fairly. Often, however, they would come to get Dr Sinkford's advice on where to apply for a residency or how to manage advanced education in conjunction with the employment of a spouse in a distant city. Additionally, students served on the school's Executive Committee. Dr Sinkford gave them her respect and support. She viewed their participation both as a way to develop leadership and to promote communication. Jeanne said that hopefully through this experience "they begin to understand that administrators aren't sitting back making rules and policies that are against them; rules and decisions are made for their benefit." Once a month she would have a bagel breakfast with an open agenda for different groups of seniors. She did this for years and never tired of it.

In addition to the cordial relationships she had with students, Dr Sinkford also enjoyed working with the support staff. In fact, they too once presented her with an award of appreciation. For years, the staff, an active group that would give Christmas parties for senior citizens and launch bake sales for stu-

Commentary

In an oft-cited interview conducted by Doris Kearns Goodwin some 20 years ago, author James MacGregor Burns[1] identified a key characteristic that distinguishes true leaders from mere power wielders. Drawing on examples from history, he showed how power wielders are guided primarily by their own objectives of control and respond to their followers' needs and motivations only when they have no other options. True leaders, on the other hand, view their charge first and foremost as the recognition and mobilization of their followers' needs. Furthermore, effective leaders reach beyond the satisfaction of basic needs to attain new and "higher" needs. They arouse hopes, aspirations, and expectations. But by arousing higher-order needs, leaders put themselves at risk. Unless the leader is exceptionally resourceful, flexible, and effective, the expectations that he or she has created can mutate into thorny, politicized demands that, in turn, may undermine the leader. When

the leader is effective in satisfying the newly aroused higher-order needs of the followers, the engagement may transform even the leader's motives and aspirations.

As we reflect on Jeanne Sinkford's account of her life's work, we see how her motives and aspirations were altered by the needs of the faculty, staff, students, and even the profession she served. For example, she began her academic career with a subdued gender-activist role, concurring that to be accepted by the community she could not "be seen as a skirt," nor did she join women's organizations. Later, as dean, when she engaged with faculty and students and began to identify with the needs of the women she was serving, her goals were transformed. Still later, in her current position, seeing the need for the kind of mentoring and support provided by women's organizations, she actively championed their development within the profession. It is fascinating to observe how her sense of responsibility to those she serves expanded. While preparing this commentary, I (MJB) received the announcement for the Second International Women's Leadership Conference

dents, had come to Dr Sinkford for advice and occasionally for money. At one point they were in a jam. They had committed themselves to join a campus union, but when they fully understood the financial implications, they questioned whether the benefits were worth the cost. They approached her once again, this time with trepidation, fearing that Dr Sinkford would be angry about their decision to enter organized labor. Although she had not been upset with them, as the school's chief administrator, it would have been a conflict of interest to offer any advice. Working with the university's general counsel, Jeanne arranged for them to get some legal advice, and ultimately the staff was able to withdraw from the union without penalty. The staff was grateful for her help and relieved that she had withstood their adventure with equanimity.

As to Dr Sinkford's relationships with faculty, she said, "I think the faculty knew that I was trying to do what was right for them also." She tried in as many ways as she could to improve their professional experiences. She decreased the number of their teaching contact hours (which were extremely high compared with other university units) so that they had more time to work on research or other academic assignments. One year when salary raises for the faculty were almost nonexistent, Dr Sinkford successfully proposed to the chairs that they, along with the deans, give up their salary increases so that the junior faculty could receive significant raises. She provided many opportunities for continuing education and conducted full faculty meetings every month and retreats each year. Furthermore, she did not meddle in academic decisions that properly belonged to the faculty. She said, "I never had a problem with the faculty, because, I don't know, I just felt that dental school faculty thought they were underdogs anyway. They felt the department chairs didn't appreciate them. They had to work long hours as compared with the rest of the university faculty. Their salaries were not comparable to private practice. So I did whatever I could to make them feel that what they did was appreciated and to try to give them the resources they needed to do a good job."

Moral Concerns

Asked what she thought were the essential qualities of a dean, Jeanne said, "Honesty and integrity, I think, first. I put [them] at the top, because you are always challenged, and you're always making decisions. And if you're not moralistic, how are you going to tell somebody else to be? How in the world are you going to implement things if you're not?" She said that in professional schools, "You're always asking people to do over and above what the job requires. If you just do what the job requires, you're not going to get things done. You've always got to be overextended." In addition to those qualities, "we have to have intelligence and diligence and 'stick-to-itiveness.' I think those would be the top things. And then I think you have to be willing to take chances. Last of all I would say you have to be a visionary." As important as these latter qualities are, a dean's

organized by Dr Sinkford and Dr Lois Cohen (of the National Institute of Dental and Craniofacial Research). The conference addresses "Global Health Through Women's Leadership." The development of women as leaders is the subtext for an expanded goal: women coming together to affect the health of all women, particularly less-privileged women.

This kind of evolving concern, as described by Burns[1] in his discussion of transforming leaders, motivates *executive integrity*. Srivastva and Cooperrider[2] describe executive integrity as "one of the key life-sustaining properties" of organizations. They define integrity as "a unifying process leading to a state of wholeness, completeness, or undividedness." For them, "organization is impossible without integrity, for by definition organization is differentiation integrated,"[2p5] suggesting that the complex interaction among the diverse strata of any organization will fail without unifying coordination. In this context, then, executive integrity is a moral orientation to leadership and decision making. When organizations have Burns-type transforming leaders, they create an environment in which integrity can flourish. Although Jeanne Sinkford does not speak of executive integrity in these terms, the elements that Srivastva and Cooperrider describe are evident in her perspectives on leadership. Jeanne believes that these elements can be learned and that she can teach them. She tacitly applies the following ideas.

Executive integrity, applied to academic leadership, is a process embedded in social *interaction*, carried forward through the initiation of mutual *dialogue*. The movement is *directional*, starting with face-to-face relationships and then widening to include more distant relationships and the societal and professional environments in which they are embedded. The presence of integrity is *consequential*, resulting in the construction of new meanings (values) and forms (social arrangements) that reduce schisms and enhance the relational life of the whole. Let's examine these processes as Jeanne employs them in her leadership roles.

Interaction. Dr Sinkford seems to take pleasure in creating opportunities for people who need help. For example, in her

business cannot be conducted properly without honesty and integrity. However, Dr Sinkford believes that these traits are no more important for a dean than they are for any other professional. "It is the public trust that we exist for. If you don't buy into that, you have no business being a professional. The public trusts us. If we tell the public something, it's not like selling them a car. We're telling them something for their benefit."

In her deanship, as in every aspect of her life, Jeanne observes that there is a moral component to each action and each decision. "Most of the time I think you do it unconsciously. You don't really think about it. Whether you recognize it or not, you're making judgments that are going to affect people's lives, how people respond, and how they accept things in a positive way versus a negative way." Sometimes, however, the decisions are weighty, and one's moral courage is challenged. The experiences of being a dean provide more difficult challenges than do most positions. Dr Sinkford said there were times when she was asked to do things in return for money. She had requests to accept money for poorly conceived or unhelpful projects. She had offers of money to accept unqualified students. Usually when money was proffered, it was the dental school that was to benefit, but once Dr Sinkford was personally offered $25,000 in exchange for the admission of a student. The latter offer was outrageous and easy to reject. Sometimes, however, Dr Sinkford said, "It takes a lot of courage to say no. I have to weigh whether I'm being too moralistic, because I know that the competition [for money] is great and it [could mean] survival. You have to think about all the other people that you are either helping or hurting with those kinds of decisions." Dr Sinkford continued, "I'm always leery of financial ventures that are presented to you as win-win. Something goes off in me that says back off and think about it and see what the bottom line is before you make a commitment. You have to sleep at night. I guess my angel is looking over my shoulder sometimes."

For Dr Sinkford, as for several deans before her, an overarching issue was "maintaining quality and excellence. Always quality and excellence." Howard University was viewed as a model for the collaboration between federal subsidies and higher education. The fact that half of Howard's budget came from the federal government meant that a national commitment existed. Each year the dental school accepted students from across the nation, usually from more than 20 different states. Dr Sinkford said that Howard University wanted to be sure that, when the students returned home, they "were able to compete with graduates from across the country. They would be practicing in communities with dentists from other institutions, and we wanted to be sure that excellence was one of the objectives that we incorporated. We have always pushed for excellence, and that's very difficult in a minority institution. The students come with varied academic backgrounds, but they are there because they have reached a certain level. They have already been screened. To get into dental school, they have already overcome a lot. And when they leave, they will be in the

role as dean, she developed multiple ways to learn about issues of concern to students, faculty, and staff. The open-door policy, the lunches without agendas, and the involvement of students on the Executive Committee were all ways of encouraging dialogue. In addition to developing leadership, she helped them appreciate each other's perspective. But as important as the opportunity for interaction is, she also respected and supported faculty decisions. She spoke of "not meddling" in faculty decisions, but also of holding people accountable for following rules. Through force of personality, she promoted respect, collegiality, and a willingness to give of herself for the good of community. Her story of motivating department chairs to give their raises to younger faculty during a time of retrenchment is a particularly telling example. Similarly, she related a story of staff who came to her for advice and counsel about joining the union. Most leaders would point out their own conflict of interest and leave it at that. Jeanne worked out a way for these colleagues to get good advice. She consistently orients herself to the others she serves.

Dialogue. Jeanne sees executive integrity as more than setting standards and promoting values, as essential as they are. She understands that the way to develop a culture of organizational integrity is through open dialogue. Jeanne exhibits a fearless trust in what true dialogue and understanding might bring to problem resolution or to the creation or revision of policies. Accomplishing true dialogue, in Jeanne's view, requires more than trust. It requires respect for dissenting voices and tolerance for candid and sometimes volatile meetings while working for "reasoned reasonableness." It requires cultivating an environment in which people would bring their problems to her rather than go to a lawyer. Reflecting on dialogue in the larger professional arena, Jeanne's report on graduate education moved the profession to "reasoned reasonableness" with respect to the proliferation of specialty programs.

Directional. Through dialogue, the executive acquires a more extended, empathic, and valid conception of the broader context in which the organization is embedded. It is interesting

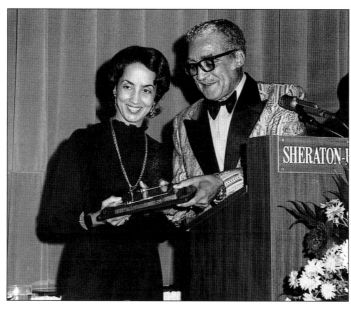

Dr Sinkford receives a Howard University Alumni Achievement Award from Dr Edward Mazinque, then president of the Alumni Association.

'upper' stratum wherever they are. So we were trying to build in a feeling of excellence for all of our graduates."

From Dr Sinkford's view, part of the concern for quality and excellence had to do with the development of sensitivity, responsibility, and concern for individual patients and a sense of obligation to the larger community as well. Jeanne had seen her own perspective about obligations to patients grow during her years as a student. As a teacher and a dean, she had observed that somewhere around the end of the junior year or the middle of the senior year, students acquire an expanded view of their responsibilities to patients. They acquire confidence in their skills and a feeling that they are in charge; they also realize that the well-being of their patient is in their

to observe Jeanne's career development with respect to this process. She began with a narrower focus—to conduct research in physiology, the area in which she received her PhD; but almost immediately, she responded to what her community needed more—the leadership she was able to provide. At various times she tried to return to her original purpose—also a community need—and made scholarly contributions to her discipline. Her scholarly output reveals how the interactional and dialogic processes of leadership have transformed her perspectives, motivations, and aspirations. Her publications demonstrate an exceedingly broad perspective that transcends her discipline and reaches to all aspects of her profession. For example, her publication record encompasses science; "nuts-and-bolts" dentistry; graduate education; manpower needs; clinical evaluation; minority recruitment; developmentally disabled children; minorities in dentistry; trends in dental education; education in dental public health; helping students who fail; strategies to achieve world dental health; the future of dentistry; oral health care needs in African Americans; impaired

dentists; oral health problems in the elderly; classification of malocclusion; women's health; women's issues; and sexual harassment.

Consequential. As dean, Jeanne understood the importance of transmitting values, especially the maintenance of professional standards and the treatment of patients with respect, compassion, and concern. She challenged young minority students to achieve those standards and to expand their frame of reference beyond their offices into their communities. Communication of aspirations such as these serves to promote unity and continuity between any academic institution and the public it serves. The force of integrity is realized each time new forms of responsiveness to students emerge; each time new systems and policies are put in place to address longstanding inequities (minority recruitment); each time complex differentiations are integrated into a coordinated unity (culturally competent care); and each time self-interest is replaced by an increased solidarity with others (the evolution of the themes for women's leadership).

hands. They come to understand that when they enter the clinic, it is necessary to put their personal problems and their daily preoccupations aside and concentrate exclusively on their patients. They begin to feel that it is an honor and a privilege to treat patients. Dr Sinkford tried to create an overall environment that enhanced those transformations. Ultimately she tried to help the students view their patients as individual people, rather than as "requirements for graduation."

Dr Sinkford also worked to help students understand their obligations to their community. Her view was that although they would probably practice in neighborhoods where patients have the financial means to pay for their care, they should also expect to provide care for the disadvantaged and to participate in "neighborhood planning programs in their churches and their schools." Jeanne believes that students take such messages to heart. Some of the school's programs were especially effective in developing sensitivity to the underserved. One was a home care health program for the elderly homebound, which involved students going to the homes of patients to provide care. Another program was at a neighborhood elementary school where students rotated to provide oral health care information. Former students often have told her how those experiences have served as models for their involvement in their own communities.

> "I just grew up feeling that whatever you had was a gift, and that you had certain talents, and you were supposed to use them."
>
> *Dr Sinkford*

Besides the aspirational aspects of the education program, it also had its problems. One thorny problem faced by all deans is the management of cheating. For example, when it is clear that a student is guilty of cheating on a major examination, how does one determine a just sanction? Opinions among faculty members range from taking the course over to expulsion. Some want to give the student another chance, while others focus first on the need to protect the public. Dr Sinkford commented, "It's difficult to say. Each situation is different. I think we certainly have to take the high road and protect the moral standards of the profession. But because of the cultural differences and the levels of acceptability [of cheating] that I found, cultural mores played an important role in how some individuals perceived cheating. I think the leader has to uphold the standards of the profession, but you've got to be flexible enough to understand that there can be extenuating circumstances, and those would mitigate discussion. And that's why you bring other groups in to talk about it. You have individuals that are hard-liners and individuals that are more flexible, and you come with a compromise solution that you can live with. But it's not easy, because sometimes innocent people get caught, and they have to suffer [too]. The academic environment is a learning environment, and some people come with beliefs and values that aren't what they ought to be because we don't pretest beliefs and values. They come

---

Although we see the elements of executive integrity in Jeanne's account of leadership, do others agree? The test of executive leadership, according to Robert Greenleaf,[3p13,14] is whether those served grow as people and whether, while being served, they become healthier, wiser, freer, more autonomous, and more likely to become servants themselves. Greenleaf's criteria have an even broader component: whether the least privileged in society will benefit, or at least not be harmed.

Our evidence of Dr Sinkford's effectiveness as a leader rests not only on her account of the processes she employed to promote the autonomy of others, but also on the testimony of others. Certainly there are her numerous citations for leadership; yet leadership, as Burns[1] points out, does not necessarily constitute true leadership or moral leadership. In our search for moral exemplars, Jeanne Sinkford was mentioned several times, especially by other women, not so much for her moral accomplishments but primarily because of her achievements in the professional world. She was as honored for her administrative

leadership as Irwin Mandel (see chapter 11) was for his pioneering research in salivary physiology. Just as it took time to become aware of the subtle moral aspects of Dr Mandel's integrity as a researcher and his warmth as a mentor, it was not until we began to explore the definitions of executive integrity, together with the qualities and characteristics that Jeanne expressed in our interviews, that we began to understand more clearly the meaning of moral leadership and its complexities and challenges.

David Kolb[4] argues, "The challenges of moral leadership are the most difficult in advanced professional life. For many, caring relationships and careful work have been continuously growing since early career. The requirements of moral leadership are often sharply discontinuous, offering difficult new challenges—to be a public person, to represent others, to serve as a model for others, to be a leader and creator of culture, to choose right from wrong in the most complex of circumstances. . . . The tasks of moral leadership are to make judgments about value priorities, to promote them in one's activi-

in with GPAs [grade point averages] and DATs [dental aptitude tests] and letters of recommendations, but all of those provide limited information. The teachers, however, who work closely with the students, begin to know which students let things slip by and which ones do not. Furthermore, the students' peers know even more. The involvement of both groups helps determine who happened to have gotten caught up and maybe is an 'innocent type' versus the person who is bending the rules all along and you just haven't caught them. These situations are rare, but when they occur, they require due process and observance of academic policies."

There were also the moral concerns that occur wherever people work together. Of these, sexual harassment was one of the most compelling. It had many variations: faculty to staff, faculty to faculty, faculty to student. Often the subtleties of the situations made equitable resolutions difficult. "Some women play games with men, so males don't really know whether it's a game, or whether they're getting into trouble. Sometimes I felt sorry for them, because they were going down the path, and it was too far. So I had to step in." At that time, there were no written guidelines for managing sexual harassment complaints. Dr Sinkford's approach was to try to cultivate an environment in which people felt that they could trust her to settle situations equitably. "I was prepared to make the difficult decisions, and therefore the individuals were willing to bring their problems to the dean rather than go to a lawyer." When complaints occurred, Dr Sinkford said she tried to foster discussions

that would lead to rational solutions without litigation. It seems that not only would she try to appraise the differing perceptions of fact, she would do it with compassion, focused observation, and an open mind–plus toughness as needed.

Reflections

In a long and illustrious career, Dr Sinkford has received many awards and much recognition. Among them, Howard University presented her with its Alumni Achievement Award at its 125th anniversary celebration. She has been listed in at least five classifications of Who's Who, and roughly 30 groups have given her awards or citations for various significant contributions, distinguished services, or outstanding achievements. Ten publications, most representing the interests of women or African Americans, have acknowledged her professional accomplishments. She has received presidential citations from the ADA and the National Dental Association (twice) and honorary degrees from Georgetown University, the University of Medicine and Dentistry of New Jersey, and the University of Detroit-Mercy.

Dr Sinkford's academic leadership has been reflected in the breadth and scope of her writing. She has authored scores of papers, with at least 30 appearing in refereed journals. An extraordinary number of the articles, more than 80%, appear with her name as the senior author.

---

ties, and to preserve these values through the creation of a culture that sustains them."[4p77] Jeanne observed that in her role as dean, as in every aspect of life, there is a moral component to each action and decision. Though courage is often required to say no, she believes that she possesses a strong sense of right and wrong that guides her in making decisions. Interestingly, Kolb[4] cites a study of advanced professionals, of whom 67% said that "a strong sense of right and wrong" was the personal characteristic that best described them. Of that group, for those rated as most highly successful, the proportion was even higher: 78%.

What were the contributing factors to Jeanne's development of executive integrity? She spoke with warmth about the early influences of growing up in an integrated neighborhood; having a grandfather who modeled a gentle nature in correcting her; and having parents who loved her and whose open-mindedness supported Jeanne's decision to convert to Catholicism. It was obvious that Jeanne grew up with a firm grounding in religious values and a strong appreciation for a

disciplined, orderly, frugal lifestyle. In later years, it was also clear that she profited from the perspective of her predecessor as dean, not only for his practical lessons in the art of deanship but also for his concern for quality and excellence. Not cited as contributors, but obviously important factors, are her intellectual precocity and her commitment to academic achievement. She actually used a sabbatical to get another specialty degree to promote her credibility.

Next, what qualities or characteristics are salient? The qualities she perceives as essential for a dean are the ones that come through in her own life: honesty, integrity, intelligence, stick-to-itiveness, the willingness to take chances, and vision. Jeanne Sinkford also has the ability to take a moral stand on questionable projects and has a deep sense of responsibility for the public good. She is enormously oriented to community—preparing students to serve and, in turn, serving hearing-impaired youth herself. Perhaps her greatest accomplishment may yet prove to be her advocacy for the interests of minority groups through culturally competent care, through minority

Overwhelmingly they focus on issues of health education that have social implications. The themes are predominantly related to minority issues, but they also discuss women's concerns and the problems of children, the elderly, and those with developmental disabilities. Also impressive is the scope of her concerns about education. She is known for her skills in identifying issues and trends and her estimates of the future. By the time most people attain a deanship, their productive days of writing are on the wane. Two thirds of Jeanne Sinkford's publications have occurred since she became dean.

Asked about her greatest achievement, Jeanne said that it depended on how she looked at it. Clearly, from a personal standpoint, "I think I'm a good mother, a good wife. I have a wonderfully supportive husband and family. And they love what I do. I think if they didn't, I wouldn't be able to do what I do. My daughter says, 'I don't know how you did all the things that you did. You went to soccer games, parent-teacher meetings, ballet lessons, and all that stuff.'"

From the standpoint of an achievement that was "against all odds," a construction project that she faced as a new dean was paramount. Her inherited top priority was to complete construction on new fourth and fifth floors for the dental school that would provide critically needed space for patient care, research, and classrooms. Eighteen months before she became dean, the project had been ready for the university to authorize funding. However, it had been dormant ever since, and many of the faculty thought the opportunity had passed them by. Her first real challenge as dean was completion of the project. She brought together all the resources she could muster, and the addition was built.

From the standpoint of something that had made an impact on others, Jeanne said that it would be a report she did on graduate education in dentistry. The report was published in 1969 as a special commission from the ADEA, the ADA Council on Dental Education, and the National Institute of Dental Research and had a widespread effect on graduate education. It was a major document that called for a halt to the expansion of advanced dental educational programs and helped focus attention instead on the need for graduate training in general dentistry. Essentially, it helped save dentistry from the overspecialization for which medicine has been criticized. Jeanne said, "If you look at the enrollments over the past 20 years or so, we have not escalated enrollments in our advanced specialty programs."

Jeanne thinks her greatest professional accomplishment in terms of personal satisfactions is "the impact I might have on young women now, who are aspiring to do things that they perceive that I have done, with all of the different challenges that face them today." People view her as a resource. Jeanne said, "I get calls all the time [from women] looking for advice." She loves the satisfaction of the personal contact and the steps forward that her policy innovations have provided. She said that her defining characteristic is that "*I like people. I like people. I really care about people.*" For Jeanne, liking and caring are the same. She goes on to say, "I like to talk to people. I like young people. I like to advise young people. They don't take your advice, but they like

recruitment to professional schools, and through recruitment of women to leadership positions.

Dr Sinkford gives the impression of having enormous confidence. Her self-assurance is the result of internally driven concerns about fairness, correct action, and the establishment and maintenance of standards. Her effectiveness as a leader is the result of a determined toughness coupled with a love of people and a gracious, respectful style of interaction. When asked if she had ever worried about what others thought of her, she said: "I was too busy plowing new ground." She seems to have achieved what Fisher and Ury[5] identify as essential qualities for effective negotiation: being soft on the people, hard on the problem. She is so confident and determined that it is hard to imagine many people challenging her unduly. Yet this confidence in herself and in her judgment is the result of "reasoned reasonableness" and persistent reflection and meditation.

The balance she has achieved between her personal, professional, and religious values sustains her focused, dedicated service to others and is the essence of this exemplary moral leader.

References

1. Burns JM, Kearns Goodwin D. True leadership. Psychol Today 1978;Oct:46–110.
2. Srivastva S, Cooperrider DL. The urgency for executive integrity. In: Srivastva S, et al (eds). Executive Integrity: The Search for High Human Values in Organizational Life. San Francisco: Jossey-Bass, 1988:1–28.
3. Greenleaf RK. Servant Leadership: A Journey into the Nature of Legitimate Power and Greatness. New York: Paulist Press, 1977.
4. Kolb DA. Integrity, advanced professional development, and learning. In: Srivastva S, et al (eds). Executive Integrity: The Search for High Human Values in Organizational Life. San Francisco: Jossey-Bass, 1988:68–88.
5. Fisher R, Ury W. Getting to Yes: Negotiating Agreement Without Giving In. New York: Penguin Books, 1981.

to talk to me, and they need someone to listen. Ten years later, they [may] say, 'Oh yeah, you told me that.' To me it is so exciting to see the challenges that young people have today that are different from ours, and that we are able to cross that generation gap by communication." She hopes that some of the things she does will help people she will never even meet.

Jeanne thinks that this nurturing quality is what those who are closest to her see. "They would say I was warm, generous; I'd give you the shirt off my back." Part of their judgment would be made with knowledge of her work in her community. Though now limited compared with previous years, Jeanne still works with the Washington, DC, chapter of Links, Inc, in programs for both children and elderly populations, and with the Chesapeake chapter, which for 15 years has helped talented deaf youth exhibit their work to the public.

Jeanne said others, however, would characterize her as "distant" and perhaps "an elitist." But, as she explained, "I had always been challenged to do more than most people I knew." No one else she knew, especially a woman, had double doctoral degrees, had been chair of a dental department, and on down the line. "I was plowing ground, and so I didn't have time to worry about what they thought about me. I was very focused and dedicated. I think those are things that they would say also."

Despite these reflections, Dr Sinkford more characteristically speaks not of the past, but of the present and the future, especially about unsolved problems. This focus reveals the true depth of her concern. For example, she feels that it is imperative, now that some states have removed race as a criterion for admission to institutions of higher education, that methods must be found that broaden the criteria beyond GPAs and DAT scores. Other characteristics that contribute to the making of health professionals must be identified.

She worries about finding ways to overcome language barriers in the provision of oral health care and wants to help talented Native American children to "get through the pipelines" to dental school. She is vitally concerned that dental schools and eventually the profession accept the concept of culturally competent care. "It's culture; it's behavior; it's language. It's all the things that make individuals understand their health situation, understand what you are trying to communicate and also how your own personal values will impact on how you assume responsibility for a part of the care and the follow-up."

Dr Sinkford is especially concerned about the public image of dentistry. Despite polls that perennially show high ratings of public trust in dentists, Jeanne said, "It depends on where you are. The 'haves' think it's great. We probably have the highest standards in the world as it relates to oral health. But the people that are beyond the margin are the ones that you don't really hear from, because they don't really understand the importance of oral health to general health. They don't have the money, and most of them are trying to live from day to day. They are worried about putting food on the table." In addition, there are influential groups that look at the profession askance. For example, Dr Sinkford said that when she talks with foundations about getting help to recruit a diverse population of dental students as an approach to improving access to care, they tell her that the profession is part of the problem. "They say that we have not allowed dental hygienists independent practice. And there are dentists who do not treat patients who cannot pay. So they're not sympathetic to the profession."

Dr Sinkford emphasizes again her concerns about minority recruitment. "Dentistry has got to take the lead in making some of these changes. Only 15 schools have significant minority enrollments. So my challenge now is to try to get the other schools to be a part of what is a national problem. We must help the deans of the other schools. If they have classes that have no underrepresented minorities in them, there is something wrong with their recruitment program. It's a matter of leadership." Jeanne believes that the profession is making progress, "but too slow. Much too slow. We need money, and we need commitment. It's not just money."

In listening to Jeanne Sinkford, it is obvious that she cares deeply about these issues. Indeed she is passionate about them and has long since taken the road to activism. "I just grew up feeling that whatever you had was a gift, and that you had certain talents, and you were supposed to use them."

Questions for Discussion

1. A striking feature of Jeanne Sinkford's career is how her sense of responsibility expanded over time. How important do you think the quality of an expanding sense of responsibility is in academic leadership? In clinical leadership?

2. What qualities distinguish Jeanne Sinkford's leadership? As described in the commentary, what is the test of executive leadership according to Robert Greenleaf?

3. Is it important for an academic leader to demonstrate moral qualities? What distinguishes moral leadership from other kinds of leadership?

4. Most dentists who run their own practices are leaders. Picturing yourself in that role and reflecting on the qualities of moral leadership, what goals would you set for yourself?

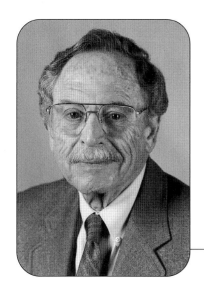

11

Irwin D. Mandel

Integrity and Mentoring in Research

In the mid-1940s at Columbia University School of Dental and Oral Surgery, Dr Irwin Mandel began a pioneering career in research on salivary chemistry in health and disease. It brought him an international reputation, an array of awards, and honorary degrees from prestigious universities. In the first half of his 50-year tenure at Columbia, he shared his commitment to research with the operation of a half-time private practice in Manhattan. Then, after giving up his practice, he became a full-time faculty member at Columbia as division head of preventive dentistry and community health and concluded his service as associate dean for research. Dr Mandel has become recognized by his peers at Columbia and by the academic community across the United States as a symbol of integrity, both in his research and as a person. Shaped in childhood by a culture of caring in a community of Jewish immigrants to which his father was dedicated, he became well known for his thoughtful mentoring of rising scientists. Additionally, for much of his life, he was a committed social activist.

In 1996 Dr Irwin D. Mandel gave the keynote speech at a symposium on research ethics sponsored by the American Association of Dental Research. According to Dr Mickey Bebeau, who had chaired the planning committee, he was everyone's first choice. The task had been to find someone who was not only an eminent scientist, but who would also be believable as the lead speaker at an ethics conference. The committee had reservations about every nominee except Dr Mandel.

Dr Mandel's speech[1] accented the changing ethical culture of science. He spoke about the burgeoning period for dental research from 1950 to the mid-1960s, a time when his own research efforts first prospered. This was the time, he said, "when the defining images for many of us in the biological and health sciences were from movies and novels: Louis Pasteur as played by Paul Muni; Paul Ehrlich as depicted by Edward G. Robinson; and Ronald Colman as the fictional Martin Arrowsmith, the hero of the popular novel by Sinclair Lewis, . . . who dedicated himself to the pursuit of scientific truth, despite social and commercial pressures for compromise." Dr Mandel went on to say, "There was a strong feeling of community among researchers–as if it were a collective–with open communication and close cooperation in the various disciplines. . . . Mentoring was a critical component in both specific research training and in the introduction to the culture of science."

The above-mentioned idealistic integrity, sense of community, and mentoring were not only expressions of what Dr Mandel saw happening those 40 years past;

they were also examples of what others saw in him. For instance, Dr Martin Lunin, who nominated Dr Mandel as a moral exemplar, saw in him "a deep altruistic feeling and a continued enthusiasm for his work and new projects. He also had a long history of helping aspiring researchers and students. I am one he helped."

The same qualities and more were seen by three colleagues who wrote a 1997 article about him that appeared in the "Discovery" section of the *Journal of Dental Research*.[2] The "Discovery" section features important contributions in oral research and the scientists who have made them. Although this section was tailor-made for someone like Irwin Mandel, there was a potential roadblock in publishing the manuscript about him: Dr Mandel was the editor of the series, and the authors knew he would be very uncomfortable. It took some creative collusion with the journal editor to publish the article surreptitiously.

The authors, two of whom had been students of Dr Mandel, described him as the preeminent "general of the salivation army." His work, they wrote, "made saliva an indispensable tool for oral medicine and preventive dentistry. His body of work during these two decades (the 1960s and '70s) set the foundation, and built the first several floors, of a research field which has blossomed in numbers, depth, and clinical relevance. From Irwin's relatively modest resources at Columbia, great things developed. Irwin is a modern Martin Arrowsmith for dentistry, for Columbia and for many young and not so young salivary researchers. He continues to set a high standard and a wonderful example."[2]

They also said that working in his laboratory was a special experience, not for its competitive, ambitious aura of productivity, but for its feeling of inclusiveness, acceptance, and refuge. The authors viewed Dr Mandel as "a tangible example that someone can be highly successful in the 'aggressive' academic community, rigorous and productive in research, and still retain humanity, humility, and compassion."[2] They went on to list 20 well-known researchers, research directors, and department chairs on whom Dr Mandel had had a major impact. They said, "The secret of this success lay in Irwin being a consummate mentor. Mentoring is an oft-used term today, quite in vogue. Teachers and scientists are expected to guide and nurture the careers of their younger colleagues. For Irwin, this was a given. He saw his teachers as helping him to develop, and the 'payback' was obvious: He was to help the next generation."[2] One of the authors of the "Discovery" article, now himself a mentor in the Mandel tradition, affirmed at a party celebrating Irwin's 60th

birthday that to have been a student of Irwin's is to have a friend forever, subject to a guarantee of interest, concern, and help, too, if needed, for the rest of your life.

What made his reputation for integrity extraordinarily appealing was his impressive reputation as a scientist. Irwin Mandel was a pioneer in the development of increasingly sophisticated methods for the study of salivary chemistry, physiology, and immunology to better understand the etiology, development, and treatment of dental caries. He published his first scientific article in 1941 while he was still an undergraduate college student, and has since published more than 200 articles, along with 17 book chapters, mostly on saliva and oral disease, especially caries, but also on systemic disease and the diagnostic uses of saliva. The organizer of a mid-1990's National Institute for Dental Research (NIDR) conference on the use of saliva as a diagnostic fluid dedicated the conference to Dr Mandel, saying it was a "unique opportunity to honor the man most responsible for the development of the field. . . . It is difficult to identify an area within the field of salivary diagnostics that has not been influenced by his studies."[3]

The excellence and importance of Dr Mandel's work has been recognized by research awards from Columbia University, the University of Connecticut, the Federation Dentaire International, and the International Association for Dental Research. He has been made a Fellow of the American Association for the Advancement of Science and was the first winner of the American Dental Association's (ADA) Gold Medal for Excellence in Research. Honorary doctorate degrees have been presented to him by the College of Medicine and Dentistry of New Jersey, the University of Göteborg in Sweden, and most satisfyingly, he said, Columbia University.

When asked how he responded to tributes such as this, Dr Mandel said, "Obviously it gave me satisfaction, and of course ego gratification. However, these honors always provoke an unwanted feeling of 'second-class citizenship,'" since he had never received a PhD the hard way. He said it made him feel "pressured to work hard to live up to the reputation. I'm afraid my ego does need bolstering, and rewards come in different forms. My income has been modest; recognition is a different form of currency." On the other hand, he receives such praise with caution: "There always is hyperbole on such occasions—not to be trusted." As to his reputation for integrity, he said, "I always felt [the need for it] was a given."

Besides his scientific contributions, Dr Mandel has to his credit another 30 articles of a different type. These articles show the breadth of his activities from researcher to practitioner to social activist and give evidence of his philosophical turn of mind. They include such diverse themes as preventive dentistry, care of the elderly, the need for clinical research, trends and transitions in the profession, environmental perspectives of dental amalgam, occupational risks, the communication of science to patients, the image of dentistry in contemporary culture, and issues of social justice in dentistry. Most recently he has authored a series of papers about dentistry as it appears in the world of arts and letters.

Before we can further examine Dr Mandel's accomplishments and his distinguishing traits, a look at his earlier years and the influences in his development is essential.

The Auto Parts Store and the Leeds Fraternal Society

Irwin D. Mandel was born in the Brownsville section of Brooklyn on April 9, 1922. His parents had immigrated as children from what was then part of Russia, and his grandparents owned a candy store in a predominantly Jewish neighborhood. Irwin said that his father, Samuel, though not formally educated beyond high school, "was an autodidact. We had a thousand books at home–he was extremely well read. I grew up on the Harvard Classics.*" Before his marriage, Samuel had dreamed of a career as a writer. Irwin recalled, "My father worked for the *Waterbury* (Connecticut) *Republican* as a cub reporter, as he called it. He left to enlist in the Army in 1917. Even during the war, he sent back articles to the paper. . . . But after the war when he came back and met my mother and they decided to keep company, there was just no future there [at the newspaper], so he took a job in what was then a big new industry–and that was automobiles–and he managed a tire store in Brooklyn. And then they were married." He opened his own automobile parts store, which prospered and expanded to include a machine shop. Irwin remembers the bustle of the store, with everyone pitching in and working harmoniously under his father's calm, low-keyed supervision. Irwin admired the relationship between his father and his customers. They would come

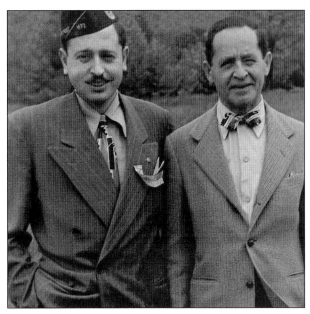

Irwin *(left)* with his father at a New York State Jewish War Veterans convention in 1948.

into the store and say with warmth, "So you're Sam's son . . ." and then extol his father. As the Mandels moved up the economic ladder, Irwin, his brother, and his parents located themselves in progressively more desirable neighborhoods.

The Depression had a major effect on the Mandel auto parts store. Irwin recalls, "There were terrible problems in surviving, but also important childhood memories. I used to work there in the summertime; I was 10 or 11 years old. And I had an opportunity to see my father with his employees and their families. He was very concerned for them. He would stick with them." Irwin remembers his father working hard to avoid bankruptcy and writing to his suppliers to request extensions of credit. Samuel's problems were compounded by the burden of his six or seven salesmen, machinists, and countermen who depended on him. Irwin also remembers an uncle who had written some bad checks. His father made the checks good and gave his uncle a job for the rest of his life. His father also gave a job to a cousin, who was at loose ends after an unsuccessful attempt to get into medical school. After World War II his father discovered that some cousins in Poland had survived a Nazi concentration camp and sponsored their immigration to America. Having expressed such concern for his extended family, it was not surprising that years later, when Samuel retired prematurely because of

*Harvard Classics: A 50-volume publication of classical works, with a copyright in 1909 to 1910, edited by Charles W. Eliot, who said its purpose was "to present so ample and characteristic a record of the stream of the world's thought that the observant reader's mind shall be enriched, refined, and fertilized by it."

ill health, he extended the same generous spirit to his employees and sold his business to them.

Samuel's auto parts store was also a center of activity for the Leeds Fraternal Society, of which Samuel was a member. It was so named because the founding members were from Leeds, England. "In fact," Irwin remembers, "I grew up drinking English tea. [Actually] it was mostly milk with a Lipton's tea bag dipped into it. . . . Fraternal organizations were very cogent in those days, and to this day, of course.

"They were also burial societies. That is, they had this function of combining resources and paying dues that included buying a plot in a Jewish cemetery. When any of the members died, [the group] took over the responsibility of the arrangements for burial. My father, who, several times over the years, was president of the organization and highly respected by this group, was also, for most of his life, chairman of the cemetery committee. He handled the mechanics of it." Irwin continued, "If you go through the Jewish cemeteries in the New York area, especially in Queens and Long Island, you will find that most of them are divided by what they call *gates*. They would buy half an acre or an acre or three acres, depending on the size of the organization. Then they would mark off the perimeter. And in the center where you walk into the plot, they would put up a modest edifice with the name of the organization. So this became the Leeds Fraternal Society plot."

Irwin remembers the societies as important for other reasons. "The social aspect was very important. They enjoyed each other's company and did many things together. They provided support systems for each other. They hired a physician for the society during the Depression and paid him a stipend of a couple of hundred dollars a year. . . . And then [the physicians] would make house calls for 2 dollars and office visits for a dollar to members of the organization. [It was] an early version of managed care. . . . Dr Teitelbaum was the guy who came to the house. The first thing he did for the first 10 minutes was tell jokes. Mostly off-color jokes that I was not allowed to hear. It was a warm relationship," Irwin said. In addition, "A good part of their activity was to raise money for charity." His father had a lot to do with this endeavor. When two brothers in their 30s died, Samuel formed the Efros Foundation in their memory. "The Efros Foundation would raise money through raffles, card parties, and theater parties," and then give the proceeds to charity.

The auto parts store with all its ramifications became a laboratory for Irwin's moral development. There he saw his father not only as a parent but as a beneficent employer and a key figure in their community. Irwin's father modeled concern for others, commitment to his community, and acceptance of responsibility. With a quiet leadership style that promoted a harmonious, supportive, smoothly functioning organization, these lessons would all be revisited in the way that Irwin lived his own life, led his own organization, and related to his own community.

Problems and Adjustments

Irwin's parents contributed equally to the intellectual climate of his childhood. His mother loved to read and had respect for learning and professionalism. They both enjoyed politics, were involved in implementing Roosevelt's New Deal in their community, and supported liberal causes, although his father was primarily a fan of Norman Thomas, the socialist leader. Irwin said his father voted for Roosevelt "because he thought a vote for Thomas would be wasted. (Ralph Nader, are you listening?)" Furthermore, both of them being writers, they had friends who were poets and writers. Writing eventually became an interest of Irwin's; in fact, Irwin and his wife, Charlotte, who is now a published poet, wrote a novel that was never published and a musical that was nearly produced.

Irwin's mother, Shirley, like his father, showed support and pride in Irwin's accomplishments, but from Irwin's perspective, "My mother was overprotective. My time in school in the early grades was not a comfortable one. I was what was called a nervous child. I remember not wanting to go to school sometimes and kind of vomiting and playing sick. I don't know why." Any physical complaint—from headaches to sinus trouble—increased his mother's anxiety. The cycle became self-perpetuating and led to an excessive preoccupation with health. Irwin called it "a kind of hypochondria [that] stayed with me all through my adolescence. God, one of the worst experiences of my life—and why I choose not to remember those days—is that my parents had one of those home health advisors with all sorts of pictures of diseases of the digestive system, excretory system, and so forth. We used to call it—a Jewish expression—the *kishka* book." The *kishka* book was his mother's doing, and over time Irwin became convinced that most of the illnesses were his personal possessions.

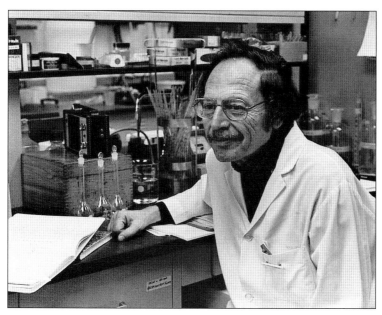

Dr Mandel in his clinical research lab at Columbia dental school (1980).

Presumably, his health concerns had no serious effect on his education. He skipped three grades and graduated from high school at the age of 16. His health probably also had a positive legacy. Irwin thinks, "[it] made me more sensitive to people's complaints—even hypochondriacs have real problems sometimes. I'm a good listener with patients. To this day, I get an occasional call from patients I haven't seen in more than 30 years; they call to seek advice." Nonetheless, it was exceedingly troubling to Irwin. His hypochondria stayed with him through high school, college, and most of dental school. It abruptly disappeared when he got married and left home. "My wife always takes credit," Irwin said.

Irwin was small as a boy and acutely aware that, unlike his brother, he was not an athlete. He found many substitutes for athleticism; his expected enthusiasm for books was but one. Using his innate verbal skills, he developed a reputation as the neighborhood comedian. Some say he still has that reputation. Irwin said, "Humor is very important to me. I enjoy finding humor in various situations. I employ it frequently in talks to professional groups. It helps me have a sense of perspective. It helps in not taking myself too seriously when I get stuffy."

Another effective substitute for sports was the Boy Scouts. It gave him great satisfaction to rise quickly through the ranks to become a Life Scout and a senior patrol leader. It was so important to him that he became a scoutmaster and stayed in scouting through college and dental school. Irwin loved to camp out and excelled at the skills of scouting, except for swimming. This lesser proficiency kept him from achieving the life-saving merit badge and the ultimate rank of Eagle. Commenting on this disappointment, Irwin said, "I have not had many defeats. I've always considered myself very fortunate. I keep waiting for the other shoe to fall, but so far, except for a heart attack in 1984, it hasn't." Scouting provided Irwin with a first awareness of his innate leadership potential and presented him his first personal mentor, Dave Block. This scoutmaster's warm relationship with young people became the standard for Irwin's own relationships. Dave Block "took an interest in the older boys, taking them camping, paying attention to their interests and schooling. It wasn't his bent to be corrective, but rather to be a friend. Despite the age difference, you could be comfortable with him and seek advice."

Intellectual and Social Growth

Irwin's social growth in scouting had an intellectual counterpart at Boys' High School. Everything about Boys' High was stimulating, but the focus on the unfolding events of the world was especially exciting, because it complemented what was happening at home around the table. His father read the newspaper from cover to cover, and everyone would discuss the news, bad though it was in that pre-war period.

The *Herald Tribune* sponsored a school-based weekly contest for the best essays on the news. Irwin was a regular contributor. It seemed that Boys' High students, including Irwin, were often winners. In truth, Boys' High students *should* have done well. Besides Irwin, there was Harry Schwartz, a future editorial writer for the *New York Times*; Robert Hankin, who became a professor of Russian studies; Isadore Diamond, who collaborated as a co-writer with Billy Wilder on most of Wilder's movies; and Isaac Asimov, the future science writer and novelist. Among the students interested in science, the competition for grades was fierce. Some students would take 2 or 3 weeks off to study for final examinations. Irwin admired their intensity but did not see it as a way of life for him. He did well, and his 92% or 93% grade average kept him on the honor roll. But he observed from afar the real competition at the 99.1% to 99.2% range–the level needed to get a scholarship to Columbia or Cornell.

Irwin graduated from Boys' High School at the age of 16 and entered the College of the City of New York, which was even more academically oriented. As expected, it provided an excellent background for Irwin in science and research, but it also made a major contribution to his later activities as a social activist. Although the seeds for his social orientation had been planted at home, City College provided, as Irwin puts it, "a lot of fertilizer." It was an extremely liberal environment, with all sorts of student political ferment: rallies opposing Franco in the Spanish Civil War, groups for socialism, followers of Marxism, speakers critical of New York Mayor LaGuardia's opposition to Bertrand Russell's appointment to City College, and protestors against the Rapp-Coudert Committee, which, a decade ahead of Joseph McCarthy,

promoted the firing of professors based on their political beliefs. Whenever Irwin left the subway and went up the hill to the school, by the time he arrived his arms were full of circulars supporting one movement or another.

Fascinated by most of the ideas, and turned off by some of the factionalism, Irwin could not participate actively in anything. He rode the subway for an hour and a half each way, continued his role as a scoutmaster, and beginning in his junior year worked 12 hours a week in a research laboratory. Nevertheless, the environment provided great substance for discussions with his father. They talked about all the tumult on campus and more, including his father's concern about the anti-Semitic diatribes of Father Coughlin and the anti-Semitic and anti-Negro activities of the Ku Klux Klan. Though not a political activist himself, Irwin's father expressly approved of what was happening on campus. For Irwin, his college years fixed his social orientation. His intellectual interest in ideas became linked with the realization that some public issues were important enough to deserve his active support.

At City College Irwin majored in chemistry and met his second mentor, Leo Lehrman, the head of the analytical chemistry department. Dr Lehrman invited Irwin to work with him, and together they published two articles in top-flight journals. By the end of his junior year, he was all but certain that a career in research was for him. However, even as early as high school, Irwin had thought about dental school. His family thought it was a good idea. Irwin said the general view was that, "Dentistry is a good thing. You never get rich, but you always make a living and it was a profession. . . . Security to a Jewish family of modest means during the Depression was very important." Also, he added, "I was undergoing orthodontic care at that time, and so I was even considering becoming an orthodontist." Because he spent his early years anguishing over one disease after another, medicine was never a serious option.

In 1942 Irwin graduated with a bachelor's degree in chemistry and entered dental school at Columbia University. By that time, he said, "I saw dentistry as pragmatically able to combine the sciences that I loved and a solid profession."

With Irwin's record at City College, getting accepted to dental school was not a problem. Once he was a den-

> Dr Mandel is "a tangible example that someone can be highly successful in the 'aggressive' academic community, rigorous and productive in research, and still retain humanity, humility, and compassion."
>
> *Former students of Dr Mandel*

tal student, being accepted for a reserve commission in the US Navy (and the financial support that went with it) was harder. Irwin said, "I was a chubby kid. I was an eater. I was a good boy, so everything my mother put in front of me I ate. I gained a lot of weight and yet I was in good shape because I used to exercise a lot." Besides his weight, he faced another problem getting into the Navy program: "I had hypertension because I was very nervous and hypochondriacal." To pass the Navy physical, from his 180-pound peak, he lost 25 pounds, which helped to stabilize his blood pressure. He is now a trim 145, the last reduction spurred by his 1984 heart attack.

Clinician and Researcher

Getting Started

Whereas Irwin's undergraduate education expanded his moral outlook toward advocacy in the larger community, his dental education was morally neutral. Just learning how to be a dentist and a researcher was challenging enough. Making progress in research was the easier part of dental school. He easily found some people to work with, and within a few years had submitted two abstracts for presentation. He said, "I got straight A's in all the science courses, but I only got a B– in dental anatomy. I got a C in prosthetics. . . . Developing manual skills was a challenge, but it was not debilitating. . . . In any event, I caught up, and I was a good dentist. But it took me a while. It was very worrisome." Even so, he said, "With enough practice over the years the lack of natural talent can be overcome."

Despite having to work hard to acquire clinical skills, Irwin enjoyed dental school and working with patients. Based primarily on the values he brought with him to dental school, concern for the welfare of patients came naturally. However, there was a constant tension between the responsibility he felt for his patients and what he calls the "terrible self-centeredness" of not feeling entirely comfortable with his hands. He felt as if he had no choice but to be completely dependent on the instructors who, in the style of the day, often acted like drill sergeants and treated students as if school were boot camp. Like many students, he quaked when he called the instructor to his chair. It is a memory that I (JTR) share with Irwin.

Dr Mandel graduated in 1945 from Columbia University School of Dental and Oral Surgery and was commissioned in the US Navy. With the war recently

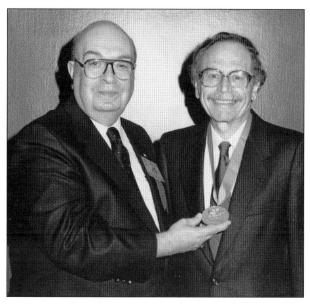

Dr Mandel *(right)* receives the first ADA Gold Medal Award for Excellence in Dental Research in 1985. With him is Dr John Bomba, then-president of the ADA. (Reprinted with permission from the ADA.)

over, and in consideration of his having been married while in dental school, the Navy discharged him after only 1 year's service. Immediately he started a half-time practice, which for most of that period was in midtown Manhattan across the street from Carnegie Hall. The other half of his time he spent at Columbia doing research. According to his nominator, "It would be unfair to say that he did either part time. Instead he did both full time and both on the dead run."

He made steady progress in both endeavors until the Navy called him again in 1952 during the Korean war to serve another 2 years. He said, "I gave up the practice. It was difficult to do, but I did it." Having previously received an early discharge, he said, "I felt that it was payback time . . . and it was a nice lifestyle. We had a small house and the officer's club and two young children and were away from parents. . . . I actually found that those 2 years in the service were very good for me and my family. . . . And so, shortly after we got home, we started to look for a house and so forth. It just changed the way we lived."

Picking up Speed

After his discharge, Irwin found another practice location and resumed his half-time position at Columbia. His practice grew because he attracted people who worked in

Manhattan, many of whom were writers, artists, or actors. Friends became patients, and patients often became friends. He received many referrals from dentists who worked at Columbia. He did a lot of fixed prosthodontics, including many full-mouth rehabilitations. Concerns about his hand skills vanished. "I was not a 'super' practitioner. I was 'good.' And I empathized with patients."

Referring dentists sent him their less affluent patients because his fees were low, and Dr Mandel was happy to get them. Commenting on his low fees, he says it wasn't that he was a soft touch: "My previous experience was with Brooklyn dentists during the Depression. Their fees were very low and, even after World War II, were much lower than in Manhattan. In addition I remember the experience in the 1930s when I was an orthodontic patient, and my father had great difficulty paying the $12 per month fee. The office assistant often gave me 'reminder' notes to take home." When Dr Mandel finally sold his practice, his successor doubled the fees within a year or two.

Besides the satisfactions gained from his relationships with patients and from the new confidence with his hands, Irwin enjoyed using innovative techniques in preventive dentistry. He was among the first in the area to use topical applications of fluoride. He formulated his own dentifrices with anticaries potential. He did dietary

> "Humor is very important to me. I enjoy finding humor in various situations. . . . It helps in not taking myself too seriously when I get stuffy."
>
> *Dr Mandel*

analyses and *Lactobacillus* counts for his patients and helped them learn methods of good oral hygiene. Within a few years he became Columbia's half-time unpaid cariologist. By 1948 he had written an article on caries prevention for *Consumer Reports* magazine, which until then had not included dental articles. After a few years, he became their dental advisor, a relationship that has now spanned some 50 years.

During the same period, Irwin's research skills also received a boost. He recalls that upon his return from the Navy, "I began to work seriously with Dr Barnet Levy. He became my model as a mentor for dental research. He was broad-based scientifically, interested in everything and everybody, and a model collaborator, both with the dental and basic sciences and with medical colleagues. . . . Under his tutelage, I really began to learn what a laboratory was like: how to ask the proper questions and how to develop a research project. I began to see how you deal with technicians and how you deal with people."

When I asked Irwin about the laboratory community he created–noted for its collaborative rather than its competitive atmosphere–he was careful to point out, "It certainly wasn't planned that way. I inherited a warm, friendly atmosphere from Bar Levy. . . . He was a wonderful guy to work with, and we're still close friends." In

Commentary

When we come to the end of our life's work, what will matter most? A legacy of professional and personal accomplishment? A trust fund for our children and grandchildren? A large endowment for our favorite educational institution or charity? For Irwin Mandel, it is not the legacy of scientific achievement but the respect of his peers that matters most. To be remembered and cherished as a person of integrity implies a completeness, wholeness, and unity achieved through sustained commitment to virtuous ends.

Irwin Mandel has achieved his goal. He is universally respected by his peers not only for his scientific accomplishments, but for the way in which he achieved them. In the final analysis, it is the method rather than the accomplishment that sets him apart as a moral exemplar. The collaborative atmosphere of his laboratory, for example, was fundamentally different from the competitive environment of so

many of today's high-powered research laboratories. It demonstrated the essence that Robert Merton[1] refers to as one of four key values essential for the pursuit of science: the communal sharing of ideas and findings. Irwin intuitively recognizes that knowledge is not private, that the generation of new knowledge should serve communal ends. Further, in a community that often argues about the relative merits of basic versus applied research, the breadth and scope of his research activities are particularly remarkable. He commits to the pursuit of knowledge for the benefit of humankind, and his concerns extend beyond pure research to translational research, to educational research, and to issues of application and policy formation. He takes on each of the roles of the scientist: creator of knowledge, collaborator, mentor, director, coordinator, and ultimately scientific leader and advocate for the interests of the larger community. What are these intangible qualities, exhibited over a lifetime of interactions, that define him as a moral exemplar, rather than "just" a highly accomplished scientist?

addition, he said, "It would take psychoanalysis to find underlying reasons for my style. There was, of course, a very good reason for the closeness: space was always minimal, so 'togetherness' was virtually thrust upon us. Collaborations came naturally. The faculty lunch room was an especially valuable resource for establishing collaborative projects."

In 1956, 11 years after graduating from dental school, with his research program underway and his publications starting to attract attention, Irwin received his first paycheck from Columbia University. Until this time his work at the university had been funded by his practice, and his research had been funded by grants from industry. His willingness to donate half of his professional time for such a long period seems extraordinary. Irwin said that he looked at it as a major opportunity to fulfill his interest in research. His practice income provided his family with comfort, though certainly not affluence. It was possible because neither he nor Charlotte expected or required large amounts of money. They were of like mind on this issue, and they both valued scholarship and academic pursuits.

Full Acceleration

By the late 1950s Dr Mandel's research had progressed nicely, and he had started to publish regularly. In fact, his publication record can serve as a scientific barometer that reflects his accomplishments of the day and predicts their consequences. In the 1950s he published 7 articles.

The number rose to 55 in the 1960s, 57 in the 1970s, and 71 in the 1980s. In the 1990s it tapered off to fewer than 50, most of them appearing after his retirement in 1992. Irwin felt obliged to comment on his publication record: "The numbers are deceiving. Most of the papers are with multiple collaborators, and I'm not the first author in many of them. With increased grant support and more collaborators, the number of papers increased. I sought out collaborators, and collaborators sought me out."

In any event, his promotions and honors reflected his publication record. In 1950 he held the rank of instructor. By 1957, he was associate clinical professor, and clinical professor in 1960. By the end of the 1960s Dr Mandel, as a half-time scientist, had established a national reputation as a leader in salivary research. In 1969 hypertension and the excitement of his successes in research led him to cut back his activities. He sold his half-time practice and joined the faculty full time as professor and director of the new division of preventive dentistry and community health. Although his position was prestigious, his full-time university salary was less than that of his half-time practice. Fortunately, the income from the sale of his practice almost made up the difference.

During the 1970s Dr Mandel began to reap the benefits of his reputation: ADA consultancies, research medals, awards for leadership, fellowships in prestigious organizations, membership on editorial boards of nine journals, and participation in NIDR study sections, including some years as the chair. He started the

Of great importance was the way in which Irwin's intellectual development was shaped with values. His family, especially his father, Samuel, respected and actively participated in learning. The family culture valued an education that was grounded in classic literature and that provided exposure to a broad range of ideas. There is considerable research evidence[2] that a broadly based liberal education promotes moral and intellectual maturity, and we see from Samuel's intellectual development (sans college) and from Irwin's own development (sans PhD) that it isn't essential for that education to occur in formal educational settings. It is necessary, however, for an individual to grapple with the intellectual and social issues of the day. Irwin's high school and college education exposed him to a wide range of ideas, but the stimulating dinner conversations at home were what made the difference. Samuel's openness to new ideas during these conversations may have been defining experiences for Irwin. Reflecting on an example that occurred later in life, Irwin was especially proud of his father's forsaking the restrictive views of the "old guard" as he became active with the Jewish

War Veterans. It was this interaction between ideas and ideals that promoted and sustained his relationship with his father.

As we reflect on Irwin's activism, his achievements in science, and what he says about these activities, we see an individual who has achieved the elements John Dewey described as the basis of practical and theoretical judgments. King and Kitchner[3] have shown how Dewey's concepts of knowledge and justification develop across one's life span, and how higher and advanced education can promote development of critical thinking and reflective judgment. Typically, the most advanced levels of reflective judgment are associated with advanced degrees (ie, PhD). However, higher education does not guarantee it. Educators, like Irwin and his father before him, must encourage and model open-minded thinking where beliefs can be revised based on new evidence, counterevidence, or new alternatives. Intelligent action, then, results from "a complex set of flexible and growing habits that involve sensitivity, the ability to discern the complexities of a situation, imagination that is exercised in new possibilities and hypotheses, willingness to learn from experience,

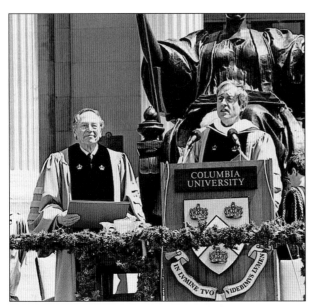

Columbia University presents Dr Mandel with an honorary doctor of science degree in 1996.

1980s as president of the American Association of Dental Research (AADR). As the decade continued, there were more awards and increasing obligations to the national community: honorary doctorates, more research awards, invited lectures, and membership on the NIDR Board of Scientific Counselors and the ADA Future of Dentistry Committee. In 1991 he was appointed associate dean for research at Columbia.

Under the requirements of mandatory retirement, he left the university in 1992 at the age of 70 and was appointed professor emeritus. During the remainder of the 1990s, his obligations to others decreased but the awards kept coming, including his most prized honorary doctorate from Columbia University.

Dr Mandel's accomplishments had all occurred at Columbia University. Add to them, from his nominator's standpoint, credit for helping to save the dental school. His nominator said, "I have for years felt that the dental school at Columbia was barely hanging on, suffering as many of the private schools did, often on the verge of closing. I think that [Irwin's work] helped to save and improve the school and allowed it to survive." Irwin said that the dental school's hardest times were from 1957 to 1969. These were years with a dean who did not support research and who was especially opposed to government grants in private schools. Irwin thinks that is what the nominator was alluding to, "that I was able to maintain a research presence in an institution where the administration was opposed to it." His strategy was to procure some small but crucial grants from industry that kept research alive and set the foundations for subsequent expansion.

Dr Mandel's reputation as a Columbia loyalist is well known among his peers. Irwin accepts the reputation as valid, explaining, "I always saw the dental school as a second home . . . I shared in the problems and the successes—very much as in a family. There are rewards *and* responsibilities."

fairness and objectivity in judging conflicting values and opinions, and the courage to change one's views when it is demanded by the consequences of our actions and criticisms of others."[3p73]

Intellectual development is only one part of the equation for effective functioning. The powerful modeling in Irwin's background also displays the elements of what Goleman[4] refers to as emotional intelligence. His father's qualities of generosity, compassion, and loyalty were illustrated by his helping his employees out of difficult situations, assuming the burial responsibilities for the Leeds Society, and, through a lifetime of interaction, the empowerment of his employees to purchase the business they had helped to build. The same qualities are seen in Irwin in his extensive social activism, the development of departmental programs for disadvantaged people, the empowerment of patients to prevent oral disease, and his loyalty to Columbia University and the students he mentored. In all of Irwin's efforts, including the collegial and cooperative environment of his research laboratory, one sees the communitarian values of his father.

Of special note is Irwin's disposition to view others positively and with compassion, as illustrated in his efforts to redirect the "long-haired malcontents" who entered his laboratory in the 1960s. Given the natural distrust so evident in the dependency relationship of that decade—teacher/student, employer/employee, doctor/patient—how did Irwin exercise compassion without compromising his responsibilites? As a virtue, compassion must strive for a mean. When the educator, employer, or healer identifies too closely with the student, employee, or patient, she loses the objectivity essential to the most precise assessment of what is wrong, of what can be done, and of what should be done to meet those needs.[5] A parallel question is, how was Dr Mandel was able to disregard the paternalistic models of his own dental education? Interestingly, Irwin saw his own dental education, in contrast to his undergraduate education, as morally neutral. Yet the educational process he and so many others describe was often anything but morally neutral. Whereas the goal of the technical side of dentistry was to promote perfectionism, the methods used often modeled the most negative kind of teacher-

One would think, given the magnitude of his reputation, that he would have had opportunities to take positions of greater responsibility. In fact, several such opportunities arose. Although Irwin does have a deep loyalty to Columbia, the reason he turned down the opportunities has more to do with family considerations. After his father died, his mother developed increasing emotional difficulties, and Irwin felt that he had to be available for her. Likewise, as Charlotte's parents grew older, they required both Irwin's and Charlotte's attention.

Social Activist

Irwin Mandel has a sustained history as a social activist. His choices of activism and activities revolved around the major issues of the day, and given his background, they were always part of the liberal agenda. He says, "Selecting an activist agenda is like selecting a research project. You feel; you read; you care; you do." Returning home from his first stint in the Navy, having at last given up the Boy Scouts, he joined the Jewish War Veterans to fight anti-Semitism in education, housing, and employment. Irwin quickly acquired a reputation as a public speaker on this issue. He led rallies, gave talks on the radio, organized symposia, called meetings, held public assemblies, helped write legislation, lobbied in Albany, New York, on behalf of state legislation, and went to Washington, DC, to lobby for national legislation. At one point he even ran for County Commander of the Brooklyn chapters.

Working with the Jewish War Veterans was particularly satisfying because his father joined him for his first direct taste of social activism. Irwin was especially pleased when his father decided that the "old guard" contingent of the organization was too conservative. Irwin still has a proud image of his father sweating in his undershirt in the hot summer sun at the state convention during the contest for leadership, producing campaign literature on a mimeograph machine. It was the last such activity they shared. Samuel Mandel died of a heart attack a few years later while Irwin was in the Navy during the Korean War.

When he returned from his Korean War duty in 1954, his practice expanded rapidly, and his spare time was constricted. Additionally, during the quiet interlude provided by the Navy, Irwin reflected that during his previous social advocacy, especially his activity at the state level, he might have "short-changed Charlotte and the children." He and Charlotte bought a house in New Jersey, where they still live today, and Irwin restricted most of his activism to local organizations to avoid the frequent runs to Manhattan and Albany. It is not clear that Charlotte and the children felt short-changed. Irwin said that Charlotte herself, while raising three children, "shared my beliefs and enthusiasm and was an active volunteer and became county chairperson of the Women's International League for Peace and Freedom."

student relationship imaginable. That example was then replayed in the kind of doctor-patient relationship that so characterized many a practitioner's dental experiences. Some even convinced themselves that shaming and blaming and other negative tactics were what patients (or students) needed in order to change their ways. Irwin, though he comments on the tactic, seems not to have adopted it. Had he done so, it is unlikely that he would have achieved the respect of his students, patients, and peers.

Irwin seems to have achieved a balance between what many in research ethics are seeing as essentially distinctive roles: advisor and mentor. An advisor is expected to devise learning experiences and direct technical and scientific activities that are goal-oriented and critical. While advisors provide supportive assistance, they also sit in judgment of the student's competence. They have conflicting responsibilities: to the institution and to the student. Mentors, on the other hand, are loyal advisors whose role is to serve as protectors as they shape character, build competence, and serve as role models. Mentors do not have conflicting loyalties. While mentors can be advisors, it is rare to see someone who is effective in both roles. To achieve the universal respect that sets Dr Mandel apart as a moral exemplar in scientific research is testimony to his ability to blend these roles effectively. But how can this be done?

King and Kitchner[3] alert us to the challenge educators face in moving young people to the levels of intellectual maturity required of the competent researcher. They point out that the evolution of knowing requires that education attend to the emotional as well as the cognitive side of learning. The educator must recognize that students' beliefs, whether about science, politics, or religion, can be grounded emotionally as well as cognitively. When educators cognitively challenge students' ideas, they may also be challenging them emotionally. Establishing supportive learning environments that are both intellectually challenging and emotionally supportive is difficult. Often the educator alienates himself/herself from the student during the educational process. Only when the educator is able to consistently provide emotional support along with intellectual challenge do we see the development of high levels of respect that engender the kinds

One of his daughters happily accompanied him on protest trips to Washington. She and his son both obtained degrees in urban planning and have been significantly involved in cultural planning and low-cost housing. Their eldest daughter is dean of libraries at New York University.

Besides working at the local level, the nature of Irwin's activities also changed. He began to work with groups that opposed McCarthyism. Instead of time spent with the Jewish War Veterans, he joined the American Veterans Committee. Instead of working against anti-Semitism, he campaigned against racial discrimination. He helped start a group called Dentists for Peace in Vietnam, an activity that caused a few rumblings from the ADA. He participated in various local activities, such as the American Civil Liberties Union and especially with the Committee for a Sane Nuclear Policy (now called Peace Action). He also worked on the nuclear energy issue with the Physicians for Social Responsibility. He even used his talents to promote water fluoridation, much more successfully in New York than in New Jersey.

> For Irwin Mandel, what matters most is not the legacy of scientific achievement but the respect of his peers.

Educator

When Irwin became division head of preventive dentistry and community health in 1969, his activities were an extrapolation of his interests and his social activism. He offered a course in cariology to provide a substantial basic science background for the disease that dental students treated the most. The division developed manuals and videotapes on preventive dentistry. He created a student extramural program that serviced the local public schools with classroom education and preventive therapy that was staffed by a team of new volunteer dentists who had preventive-oriented practices. He worked with the School of Public Health to help develop a joint DDS and master's degree in public health.

When Dr Mandel was president of the AADR, he promoted the establishment of student research groups at dental schools all across the country and a student summer fellowship program. He also initiated a health promotion committee whose mission was to make

of lifelong friendships that have characterized the relationship between Dr Mandel and his students.

In the end, what can we learn from the example of this remarkable person? One message is that what matters most is the method by which we achieve our ends, rather than the end itself. Whereas Irwin, having simply fashioned himself and his patterns of interaction after what was modeled in his earlier years, seemed not to be particularly conscious of the values that are central to the role of the researcher in contemporary society,* those of us who are about to embark on a career as a scientist or dentist can see what qualities are most admired in the end. We can then consciously decide how we will conduct our personal and professional interactions. Further, we can take advantage of opportunities not present in Irwin's time: to engage in course work that provides guidance, practice, and feedback on essential professional ethical behaviors. Today, educators need not rely only on the modeling of their predecessors to develop effective and stimulating learning environments. There is now greater understanding of the methods that are effective to promote intellectual and emotional maturity.

References

1. Merton RK. The Sociology of Science. Chicago: University of Chicago Press, 1973:267–278 (original work published in 1942).
2. Pascarella ET, Terenzini P. How College Affects Students: Findings and Insights from Twenty Years of Research. San Francisco: Jossey-Bass, 1991.
3. King PM, Kitchner KS. Developing Reflective Judgment. San Francisco: Jossey-Bass, 1994.
4. Goleman D. Emotional Intelligence: Why It Can Matter More Than I.Q. New York: Bantam Books, 1995.
5. Pellegrino ED, Thomasma DC. The Virtues in Medical Practice. New York: Oxford University Press, 1983.

*When I (MJB) first asked Dr Mandel to be the speaker for the AADR symposium on research ethics, he initially declined, saying he really had no expertise on the subject. It took considerable effort to persuade him that while he may not have the discipline-specific expertise of one who is able to articulate the values that guided the research enterprise, he had lived the values and was regarded by his peers as a person of the highest integrity.

the results of research useful to the profession and the public. Unexpectedly, this turned out to be controversial. Many of his colleagues did not see this form of education as an appropriate function of a research organization. He finally obtained approval by calling it a science transfer committee. Because of such activities, he has become somewhat of a national spokesman for bridging the gap between science and clinical practice.

Education has likewise been a key aspect of Dr Mandel's research program. In the early 1970s his research activity developed rapidly, aided by a 3-year Career Scientist award from New York City. In the research labs, as in the clinic, Irwin developed teams of scientists and technicians. They approached salivary research from different standpoints. Some focused on its relationship with calculus formation; others on its connection with caries; still others on its correlation with various systemic diseases, or its composition under the influence of various drugs. With the formation of a full academic program in preventive dentistry and community health, several full-time academic positions for researchers in related fields became available. It was an exciting time. Dr Mandel also attracted volunteer clinical faculty who worked on projects a day or two a week. Dental students and children of faculty members, even high school students, came in to work after hours, on school holidays, or during summer vacations. Irwin always had something for them to work on, according to their abilities and interests.

In the 1960s his laboratory was a refuge for unhappy, long-haired students who were having difficulty with the regimentation of dental school and were considering quitting the profession. In Irwin's lab their perspectives were restored, and some who initially had wanted to leave school eventually distinguished themselves in the profession. Irwin stopped doing bench research himself and became a laboratory director. In terms of the volume of activity, it was the most productive period of his life. People enjoyed themselves in Irwin's lab. Students and technicians from Cuba, the Philippines, Hungary, Russia, and a variety of other places would prepare their ethnic dishes to share in potluck meals. It was like an extended family for Irwin, and he loved the buzz of activity.

Reflecting on those years, Irwin now realizes that in his laboratory he had unconsciously duplicated his father's automobile parts store. His father had formed close and lifelong relationships with many of his employees. Some had even joined the Leeds Fraternal Society. When he retired, they bought the business. Irwin likewise has formed close friendships with his former students, who are now in diverse locations from coast to coast. The only difference was that Irwin worked with technicians, students, and volunteer faculty instead of salespeople, countermen, and machinists. The important part was that everyone worked together harmoniously and productively. Privately, Irwin called this "the harmonics of research." He said, "It's like conducting an orchestra. Orchestrating multiple projects and being involved with multiple people and keeping them going . . . It was one of the most exciting periods of my life."

Mentor

Irwin Mandel's concept of mentoring was based on doing for his students what his mentors had done for him. He credits his own chief mentors: Dave Block, his scoutmaster; Leo Lehrman, his department chair at City College; William Lefkowitz, his student research advisor at Columbia; and Bar Levy, who introduced him to the merits of extensive hands-on mentoring while he was a young scientist just out of the Navy for the second time.

In Irwin's view, "If I look at a laboratory as an extended family, then the mentor has much of the same role as a father. Mentors have to show confidence in their students and associates, appreciate their difficulties, and be available to help when needed." He said that while students needed to be treated like colleagues and given all the responsibility they can handle, "You just don't let them go along on their own. There has to be some checking on what they're doing, including how they keep notebooks, and how they record their data . . . everything has to be written down." A mentor needs to know how students evaluate their work and whether they can make mature judgments about the validity of the data. Mentors need to help students learn how to acquire the relevant scientific literature and evaluate it critically. Every afternoon, over a cup of coffee, Irwin would have group discussions on the problems of the day.

Mentors should work closely with their students as they prepare their papers for publication. "I would encourage them to do the first draft and work with them and check it very carefully. I was also very careful to give adequate credit. For many of the papers, a student was the senior author." In all of his efforts, he worked toward creating a supportive and comfortable atmosphere. He encouraged them to appreciate the contributions of others before them and to respect the integrity of data; and he gave them as much day-by-day, practical, concrete instruction as he could. All of these things had been done for him by others, but he has added a few touches of his own. For Irwin, mentoring does not end when the students leave his laboratory. The need for his advice continues, and so does the friendship. Today, many of those whom Irwin mentored have become mentors themselves.

Irwin sees several thorny challenges in mentoring. "I think the hardest thing is dealing with failure. I used to use the slogan, 'Disappointment is the daily bread of the investigator.' [It is very difficult to help students to accept] that if things don't work out, you've got to do them over and over again." Students tend to be overly impressed with their early data and jump to conclusions about its merits. It is a great challenge for the mentor to get the point across that they need to 'verify, verify, verify.' Another difficult concept for students is that, "It takes time to get good at what they are doing. It doesn't happen right away."

> In Irwin's view, "If I look at a laboratory as an extended family, then the mentor has much of the same role as a father."

Sustainability

There is such diversity in the scope of Irwin Mandel's accomplishments and values that the juxtaposition of some components is surprising. Even considering the fact that people can have exceedingly diverse values, it is difficult to find a link that connects, for example, his work in salivary chemistry, his role as advisor to *Consumer Reports*, and his participation in social activism organizations. Irwin himself sees everything as a continuum: practice, research, mentoring, administration, activism, and his role in national organizations. He said that the unifying idea, one that is so characteristic that he would not be himself without it, is the concept of sustainability. Usually this word is used in discussions of how to maintain environmental resources. For Irwin, however, human rather than environmental resources are at stake; and they should not only be sustained but enhanced. He said, "There is a responsibility of one generation for another in all spheres."

For Dr Mandel, the concept of sustainability is not new, nor is it unique to him. It has been a consistent guiding principle for his actions. He said, "If we are really to sustain the ethical basis of research or of clinical practice, then [each of us] must go beyond the technical aspects of training and transmit ideas and

values." As a university scientist, he has been the mentor of another generation of mentors. As a clinician, he not only treated disease, he tried his best to prevent future disease, emphasizing the patient's role. As a division head, he fostered a broad-based understanding of oral disease and promoted programs that helped students see themselves as part of the larger community. As a social activist, he worked to promote human equality. As a national leader in science, he promoted educational programs that benefited both students and the public. Although Dr Mandel's reputation, for the most part, is based on his research, his life-guiding principles have been expressed primarily through education, with emphasis always on a respect for the scientific process, a respect for people, and a broad acceptance of responsibility by the clinician. Furthermore, in all of his efforts, there is a conscious concern for the future.

During my interview with Irwin, I asked him what he thought had been his greatest accomplishments. The frame of reference for his answer was a movie he had seen the day before, *The Crucible*, based on a play by Arthur Miller. In an especially dramatic scene in the movie, set in the late 17th century, the protagonist chose to be hanged rather than to lie about his relationship with a certain woman. The lie would have allowed him to live, but it would have meant giving up his good name. Irwin feels that his most important accomplishment is earning the respect of his peers. He is compelled to offer the modest assessment that his research, though much lauded and significant in its time, now seems a limited accomplishment.

Currently

Not surprisingly, Dr Mandel continues to be active. He keeps his friendships intact, both with colleagues and former students. He still consults with the ADA and maintains his position as the dental advisor for *Consumer Reports*. He played a role in writing the initial draft and reviewing the final phases of the surgeon general's 2000 report on oral health. He continues to spend a day a week at Columbia University and preserves a minor presence as a social activist on the Executive Committee of the New York chapter of Physicians for Social

Responsibility. As to other forms of social activism, he said, "Now that I have much more limited energy, I give money instead of time."

He perseveres in thinking about the future, and in that respect, his latest opportunity is made to order. He is one of several members of a panel whose mission is to plan and establish health considerations for a manned expedition to Mars.

References

1. Mandel ID. On being a scientist in a rapidly changing world. J Dent Res 1996;75:841–844.
2. Baum BJ, Fox PC, Tabak LA. Columbia, salivary research, plus Irwin Mandel equal a special combination for dentistry. J Dent Res 1997;76:631–633.
3. Malamud D, Tabak L (eds). Saliva as a diagnostic fluid, vol 694, Annals of the New York Academy of Sciences. New York: New York Academy of Sciences, 1993:ix–x.

Questions for Discussion

1. Many of Dr Mandel's peers describe a dental education process that featured negative modeling. Yet his interactions with dental students and dental researchers stand in stark contrast to this model of interaction. How do you think he was able to overcome the negative models of his own dental education?

2. Whether consciously or unconsciously, Dr Mandel seems to have set long-term aspirations for who he wants to be and how he wants to be regarded by others. Have you set such goals for yourself? At the end of your life, how do you want to be remembered?

3. To achieve universal respect, Dr Mandel has had to blend two conflicting roles: advisor and mentor. What is the nature of the conflict between these roles, and how has he managed to resolve it? Do you see any similarities between the different and conflicting roles that dentists may have to play with their patients?

4. As described in the commentary, King and Kitchner alert us to the challenges educators face in moving young people to levels of intellectual maturity required of the competent researcher. Reflect on this challenge as they describe it. Do dentists who interact with patients who hold beliefs about oral health (eg, soft teeth run in my family; my amalgam fillings are exacerbating my multiple sclerosis; every time I had another child I lost another tooth) face similar problems? Are there lessons in Dr Mandel's story that can help them address such issues?

12

Dentists Who Care: What Stands Out?

What Stood Out for Us

Having written the narratives of 10 exceptional dental professionals and reflected on each individually, we reviewed the stories and their commentaries as a whole in order to formulate some general observations. As we reflected on the stories, the following eight conclusions stood out for us. After each of them, we indicate the implications these observations may have for you.

1. The interview process promoted self-examination and reflection.

Many of our exemplars commented on the value of the interview and story development process in helping them clarify their values and the forces that shaped their identity. The most stunning example of this was Dr Echternacht's delight in discovering the powerful effect his father's activism while he was a child had on him as an adult. At the same time, his own activism, including the community resistance and retaliation he endured, had been tempered by his mother's acceptance of her husband's activism and its consequences as well as her more general examples of compassion and caring for others. Similarly, Dr Rumberger expressed an appreciation, upon reflecting on her life story, for the roles her controlling father and subservient mother played in her eventual development. Dr Owens also seemed to discover, in the telling of his story, the power of contrasting models for addressing racial injustice. He says that from his Uncle George Melvin, he learned to take a stand; from his father, he learned to avoid a bad stand. Likewise, Dr Mandel came to see how his father's treatment of employees in his auto body shop during tough economic times served as a model for the way he organized his research laboratory.

Implications

The research literature[1] indicates that self-reflection and self-assessment are important dimensions of professional growth. Just as our exemplars benefited from examining the forces that shaped their identity and developed insights about the role of moral models in their lives, we believe individuals at other stages of life can benefit from such examination. Consider using some of the interview questions in Appendix B to reflect upon your own life or to assist someone else in self-examination.

Consider also looking at the descriptions of stages of identity formation (Appendix E) to determine where you see yourself fitting. When considering professionals you admire, consider how their admirable qualities reflect the expectations of a professional (Appendix C) or the virtues of the good professional (Appendix D). Appendix A also contains suggestions for facilitating this examination in the classroom or dental study group.

2. One mark of the highly developed moral self is the reconciliation of internal conflicts.

At times, our exemplars spoke of negative influences that needed to be overcome—a controlling father, a mother's negative and hurtful criticisms, growing up in poverty, or cultural or gender biases that interfered with attainment of goals. What stood out for us in negotiating the telling of their stories is that, upon reflection, most of the exemplars decided not to make public some details of their personal story that would reflect negatively upon another—for example a parent, sibling, spouse, or child. In the case of our whistle-blower, this decision protected her identity and thereby the identity of the professional who had been disciplined. This restriction caused us some dismay because in every instance the conflict had been central to an aspect of the exemplar's development. In particular it prevented us from showing the power of negative role models on our exemplar's development. However, as we now consider these restrictions (including a story that was withdrawn from the book because we could not resolve issues in its telling), we wonder whether they may signal a reconciliation of internal conflicts experienced earlier in life and thereby serve as a mark of a mature moral identity.

Where once a parent, sibling, spouse, or colleague had been marked for perpetual criticism, the exemplars now came to see them as problems, not unlike competing commitments that one learns to manage. Thus, unlike the individual who feels the need to expose a famous parent by alleging physical or mental abuse, our exemplars seem to have reconciled or moved beyond these stumbling blocks to their own development. Reflecting on our first observation about the power of the process, it appeared that telling their story somehow cemented the reconciliation of conflict.

Implications

Most of us have negative experiences that challenge us and seem to get in the way of achieving our ends, or at least get in the way of living a stress-free life. It might be easy to imagine our exemplars as perfect people—free of adversity or interpersonal struggles. This is not the case. What we notice, however, is that moral maturity seems to be marked by a resolution of some of these struggles. This is not to say that adversity disappears, but people like our exemplars no longer feel that they are defined by what others think of them and are not torn among multiple shared identities,[*] as is characteristic of those in professional schools or in their early years of professional practice. When I am no longer defined by a parent's or friend's negative perspective of me, I am able to move beyond or even see the positive side of that negative assessment. Consistent with a stage 4 identity (Appendix E), our exemplars have constructed a "self-system" that provides an internal compass for negotiating and resolving tensions among these multiple, shared expectations. By adhering to an internally constructed set of standards and values that embody the profession's values, the stage 4 professional is able to negotiate the conflicting roles and obligations that are inevitable in their working lives. To successfully balance these competing claims is the challenge for all developing professionals.

3. Competence and the will to succeed distinguish the exemplar from the ordinary good person.

Most of our exemplars described a childhood marked by an emphasis on academic achievement and the expectation that they would excel. This is not to suggest our exemplars did not have competing interests—sports dominated Dr Whittaker's early life, and the backbreaking requirements of dairy farming competed for Dr Capdeboscq's attention—or that everything came easy for them. Dr Mandel was brilliant academically but had to work hard to improve his clinical skills. In addition to an emphasis on academic achievement throughout their lives, our exemplars appear to have had a lot of innate talent, more so than most dentists and most people in general: Dr Echternacht was first in his dental school class and loved dentistry. Dr Benkelman enjoyed exceptional success in reducing the stress of his patients. Dr Sinkford always excelled in academics. Dr Owens loved to be competitive, particularly in clinical issues. Dr Capdeboscq had the reputation for being the

---

[*]Recall that moral identity shares features with other identities. For example, as a dental student, one may also be an employee, an athlete, a spouse or friend, a child, a sibling, or perhaps even a parent.

best around in gold work. Dr Rumberger received an important clinically based award upon graduation.

Despite the exemplars' academic achievements and their recognition that technical competence is an essential virtue for a professional, they were competent in other areas as well. We found them to be exceptionally skilled in interpersonal communication and in figuring out the steps necessary to solve problems. But beyond that, and at least as importantly, they also knew what to say and how to say it. Often we know the right thing to do in morally difficult situations and want to do it but fail because we are uncertain about how to manage the inevitable sensitive obstacles that we face. Competence, so defined, appears to be a powerful source of self-motivation. Dr Owens, for example, remarked that "It was enormously satisfying to do things that others thought needed to be done but couldn't do themselves." As for the importance of achieving professional competence, he advised, "First excel, then help others." We see in the examples of Drs Mandel, Sinkford, and Capdeboscq how interpersonal, professionally based competence can be used as a guide to approaching and influencing students. We see how Dr Echternacht used his ability to inspire others for the betterment of the community. We see how Dr Lowney's extraordinary drive to create helping projects ultimately inspired others to become involved in them. We also see how Dr Rumberger turned her organizational skills into examples of influential leadership. In all cases, the exemplars demonstrated uncommon perseverance.

The incorporation of moral values into the development of what Blasi[2] refers to as the "moral self" is an obvious requirement for the moral exemplar. However, without competence and motivation to achieve, one may be a kind and nice person but is unlikely to be effectual. In such cases, the moral self achieves only what Jon Hassler[3] refers to as *dispositional goodness* but lacks the goodness of activity that is characteristic of the moral exemplars we have studied. Mobilizing a large group of independent practitioners to achieve a common purpose (eg, as did Drs Rumberger and Lowney) when the purpose is purely service to others requires enormous competence and a range of skills that flourish only when accompanied by a strong drive to succeed.

Implications

Competence is an essential virtue for the professional, and the development of competence must be the aspiring professional's primary goal. Yet along the way, each aspiring dental professional will need to determine whether the pursuit of competence has motivational power for the self. If it does, the individual will happily complete professional education and pursue professional practice. If not, reevaluation is required. There is nothing worse than trying to achieve something to which one is not committed or that does not play to one's talents. Perhaps entering professional school ought to be viewed only as a tentative decision to become a dentist. Who can know before actually experiencing the educational process and attempting to succeed within it whether pursuit of competence–not just to a minimally acceptable standard, but to one that is personally and professionally gratifying–is the right decision for an individual? Who can know whether the lifelong pursuit of all the additional competencies required for effective practice will have motivational power? It is no disgrace to decide that one's talents lie elsewhere, but it may take an act of moral courage to withdraw from the profession. This is especially true if family members and friends are invested in the person's choice of profession.

4. The concept of service unfolds as exemplars move through various stages of life.

Consistent with developmental theory[4] (Appendix E), our exemplars' concept of service underwent transformations during and after professional education. The story of Donna Rumberger provides a particularly rich example of this phenomenon, as her competitiveness became transformed in its orientation from self to other–first in dental school and later, more extensively, in her work with dental societies. This type of transformation is also evident in the story of Jack Whittaker, who says that taking care of children who really needed his help resulted in a deeper meaning of caring for his patients. Most of the exemplars, but especially Drs Echternacht, Owens, and Mandel, had childhood role models who engaged in altruistic service activities. Yet early in their professional lives, our exemplars focused on the development of competence and on satisfying their own basic human needs. Whereas they initially engaged in service because that's what a professional does (Appendix E, stage 3), they report that their sense of service deepened. Their values became internalized so that their professional and individual values were one and the same (stage 4). Both Drs Lowney and Echternacht noted that only after fulfilling personal needs did they turn their attention to "sharing my good fortune somewhere else." Lowney distinguished real service from service that is self-serving: "Real service is the kind of giving where the only return is the personal satisfaction derived from helping someone who is really in need." He believes that, "To whom much is given, much is expected." We noticed that the exemplars expressed a kind of gratitude for what has been "given" to them, rather than a sense that their good fortune is the "just dessert" that results from hard work.

Implications

One of the most important discoveries from the study of our exemplars is that the concept of service develops over time. Let Dr Owens' invective be your guide: "First excel, then help others." Dr Owens' words point out the responsibility not only for competence to benefit others but also to oneself to first satisfy basic needs. It is important to understand that the concept of service to others has boundaries. Sometimes young professionals come to professional practice with great enthusiasm for helping others but do not look after the economic stability of their practice. Without a bounded sense of service, they become resentful. Set realistic aspirational goals for helping others. Create a balance between altruism and self-orientation, and the satisfactions will be worth it.

5. The exemplars inspired others and respected the people they served.

Exemplars seem able, by the power of their personalities, to inspire others. They find great joy in creating support networks that further their cause—whether it is to develop an effective care team (Drs Benkelman and Whittaker), mobilize experts to solve a sanitation problem in Haiti (Dr Lowney), support opportunities for women and minorities (Dr Sinkford), promote civil rights (Drs Owens and Mandel), recruit professionals to help the disadvantaged (Dr Rumberger), increase funding for Medicaid (Dr Whittaker), promote fluoridation (Dr Echternacht), or simply show care and concern for their patients (Dr Benkelman). Commenting on Dr Mandel's ability to break new ground in science while promoting collaboration rather than competition in the research environment, a colleague said, "Working in his laboratory was a special experience, not for its competitive, ambitious aura of productivity, but for its feeling of inclusiveness, acceptance, and refuge."

Such feelings of inclusiveness and acceptance are the byproducts of Dr Mandel's remarkable capacity for demonstrating respect for others, a quality for which he is much admired. Yet without this quality, one could hardly inspire others. Each of our exemplars demonstrates this generalized respect for humanity. This quality is particularly well illustrated by Dr Lowney's responses to questions about his ability to persevere under conditions most would find repugnant and hopeless. It is essential, he feels, to treat the Haitian people with dignity, regardless of their circumstances, and he warns his associates neither to criticize their cultural practices nor to proselytize. This same respect must be extended to those whom he asks for contributions to the Haitian Health Foundation. He is very conscious of his need to be viewed as authentic, not as a hustler. The same kind of generalized respect, this time for colleagues, is also evident in Dr Johnson's unwillingness to further publicize her disciplined colleague's transgressions, as well as in Dr Echternacht's yearly hunting parties to maintain collegial relationships, even with dentists in the community who failed to cooperate to promote community health.

Implications

One of the hardest challenges for the beginning professional is to overcome the repugnance one may feel for a person whose personal demeanor, oral health, and/or personal appearance are offensive. How do our exemplars manage to demonstrate respect for others who so deviate from the standards they hold for themselves? What we see in them is an ability to truly take a broad perspective, that is, to see the world from the perspective of the other. To understand how another might perceive his or her circumstances, the professional must learn to elicit the real concerns of the other. Kay Toombs,[5] a philosopher suffering from chronic illness, interviewed people who were similarly situated. Chronicling the frustration that patients experience as their physicians focus on curing when curing is not possible, she offers caregivers this advice: "If one is to understand the lived experience of illness, comprehending what the disorder means to the patient, then it is clear that one has to go beyond objective, quantifiable, clinical data and elicit the patient's illness story." Relating her own experiences and those of many chronically ill patients, she observed that no physician ever asked, "What is it like for you?" or "What are you afraid of?" These are questions that could elicit the patient's real concerns and connect the patient to the caregiver. By connecting with the lived experience of the patient, the physician can shift his or her focus from curing to caring. As we see from the witness of our exemplars, the true joy of helping emerges when the professional truly connects with the one being helped.

The same example applies to dentistry when we encounter patients whose appearance, outlook on life, oral health practices, or potential for personal growth are different from ours. Jack Whittaker, for example, discussed the problems that some dentists have with treating Medicaid patients. He said that dentists sometimes complain to him that poor patients are late for appointments or don't keep them at all, and that when they do show up, their clothes are dirty and their oral hygiene poor. Jack said that these complaints are exaggerated but sometimes accurate. For him, however, it doesn't make any difference. He listens to the frustrations of the mothers whose children are in pain but cannot find dentists to treat them. He has become protective of these children and is proud of their parents. As Toombs suggested above, he has connected with them. He knows their fears, and he understands their answer to the question, "What is it like for you?" Jerry Lowney arrived at the same kind of understanding in an instant during his first visit to Haiti, when a hopelessly sick and malnourished infant died in his arms. It opened his eyes forever to the health-related desperation of a huge segment of the Haitian population. Knowing "what it's like for you" can become an important bridge between a dentist and other kinds of patients as well, from elderly patients in nursing homes to victims of HIV and AIDS.

6. The exemplars show a willingness to do the "harder right."

Each of the exemplars, though in varying degrees, is engaged in some form of social activism. Four of our exemplars (Drs Echternacht, Whittaker, Owens, and Johnson) were nominated specifically because they had engaged in actions to right an injustice. In each case, they did so at considerable personal risk and without active support from their colleagues. For Dr Whittaker, whose actions righted injustice but ultimately exposed his colleagues' less altruistic motives, or for Dr Johnson, whose actions exposed a colleague's incompetence, their efforts had acutely distressing consequences. What sustained them was a set of goals that were consistent with the moral ideals espoused by their profession—to serve society and to monitor their profession. Whereas we might see their actions as requiring tremendous courage or fortitude as Pellegrino and Thomasma[6] would describe it, they (like Colby and Damon's exemplars[†]) simply saw their action as something they must do. Janet Johnson, reflecting on other professionals who had quit their jobs rather than challenge a superior's

mistreatment of patients, said, "There was no way I could leave the situation the way it was." Jack Echternacht, thinking about his 30-year battle with antifluoridationists, remarked, "I'm basically peace-loving, but if there's a just cause involved, that's another matter. Then, we go to war."

Implications

Despite the fact that our exemplars viewed their actions as simply "doing the right thing," rather than as acts of courage, we know that this is often easier said than done. Studies from the psychology of morality[8] help us to see why this might be so. To do the right thing, one must: *(1)* recognize a moral problem when it exists, *(2)* reason through what ought to be done, *(3)* see oneself as responsible for doing something, and *(4)* put in place an effective action plan.

Failure to do the right thing can result from a deficiency in one or more of these processes. Also, although these processes appear to form a linear decision model, arriving at an effective action plan actually requires cycling back through these processes in order to test ideas to ensure the effectiveness of the plan.

Janet Johnson's actions followed these precepts, except perhaps for cycling back to see whether her proposed action plan was likely to work. Let's think about her action in terms of the four processes. Initially, she recognized that Dr Cross's actions were causing harm. Further, she substantiated her assessment by reviewing records and the testimony of the dental assistants (component 1). She reasoned that something ought to be done to stop further harm to patients (component 2). She clearly saw herself as responsible (component 3), and she developed an action plan—direct communication and internal reporting (component 4). With the benefit of hindsight, we are now able to see what she missed in projecting the likely effectiveness of her action plan. Recycling her thinking through component 1 may have helped her recognize the full extent of the moral problem, which included Dr Cross's serious character flaws. In addition, it appears that she underestimated the negative aspects of the prevailing moral climate in the hospital and failed to project the likely troublesome consequences of action—either to herself or to the institution. The failure to recognize these things interfered with the development of an effective action plan. These comments notwithstanding, her actions

---

[†]Colby and Damon[7] observe that the notion of courage simply did not capture anything that their exemplars had felt or done. Feelings of moral necessity had given them a sense of certainty that relieved them of fears and doubt.

cannot be said to represent failure; they resulted in many favorable outcomes. The challenge is to develop an action plan that resolves a problem effectively while minimizing negative consequences.

As we see from the studies of medical students' perceptions of their role in regulation of the profession, perhaps the greatest detriment to implementation of an action plan are external circumstances–that the plan will not go well and we will experience retaliation, as Dr Johnson did. With the benefit of the whistle-blowing literature, we are now able to see the significance of factors of personality and of institutional climate that made the strategy Dr Johnson selected (direct communication and internal reporting) unlikely to succeed without serious personal repercussions. In contrast, we see that Dr Owens learned from the experiences of others–his Uncle George Melvin and his father–and managed to avoid a "bad stand," as he put it. Dr Owens appears to have been particularly skillful in cycling through each of the processes and projecting cause-consequence chains of events to ensure success.

The implication for each of us who wishes to "do the right thing" is to develop the skills needed for effective moral action. Certainly such skills will not protect a person from all possible repercussions, but they can help us to deal effectively with the garden variety challenges professionals face. How are such skills developed? Ethics courses may be useful in helping us to reason through what we ought to do, to at least name the moral issues at stake and, perhaps, to apply moral ideals to their resolution.‡ However, moral sensitivity, as psychologists describe it, requires much more. Morally sensitive professionals are able to interpret problems–sometimes from seemingly ambiguous clues–and to project cause-consequence chains of events. Empathy, perspective-taking, and an awareness of professional expectations are critical dimensions of sensitivity. Ethics courses usually address professional expectation (component 3) but are typically of insufficient duration to really foster identity development as we have described it. Ethics courses also often stop short of providing practice in actually implementing action plans, as would be required of role playing. Many of us have learned from experience that the words we choose and the

strategies we use can undermine our best intentions. To hone skills in problem solving and interpersonal communication (aspects of component 4), we recommend the widely regarded book on negotiation by Fisher and Ury[9] cited often in this volume.

7. What sets the exemplars apart from ordinary good people is a unity of the self with moral concerns.

As Colby and Damon[7] observed with their exemplars, none of our exemplars saw their moral choices as an exercise in self-sacrifice. Rather, their moral goals were in harmony with their personal goals, and vice versa. None of them saw unremunerated service as self-sacrifice; rather, it was viewed as a core activity that sustains them. Dr Whittaker, who promises never to retire, says, "Work is so rewarding to me. I take care of some of the most seriously ill children. I affect their lives. I make them feel better. I keep them healthy." And Dr Rumberger says: "Doing good for others is doing good for me."

Implications

We think our exemplars illustrate something we all strive for–an integration of personal and professional values. According to developmental psychologists, this is what characterizes the moral self. If moral considerations are self-defining, then not to act in accord with one's identity is to risk losing the self. So, personal distress is experienced when the stage 4 individual (Appendix E) senses that his or her internal compass has been revealed to be flawed. Stage 3 individuals–those who define themselves in terms of how they experience themselves being experienced by others–are vulnerable to feeling torn by competing, incompatible expectations. Personal setbacks are experienced in terms of failing to meet shared, collective obligations–not merely a failure to enact certain concrete role behaviors. When such failures occur, they evoke feelings of guilt over having let both the self and others down. Consider how the reflections of the following individual illustrate what psychologists describe.

In my early years structuring professional ethics curricula, I (MJB) encountered a dentist who had been disciplined by the state board of dentistry, had been married and divorced, had had several affairs, and so on. At the time I met him, he was studying to become an Episcopalian minister. He recounted how earlier in his life, he used to continually argue with himself. "If I had my assistant mix up one shot of amalgam and noticed the filling was a little short, I found myself justifying

‡Ethics courses typically employ structured problems in which the issues essentially have been defined. The task for the learner is to name the moral conflict and then apply some framework to determine what ought to be done. To really promote ethical sensitivity, learners need unstructured problems, in which there are merely clues that something is amiss. Learners must recognize that some characteristic of the patient is likely to interfere with acceptance of treatment recommendations and that the practitioner has a responsibility to address the ethical issue this presents.

that an underfilled restoration was less likely to crack, or that this was a good patient and I could always correct this later if need be. Similarly, if I saw an attractive woman, I asked myself, 'Why not?' After my experience with the board, I found myself asking, 'Who am I? How do I want to be regarded?' I decided that I wanted others to think of me as a good dentist, and my family to think of me as a loyal parent and spouse, something they did not now think. I decided that I would no longer argue with myself, but instead consider how I wanted to regarded."

8. Each exemplar came to view service to society as obligatory rather than supererogatory.[§]

What we noticed in the character of Dr Echternacht (our first exemplar), we came to see as true of our other exemplars as well. The disposition to habitually act to benefit others extended beyond their role as dentist and member of a profession. Many ethicists (eg, Frankena[10]) argue that beneficence is supererogatory rather than obligatory. Our exemplars see beneficence as obligatory. For example, Dr Echternacht conceptualizes as obligatory what others might characterize as "beyond the call of duty." He says, "I believe that if one lives in a community and makes his livelihood from it, he should return that benefit by participating in the activities of the community to better it in any way that he can." At the end of the story, when commenting upon the Salvation Army's request for bell ringers, he again uses the language of obligation: "Don't you think I ought to do that?" In response to his wife's objection, he says "No, really, don't you think I should?" Similarly, Dr Mandel used the language of obligation to describe his responsibility to young scholars and scientists in his laboratory, as does Dr Capdeboscq to describe his responsibility to students. Dr Sinkford says, "I just grew up feeling that whatever you had was a gift, and that you had certain talents, and you were supposed to use them."

In summary, we see that our exemplars fulfill Pellegrino and Thomasma's[6] characterization of a virtuous person. They separate what is morally acceptable and not acceptable "at a different place than would one who acts solely from principle, rule, or duty. The virtuous person will interpret the span of duty . . . more inclu-sively and more in the direction of perfection of the good end to which the action is naturally oriented." And they are impelled to strive for perfection, not because it is a duty, but because they cannot act otherwise. It is part of their character. They strive for perfection, "realizing all the while that [they] cannot get there and, in that realization, being prevented from the vices of self-righteousness and hubris."[6p166]

Implications

Who am I? Who will I become? What is my purpose in life? What do I strive for? Who do I want to be? These are old, old questions that have been asked and answered throughout history. They are questions each of us must ask and answer for ourselves. It is our hope that the stories we have developed and explanations we have provided will help you, the reader, reflect on your life experiences and consider who you are and what you will become.

Exemplars and the Education of Professionals

Life is a developmental journey that proceeds in phases and stages. We are indeed fortunate if, like most of our exemplars, we have parents who support our academic achievement. But we are even more fortunate if they, along with our teachers and religious leaders, serve as models for goodness of activity as well as of disposition. Our exemplars and other role models are also part of our developmental journey. They can make important contributions to our understanding of identity formation and moral motivation.

Young professionals need not view service as obligatory in the same way our exemplars have come to view it, but rather may view it as something that would be good to do and that may even bring personal and professional satisfaction. All professionals need to be aware of the challenges they will face at various stages of their developmental journey. At the same time, it should be instructive for them to see how our exemplars have worked through conflicts of commitment and negative modeling, including how they have come to see their profession's values and their personal values as one and the same. Further, we hope the readers will experience, through the telling of our exemplars' stories, the joy that is derived from a lifetime of good work. Finally, all pro-

[§]*Supererogatory* means doing more than is morally required under the circumstances. The circumstances here are those that place the person contemplating an act at risk for unusual adversity. No one thinks that individual is required to perform a certain act, but he or she chooses not to take the easy way out.

fessionals, fledgling and experienced alike, should be helped to consider what will matter most when the end of life's work is at hand. For Irwin Mandel, it is not his legacy of scientific accomplishments that matters most to him, but the respect of his peers. To be remembered and cherished as a person of integrity implies completeness, wholeness, and unity achieved through sustained commitment to virtuous ends.

Gardner and colleagues[11] suggest that optimal development requires character and competence, but that character and competence are not quite enough. Optimal development involves fulfillment of two potentials: differentiation and integration. A differentiated person is competent and has character but also experiences life as a wholly self-directed individual. In other words, the differentiated person is not only capable and guided by integrity, but also knows what he or she wants and how to get it. An integrated person "is someone whose goals, values, thoughts, and actions are in harmony; someone who belongs to a network of relationships; someone who accepts a place within a system of mutual responsibilities and shared meanings."[11]

Our exemplars appear to have achieved character, competence, differentiation, and integration on an informal basis. There has been no explicit teaching of what moral models of professionalism to follow and what behavior is expected of them, nor have they been exposed to the structured opportunities for self-assessment and reflection that are thought to be linked to the development of the moral self.[1] However, this does not mean that such standards should not be part of the educational endeavor. There is plenty of evidence that aspiring professionals do not intuit the values of their profession[12] or learn them by osmosis.[13] They need to be explicitly taught. Further, even though identity formation is apparent during college and beyond,[14,15] lessons from our exemplars suggest that students would benefit from opportunities to reflect on their goals, their values, and the role that models (both positive and negative) play in their development. The job of educators is to facilitate self-assessment and reflection, tied to explicit and public criteria.[1]

Finally, professions face uncertain times. Market forces and technological advances challenge the very foundation of a profession's value systems. All professionals need to be alert to phases of what Gardner et al[11] refer to as alignment and misalignment. Members of each profession need to consider their collective responsibility not only for the education of future professionals, but also for the policies and practices that promote and maintain public trust.

It is our intent that the stories of outstanding professionals will serve as models for aspiring and established professionals. We also hope that the lessons we have drawn from them will serve as guideposts for educators who are engaged in the development of future caregivers. Gardner and colleagues[11] suggest that the following educational processes will increase the likelihood of good work—"work of expert quality that benefits the broader society": (1) ensuring a favorable moral milieu (or climate) in professional school and in the professional's first job, (2) passing on the beliefs and practices associated with exemplary professionals, and (3) offering opportunities to experience admirable mentors or paragons. To these, we would add (4) explicit teaching of the expectations of professional practice and (5) the importance of opportunities for self-assessment and reflection to promote the development of the individual.

References

1. Mentkowski M, et al. Learning That Lasts: Integrating Learning, Development, and Performance in College and Beyond. San Francisco: Jossey-Bass, 2000.
2. Blasi A. Moral identity: Its role in moral functioning. In: Krutines W, Gerwitz J (eds). Morality, Moral Behavior, and Moral Development. New York: Wiley, 1984:128–139.
3. Hassler J. Good People. Chicago: Loyola Press, 2001.
4. Kegan R. The Evolving Self: Problem and Process in Human Development. Cambridge, MA: Harvard University Press, 1982.
5. Toombs K. The Meaning of Illness. Boston: Dordrecht, 1992.
6. Pellegrino ED, Thomasma DC. The Virtues in Medical Practice. New York: Oxford University Press, 1983.
7. Colby A, Damon W. Some Do Care: Contemporary Lives of Moral Commitment. New York: Free Press, 1992.
8. Bebeau MJ, Rest JR, Narváez DF. Beyond the promise: A perspective for research in moral education. Educ Res 1999;28:18–26.
9. Fisher R, Ury W. Getting to Yes: Negotiating Agreement Without Giving In. New York: Penguin Books, 1981.
10. Frankena W. Ethics, ed 2. Englewood Cliffs, NJ: Prentice-Hall, 1975.
11. Gardner H, Csikszentmihalyi M, Damon W. Good Work: When Excellence and Ethics Meet. New York: Basic Books, 2001.

12. Bebeau MJ. Influencing the moral dimension of dental practice. In: Rest JR, Narváez DF (eds). Moral Development in the Professions: Psychology and Applied Ethics. Hillsdale, NJ: Lawrence Erlbaum, 1994: 121–146.

13. Anderson M. What would get you in trouble: Doctoral students' conceptions of science and its norms. In: Proceedings of the ORI Conference on Research on Research Integrity. Washington, DC: Office of Research Integrity, 2001.

14. Forsythe GB, Snook S, Lewis P, Bartone PT. Making sense of officership: Developing a professional identity for 21st century Army officers. In: Snider DM, Watkins GL. The Future of the Army Profession. Boston: McGraw-Hill, 2002:357–378.

15. Rogers G, Mentkowski M, Reisetter Hart J, Schwan Minik K. Disentangling related domains of moral, cognitive, and ego development. Presented at the American Educational Research Association Annual Meeting, Seattle, 10–14 April 2001.

Appendix A

Getting the Most From This Book

The goals of this book as stated in the preface pertain both to those who are new to the profession and to those who are well established. For both groups, we hope the stories will be a source of inspiration about what can be accomplished for others by caring and energetic people. For the newcomers, we hope that learning about exemplary colleagues will foster a fuller understanding of the scope of professional responsibilities. And for the veterans, we are convinced that the stories can serve as a source of renewal—if not an expansion—of the concept of service for others. One of the joys of being a professional is the opportunity to continue to develop our expertise. Another is the developmental benefit that comes from working out the problems we face at one stage of our lives so we can go on to greater challenges in the next. Achieving a degree and obtaining a license are but the first steps along a developmental trajectory. At each stage of life there are new challenges to work out, and our colleagues are there to help us. Responding to these challenges is essential for our personal growth. With stagnation comes despair. We need to see ourselves as developing humans, with goals to accomplish and a long-term goal in mind.

How can this book be used to foster these expanded concepts of obligations and service? For the goals to be at least minimally successful, readers need to reflect productively about the meaning of the stories. To this end, we offer the following seven suggestions, which cover a broad range of applications that can be of use to practitioners, students, teachers of dental ethics, and dental school administrators.

1. Think about the questions for discussion at the end of each story.

Discussion questions can be found at the end of each chapter. They explore the exemplars' views of their profession, the motivations for their accomplishments, the factors in their lives that made their accomplishments possible, and, most importantly, the implications of the stories for you.

We believe that the primary goal of this book is to help us think about lessons that the experiences of the exemplars provide for our own professional journey. If we are just embarking on our professional studies, what should we aspire to? What goals should we choose? What struggles should we anticipate? If we are well along in our professional lives, are we satisfied with where we are going? Have we lived up to our ideals? Are we pleased with how our colleagues view us? Do we need a mid-course correction? How can the stories of these dentists' lives enrich our own?

2. Reflect with us across the stories as you read chapter 12.

Chapter 12 brings the entire book together. It presents our conclusions about the most important lessons to be learned from the lives and experiences of the exemplars. After each conclusion, we indicate what we think the implications are for you. At the end of this chapter, we draw together our observations from studying exemplars with the broader recommendations for the education of professionals. As you read this chapter, keep in mind that we derived meaning from the stories of the exemplars through the use of the three different lenses. These are briefly described in chapter 1: the special characteristics of professions and the expectations that follow (Appendix C), the virtues that are important to medical practice (Appendix D), and the age- and stage-related shifts in indentity formation that educators are likely to encounter (Appendix E).

3. Use the stories to promote understanding of professional expectations.

There are various formats for conducting small group discussions. Here is one that has been useful in discussing the stories of the exemplars:

When applying for dental school, most students write a statement of their commitment to becoming a professional. These statements reveal their ideals and seldom are referred to again, which seems to us to be a missed opportunity for moral reflection.* At the very beginning of dental school, ask your students to reflect upon their personal statements and, perhaps, what they

have come to understand based on observations in dental offices (which most schools now require prior to admission) as well. In addition, have them respond to some general questions, such as: What do you think society will expect of you as a health care professional? What do you think the dental profession will expect of you? What will you expect of yourself?† After students have written about and perhaps shared their perceptions with one another, make them aware of the characteristics that distinguish professions from other occupations and the expectations of a professional. In this book, the expectations are presented in Appendix C; for a good overview of the characteristics of professions, see Hall.[2] Then ask them to select and read one of the stories and come to the class prepared to discuss something about the exemplar that relates to the expectations of a professional as mentioned above. The discussion could move to a review of their responses to the open-ended questions at the end of each chapter.

When such discussions are part of formal classroom activities, it is useful to incorporate an essay on the expectations of a professional as a culminating activity in which students can exhibit what they have come to understand. See Bebeau[3] for detailed suggestions on the use of such essays.

4. Use the stories to enhance dental study club discussions.

For established members of the profession, the stories in this book are well suited for use as a short series of topics for discussion by dental study clubs. Discussion leaders can come from the ranks of interested study club members themselves or from invited guests who have experience in leading discussions. Invitations could be extended, for example, to faculty of area dental schools, especially those who teach professional ethics. In addition, discussion leaders could also be faculty members of nearby colleges or universities. Of particular value in this regard might be members of English, psychology, or philosophy departments. Finally, discussion leaders may be people in other professions with interest and experience in using literature as a vehicle for exploring issues of their professions, such as medicine, theology, and law.

5. Discuss the stories in postgraduate seminars.

For dental residents and graduate students we suggest a discussion series similar to that proposed above for study clubs. It would be best presented as part of an

---

*Bertolami[1] speaks eloquently about the need to promote such introspection as a preamble to professional life.

†If the instructor is able to develop good rapport with students, it is also helpful to ask them to write about the following questions: What are you afraid of? What would be the worst thing for you if you failed to meet your expectations of yourself or those of others?

informal, voluntary evening program designed to discuss literature that has relevance to issues of the particular discipline involved. Such a program has been reported in a pediatric dentistry specialty program.[4] Its primary focus has been to assist in the development of empathy for children, especially those who are disadvantaged. The inclusion of discussions of these stories could be easily adapted from a thematic standpoint.

6. Suggest this book to students considering a career in dentistry.

Most college students who are considering a career in dentistry have an incomplete picture of the profession. Their lack of information includes not only the clinical aspects of dentistry but also the special obligations of professionals and the ideals of their particular profession. This book can be helpful in correcting part of that deficiency. To this end we make two suggestions:

1. Pre-professional advisors at the college and university level could recommend that students contemplating a career in dentistry read these stories.
2. Dental schools could recommend that newly admitted dental students read this book before beginning their regular dental curriculum.

7. Incorporate discussions of the exemplars into dental school orientation or ethics programs.

Most dental schools provide first-year orientation programs that focus on developing an understanding of the nature of dentistry and the responsibilities of its professionals. Following the "summer reading" recommended above, small group discussions of the stories in this book could be very useful in the development of a professional identity for the young student. See suggestion 3 above for suggestions for making this a more formal part of instruction. See also Appendix E for insights into how students may view professional expectations, and the commentary in chapter 6 for insights into how medical students view the expectation for professional self regulation.

In addition, all dental schools now require ethics programs, most of which utilize small group discussions of ethical issues. Some of the stories in this book could be incorporated into such a discussion series.

References

1. Bertolami CN. Why our ethics curricula don't work. J Dent Educ 2004;68:414–425.
2. Hall RH. The professions. In: Occupations and the Social Structure, ed 2. Englewood Cliffs, NJ: Prentice-Hall, 1975: 63–135.
3. Bebeau MJ. Influencing the moral dimensions of dental practice. In: Rest JR, Narváez DF (eds). Moral Development in the Professions: Psychology and Applied Ethics. Hillsdale, NJ: Lawrence Erlbaum, 1994:121–146.
4. Balis SA, Rule JT. Humanities in dental education: A focus on understanding the child. J Dent Educ 1999;63:709–715.

Guidelines for Exemplars Interview*

I. A General Life Narrative

Rationale

The generation of foundational information provides a basis for further conversation and establishes working relationships between informant and interviewer.

Main Questions

- Tell me about yourself.
- What stands out as your greatest personal achievement? Your greatest professional achievement?

Topics for Probe Questions

- Current activities
- Career
- Family
- Education
- Circumstances of growing up

II. Influences on Moral Development

Rationale

Acquisition of the subject's experiences both as a child and as an adult, including those of professional life, permits the development of the project's primary theme.

Main Questions

- How would you describe yourself from a moral standpoint? Perhaps in relation to the virtues?
- How did you come to be the person you are today?
- How do you feel about the things that influenced you the most?
- How do you see yourself in relation to others? In your family? Your community?
- Were there people at any period in your life whom you think of as moral heroes?

*Adapted from an interview developed by Ann Higgins-D'Alessandro, professor of psychology, Fordham University.

Topics for Probe Questions

- Expectations of the subjects as children
- Effect of primary and secondary education
- Role of religion
- Effect of college experiences
- Challenges of professional education
- Continued changes in moral perspectives after graduation from dental school

III. How Moral Issues and Questions are Experienced

Rationale

An exploration of how the subjects actually experience and deal with moral issues is essential, particularly because questions exist about the determinants of moral action. What are the contributions to moral behavior or moral reflection as opposed to the intuitive following of previously established patterns?

Main Questions

- As a very young child, do you have memories of being concerned about right and wrong?
- When you think of your early life, are there any instances that stand out in which you became aware that others (parents, teachers, peers) did not approve of your behaviors or actions? What was that like for you? How did you resolve that conflict?
- Were there periods of your life where concerns about moral issues or moral behavior were an especially important part of your life? Why were those issues important then? How did they affect your behavior?
- Were there any periods in your life where your views or actions about moral issues changed? What were the circumstances that influenced the changes? Were the changes rapid or gradual?
- You are thought of as being an exemplar with respect to morality. Thinking about the actions in your life that have led to that assessment by others, were those actions difficult for you in any way? Was it hard to decide what your actions ought to be?

- What are the circumstances under which a moral choice becomes a difficult dilemma for you? When conflicts exist between moral conviction and moral action, how do you resolve them?
- Do you personally experience conflicts of interest in your professional life with respect to your self-interest, caring for the needs of your patients, and upholding the ideals of the profession? How do you manage those conflicts?
- How do you view your profession's philosophy about caring for patients and obligations to patients?

Topics for Probe Questions

- Barriers that prevent consistency in moral action
- Consequences of disagreement over moral issues
- Managing conflicts in the face of adversity
- Importance of recognition from others in making moral choices
- Everyday expression of moral choices in personal and professional life
- Conflicts between caring for individuals and caring for community

IV. Interviewee's Views on Developmental Issues of Morality

Rationale

A pursuit of themes, an elaboration of the context of previous answers, and an exploration of implications.

The open-ended questions and the probe questions will be formulated based on the experiences during the previous parts of the interview. Expected avenues of discussion include the relationship between a well-developed conscience and the demonstration of moral courage; the role of moral reflection and analysis in relation to moral action; what makes someone a "person of character"; the role of disaster, pain, or difficulty in fostering admirable human qualities; relationships between morality and self-discipline; and why moral choices are reflexive for some people and dilemmas for others.

Expectations for and Obligations of the Dental Professional*

1. To acquire the knowledge of the profession to the standards set by the profession.
2. To keep abreast of changing knowledge through continuing education.
3. To make a commitment to the basic ethic of the profession—that is, to place the interests of the patient above the interests of the professional and the oral health interests of society above the interests of the profession.
4. To abide by the profession's code of ethics, or to work to change it if it is inconsistent with the underlying ethic of the profession.
5. To serve society (ie, the public as a whole), not just those who can afford one's services.
6. To participate in the monitoring and self-regulation of the profession.

There are at least three dimensions to this last expectation: to monitor one's own practice to assure that processes and procedures (including the daily requirements of such things as record keeping, sterilization, and informed consent) meet ever-evolving professional standards; to appropriately report incompetent or impaired professionals; and to join professional associations in order to participate in the setting of standards for the continuation of the profession. The latter is not a legal responsibility, but rather an ethical one. However, it is no less important, because actions taken by dental associations collectively have a great impact on the direction of the profession and, therefore, its ability to position itself for long-term sustainability.

*Adapted from Bebeau MJ, Kahn J. Ethical issues in community dental health. In: Gluck GM, Morganstein WM (eds). Jong's Community Dental Health, ed 5. St Louis: Mosby, 2003:425–445.

Appendix D

Virtues Exhibited by the "Good Health Professional"*

1. *Fidelity to trust:* An indispensable virtue of the good professional.
2. *Compassion:* The character trait that shapes the cognitive aspect of healing to fit the unique predicament of the patient.
3. *Phronesis:* The virtue of practical wisdom, the capacity for moral insight, the capacity to discern what moral choice or course of action is most conducive to achieve the goal.
4. *Justice:* The habit of rendering what is due to others.
5. *Fortitude:* Considered coextensive of courage, fortitude represents moral rather than physical courage, ie, the willingness of an individual to suffer personal harm for the sake of a moral good.
6. *Temperance:* Maintaining vigilance about protecting persons from undertreatment, abandonment, and inappropriate overtreatment. Shepherding our technology to good human aims is medical temperance.
7. *Integrity:* Wholeness and unity. Two senses are of significance: *(1)* the integrity of the person (patient or physician), the claim that belongs to every person by virtue of their personhood even as illness assaults the unity of the self and its relationship with the body and *(2)* being a person of integrity, the physician's habitual disposition to fidelity to the fiduciary nature of the healing relationship.
8. *Self-effacement:* Putting others and their needs first. Striking the morally defensible balance between self-interest and its effacement recognizes the primacy of altruistic beneficence. Professionals cannot displace the moral failings of the professions onto others–on society, other professions, government, economics, the marketplace, and so on.

*Adapted from Pellegrino ED, Thomasma DC. The Virtues in Medical Practice. New York: Oxford University Press, 1983.

Kegan's Stages of Identity Formation*

Robert Kegan[1] suggests that all human beings are continuously involved in a process of constructing meaning. Rather than responding immediately and directly to external events and internal experiences, all individuals (with the possible exception of newborns) organize experiences into a meaningful whole, and it is that constructed whole to which they respond. Kegan further suggests that as individuals gain an increasing amount of experience in an extremely complex world, they construct progressively more complex systems for making sense of that world. These progressive shifts in complexity are most easily recognized by comparing a young child's understanding of the social world with an adult's understanding. It is not merely that adults know more than children. Adults also possess a more complex system of thought than do children. They see and understand things that children may not see and certainly do not understand. Similarly, each dentist constructs an understanding of what it means to be a professional, and a dentist's understanding may be qualitatively different from that of the public in general.

But rather than postulating a gradual shift in constructed meaning across one's lifespan, Kegan identifies five major shifts in the complexity of meaning-making. This results in five numbered stages from early childhood through adulthood.

Brief descriptions of the stages and transitions the reader is likely to encounter among dental students and practitioners are included below. These descriptions (stages 2 through 5 and the transitions from stages 2 to 3 and stages 3 to 4) are based on Kegan's theory of the development of the self[1] but were adapted to focus on issues of professionalism. As we hope to make clear, the way in which a young professional understands moral and ethical issues is profoundly influenced by his or her stage of identity development.

Stage 2: The Independent Operator

Stage 2 individuals look at themselves and the world in terms of individual interests (eg, their own, their employer's, others') and in terms of concrete, black-and-white role expectations. Personal success is paramount and is measured by concrete accomplishment of individually valued goals and the enactment of specific role behaviors.

*Adapted from Bebeau MJ, Lewis P. Manual for Assessing and Promoting Identity Formation. Minneapolis: University of Minnesota Center for the Study of Ethical Development, 2003.

How the Typical Stage 2 Individual Understands Professionalism

Stage 2 individuals understand professionalism as the meeting of fixed, concrete, black-and-white role expectations. They are, of course, narrowly correct in their assessment, but they lack a broader understanding of what it means to be a professional. Their motivation for wanting to meet standards is wholly individual; it expresses a personal desire to be correct and effective. As one stage 2 aspiring professional put it, "There are professional guidelines and codes that shape your life."

Stage 3: The Team-Oriented Idealist

Whereas stage 2 individuals view themselves and others as independent operators, each with his or her own agendas and interests, stage 3 individuals view themselves and others in terms of their shared interconnections. They do so by considering multiple perspectives simultaneously. The capacity to make sense of the world by simultaneously considering multiple perspectives profoundly changes the extent to which both the sense of self and the understanding of social reality can encompass shared experiences, psychological membership, and the internalization of social expectations and societal ideals. While stage 3 individuals still possess and can articulate individual interests and specific behavioral goals, these individual interests are no longer central to how they define themselves. Stage 3 individuals look at themselves and the world in terms of shared values, mutual expectations, and identification with institutional ideals and principles. They are oriented to shared experiences, societal obligations, and internal qualities.

How the Typical Stage 3 Individual Understands Professionalism

Unlike stage 2 individuals, stage 3 professionals are both idealistic and internally self-reflective. They understand and are identified with (or worry that they are not yet fully identified with) their chosen profession. Rather than seeing professionalism as enacting certain specific behaviors or fixed roles (the stage 2 view), stage 3 indi-

viduals see professionalism as meeting the expectations of those who are more knowledgeable, more legitimate, and more professional. As one stage 3 professional remarked, "We must always hold ourselves to the highest expectations of society."

Stage 4: The Self-Defining Professional

If stage 3 individuals are characterized by their embeddedness in and identification with a set of shared or collective identities, stage 4 can be understood as the forging of a personal system of values and internal processes for evaluating those shared identities. Stage 3 individuals often find themselves torn among multiple, shared identities (eg, dentist, parent, spouse) with no easy way of coordinating those identities. As one's responsibilities multiply, life at stage 3 often becomes one of constantly trying to balance the perceived obligations of multiple stage 3 identities. The self system of the stage 4 individual provides an internal compass for negotiating and resolving tensions among these multiple, shared expectations. Conflicts among the inevitable competing pulls of various roles and their attendant obligations are negotiated by adherence to one's own internal standards and values.

How the Typical Stage 4 Individual Understands Professionalism

Unlike stage 3 individuals, stage 4 individuals are no longer identified with their professional role. Instead they have a sense of having freely committed themselves to being, for example, a member of the profession. They have constructed a self system, and it is that self system, with its personal values and principles of living, that is self-defining. Because they are not embedded in their profession, stage 4 individuals have greater freedom to criticize aspects of the profession with which they do not agree. They remain committed to the profession because it permits them to be themselves and be recognized as themselves within the profession. Because they are not identified with the profession, the stage 4 individual can "think outside the box" and become a change agent for the profession.

Transitions

In the lifelong process of identity development, individuals spend a considerable amount of time (typically many months) in the transition between stages. Transitions are characterized by the process of encompassing one's current way of making meaning within the broader and more complex framework of the next developmental stage. Both stages may be demonstrated, with the higher stage expressed in a tentative and less well-articulated manner. Research by Forsythe and colleagues[2] suggests that many college-age students are in the transition between stages 2 and 3, whereas the stage 3 to 4 transition is more typical of early- to mid-career professionals.

Stage 2 to Stage 3

During this transition, there is a growing awareness of the profession as a kind of generalized other through which individuals begin to experience themselves as future professionals. Students may express a kind of excitement about having an obligation to this abstract, collective entity. The growing emphasis on a shared identity is accompanied by a decreasing emphasis on acting in certain concrete ways to meet requirements or enact specific, prescribed behaviors. Individuals in transition often feel conflicted between an emerging sense of obligation and loyalty to the collective set of stage 3 expectations and the all-too-familiar individual interests that are a hallmark of stage 2. Embeddedness in self-interest may still be evident, but it is now seen as a shortcoming that must be overcome. There is also an increasing focus on internal feelings of guilt for failures to be the sort of person the profession expects.

Stage 3 to Stage 4

During this transition, individuals are in the process of making their shared obligations and identities secondary to a process of self-definition. It is a process by which one's *received* values are examined to determine which of those values and principles make the most sense for the self. Individuals slowly develop a sort of internal compass for conducting a meaningful life. Rather than being able to fully articulate those internal principles and values, the transitioning individual is working out those values and actively using them to examine the obligations that were so much a part of the stage 3 identity. During this transition individuals begin

to understand professionalism as an evolving set of freely chosen personal commitments and life decisions. They are engaged in a process of making the values of the profession their own and are self-consciously aware of doing so. Individuals may also begin to struggle self-consciously with the implications of having internal values that seem to be in conflict with conventional professional values. Distress is experienced when these self-reflective individuals encounter instances in which they have failed to take responsibility for their own actions or have discovered that they were engaging in self-deceptive practices or in actions that run counter to their own emerging values of professional conduct.

Stage 5: The Humanist

Few individuals appear to achieve Kegan's stage 5, but it does offer a hypothetical endpoint for identity development. As with all the earlier identity stages, achievement of stage 5 makes the centrality of the previous stage's way of constructing meaning secondary to a broader understanding of the self in relationship to the world. At stage 5, the individual is no longer identified with the self system, that carefully constructed system of values, principles, and commitments that defines the self at stage 4. As stage 5 unfolds, the individual gradually comes to see the stage 4 self system as only one of many possible ways of being in the world. The stage 5 individual begins to see the self as a set of universal, deeply humanistic longings and sensitivities, qualities that are shared by all humankind. Identities become like different suits of clothing, personae that can be put on or taken off as circumstances dictate. No longer is there a need to defend a particular identity or to demand that others relate to one through one's stage 4 identity. Instead, deeply intimate contact with other human beings becomes possible (though it is probably rarely achieved) through direct contact between fellow human beings.

Age- and Stage-Related Change

Until recently, descriptions of age- and stage-related changes were based on clinical evidence rather than longitudinal or cross-sectional studies of adult development—studies that would be of interest to educators concerned with professional socialization. Kegan[1] described stage 2 as characteristic of early adolescence, with stage 3 emerging in late adolescence and stage 4 descriptive of the well-adjusted adult. However, longitudinal and cross-sectional studies of college-age students enrolled in a highly selective military academy[2] suggest that the transition from stage 2 to stage 3 occurs somewhat later, during the late teens and early 20s. For example, 63% of entering cadets (college freshmen) function in the stage 2 to stage 3 transition, with 21% still functioning at stage 2 and 16% at stage 3. By graduation, only 6% of cadets—entry-level leaders in the military profession—are still at stage 2; 28% are still negotiating the stage 2 to stage 3 transition; and 47% are a full stage 3. A few graduates (19%) appear to be involved in the transition beyond stage 3 to stage 4. Assuming that college would have a similar effect on students entering the dental or medical profession, we could expect a few students at stage 2, a few to be negotiating the stage 2 to stage 3 transition, nearly half at a full stage 3, and some involved in the stage 3 to stage 4 transition. If the identity transformations of mid- and later-career medical and dental professionals mirror those of mid-career and senior military leaders, we would not expect a full stage 4 identity until mid-career. In a cross-sectional study of military leaders, Forsythe and colleagues[2] observed the following: By mid-career, 43% had attained a full stage 4, 28% had attained a stage 3, and 28% were still negotiating the stage 2 to stage 3 transition. For senior leaders, 50% had attained a full stage 4, another 18% were nearly a stage 4, 22% were in the stage 3 to stage 4 transition, and none were below a stage 3. These findings seem to support Kegan's observation[1] that advanced levels of identity are rarely achieved before midlife and then not by everyone. The stage 5 individual is the rare and exceptional person—perhaps someone like our exemplars or those identified by Colby and Damon.[3]

References

1. Kegan R. The Evolving Self: Problem and Process in Human Development. Cambridge, MA: Harvard University Press, 1982.
2. Forsythe GB, Snook S, Lewis P, Bartone PT. Making sense of officership: Developing a professional identity for 21st century Army officers. In: Snider DM, Watkins GL. The Future of the Army Profession. Boston: McGraw-Hill, 2002:357–378.
3. Colby A, Damon W. Some Do Care: Contemporary Lives of Moral Commitment. New York: Free Press, 1992.